What Doctors Must Learn....

What Doctors Must Learn....

Y. K. Amdekar
MD, DCH, FIAP
(Retd) Professor of Pediatrics
Grant Medical College and J. J. Group of Hospitals
Mumbai
Practicing Pediatrician for 53 years

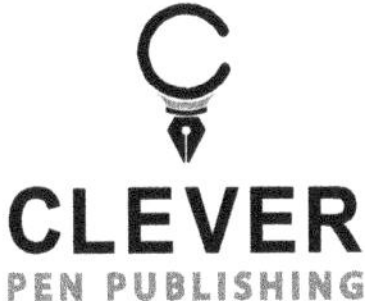

First Edition: 2023

Published by:

Clever Pen Publishing
D-2 Neelkanth Business Park Co-op. Premises Society Ltd.
Nathani Road
Vidyavihar (West)
Mumbai 400086
Mob.: 09867214519

Email: cleverpen9@gmail.com

ISBN 978-93-92215-00-1

Printed & Bound in India

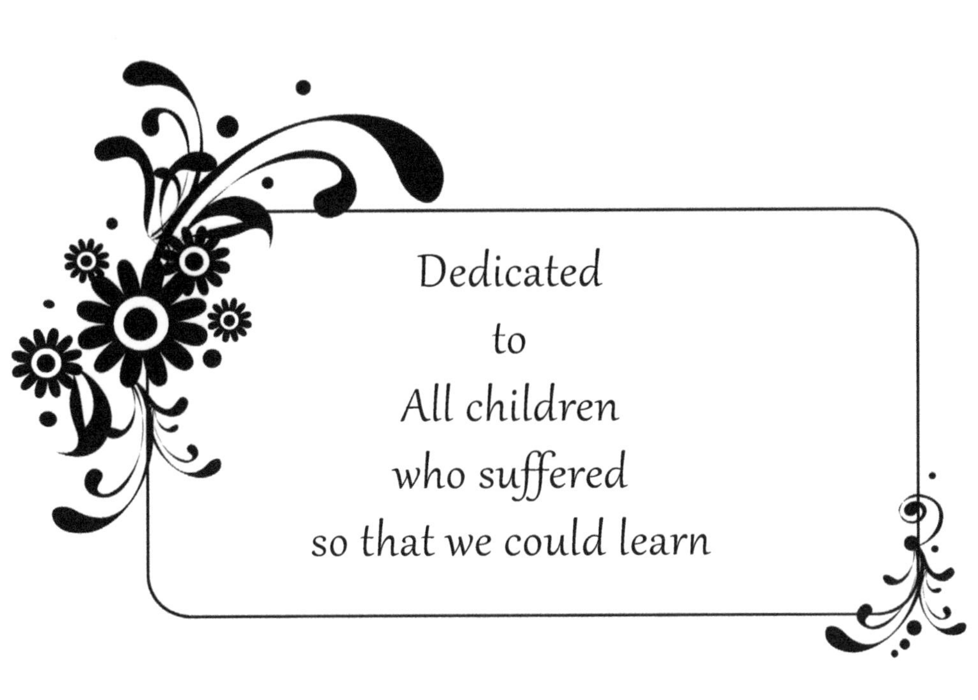

Dedicated

to

All children

who suffered

so that we could learn

PREFACE

After completing medical education in the mid-sixties, I realised that there was much more to learn. I was taught the science of medicine as it existed then but constantly changing trends were a challenge to the already trained. Uncertainties in medicine existed in spite of advances. William Osler said, "medicine is a science of uncertainty and art of probability". The art of medical practice was never given importance in medical colleges. One had to learn it by oneself. "high-tech" medicine is fast replacing "high-touch" medicine. Medical science without art falls short of the desired outcome. Ignoring the art of medical practice has led to a decline in the doctor-patient relationship. The first section of this book reminds the doctors to look beyond science.

History-taking is an art and a detailed history contributes to a provisional diagnosis to an extent of more than 80%. It helps to anticipate abnormal physical findings and nearly confirms the final diagnosis, if need be, with relevant tests. The second section of this book covers the analysis of all common and not-so-common symptoms met in practice along with case scenarios and MCQs. This should help the doctors to strengthen their skills in history taking to arrive at a provisional diagnosis.

Observing the patient, the way Sherlock Holmes used to do, is the most important part of physical examination. Doctors must develop the power of observation. The third section of this book discusses how mere observation can add so much value to arriving at the final diagnosis. Advances in medical investigatory technology and ease of availability of tests have led to their misuse. Doctors must consider the specificity and sensitivity of tests as no test is 100% specific and sensitive. Besides, the tests should be cost-effective. The fourth section of this book addresses this issue under the title "testing a test".

I am grateful to Lt General (retired) Dr Madhuri Kanitkar, the Vice-Chancellor of Maharashtra University of Health Sciences for readily agreeing to write the foreword to this book. It has been moments of pride and happiness for me when many of my students have surpassed me and the most notable amongst them has been Dr Madhuri Kanitkar.

I was inspired to write this book by my colleague and friend Dr Hrishikesh Thakre, an excellent academician and a teacher who also offered suggestions for improvement. I am indebted to Drs Hemant and Archana Joshi as well as Drs Raju and Rita Dhamankar for their suggestions and help. My colleagues in joint practice – Dr Rajaram Khare and Dr Rajesh Chokhani have been a constant support to building the concept of rational practice. Finally, I thank M3 digital platform for allowing me to reproduce partly my own contribution.

Dr. Y. K. Amdekar

FOREWORD

I consider it a privilege to write a foreword for the book 'What Doctors Must Learn' by Dr YK Amdekar. I wish to start by looking beyond the title and the cover with a reflection on my student days as a post-graduate student at a Naval hospital in Mumbai. I found myself rushing to JJ hospital for the grand round by the honorary consultant Dr YKA (as we called him with the utmost respect) not only because I wanted to learn pediatrics, but because I soon realised that on those grand rounds, I was learning to be a good pediatrician. The exemplary clinical acumen through detailed history and interpretation of symptoms and signs was a treat to hear, see and emulate. Action spoke louder than words and practice was valued more than preaching! Reaching the dot on time and giving full attention to residents and patients was the first lesson we learnt. This Dronacharya had many an Ekalavya on those rounds and clinics.

This book is exactly on the same principles. I would strongly recommend it for every student aspiring to train as a doctor who would like to Care always and Cure, when possible, in the author's own words. The personal glimpses and snippets drive home the point in easy-to-digest bites. Every chapter and story end with a message which helps consolidate the thoughts.

In recent years the art of healing has been lost in the science and evidence-based guidelines that drown the clinician in a sea of information. He or she needs a curated path to turn this information into knowledge and add experience to inculcate a pearl of wisdom beyond textbooks. This book helps the reader navigate through the maze created by pure science being taught and evaluated.

Today Medicine itself is ailing and needs someone to treat it. This has to be done quickly before it reaches the ICU! The starting point must be medical education. The first section 'Dr Look Beyond Science' is an important first step for any learner who seeks to care for this patient. Teachers have to shoulder the responsibility of guiding students to cure Medicine through the art of healing. We need many Dronacharyas and till then this book can awaken the passion in teachers and reach many Ekalavyas as well.

The second section 'History is not His Story' explains the importance of listening and how to hone the skill of taking a good history. While it reinforces the basics one learns in a standard book such as Hutchinson's Clinical Methods, it does much more by explaining the physiological basis of the symptom and sign as well as the clinical relevance. It explains the art of taking history leading to localising the anatomical system or microsystem, the physiological basis, the pathology, and the possible etiology. The best part is the use of MCQ at the end of each symptom which helps recapitulate the take-home message and helps prepare students for the ubiquitous MCQ evaluation process.

The third section 'Power of Observation' makes a powerful case for "take time to see properly and register all, not just look before you leap!" Each sign has been explained with the keen observation that is required to reach a possible etiology. The tables provide a systematic checklist of the associations clubbed together that help diagnose common causes. This can prove extremely useful to students to train themselves to arrive at a diagnosis when a symptom or sign has multiple differential diagnoses.

The best of all is the last section 'Testing a test'. In present-day practice when often investigations are ordered indiscriminately with a possibility of finding something not necessarily the needle in the haystack; this section is most enlightening to a doctor wanting to get back to the basics and the rationale of investigating an ailment through laboratory tests. The clinician needs to be able to read between the lines of a report including the very basic CBC. An astute interpretation of the laboratory report helps narrow down the diagnosis and avoids an unnecessary battery of tests in a case of fever or anemia etc. The section provides food for thought by presenting similar case scenarios with variable baseline investigations and analysis of the interpretation of the test results. The MCQs add value to a self-assessment of the learning points.

Overall, this book is strongly recommended for the teacher and the student of medicine wishing to go beyond bookish knowledge.

"A teacher affects eternity,
he can never tell where his influence stops"
– Henry Adams

Lt Gen Madhuri Kanitkar
PVSM AVSM VSM (Retd)
Vice Chancellor
Maharashtra University of Health Sciences
Senior Pediatrician and pediatric nephrologist

CONTENTS

PART 1 - DOCTOR, LOOK BEYOND SCIENCE

PART 2 - HISTORY IS NOT HIS STORY, BUT MUCH MORE ANALYSIS OF SYMPTOMS WITH CASE-BASED DISCUSSION

Section 1 – General view

Section 2 - Analysis of common symptoms with case-based discussion

Section 3 - Analysis of other symptoms seen at times in office practice

PART 3 - POWER OF OBSERVATION

PART 4 - TESTING A TEST

Section 1 – General view

Section 2 – Commonly ordered tests

Section 3 – Other tests

PREFACE TO PART 1

It is said that change is the only constant. I joined medical college more than six decades ago and I have noticed a sea-change in the science of medicine, medical teaching, and medical practice. The science of medicine has advanced so much that it is impossible to keep pace with it and no doctor can claim to know everything. It has paved the way to specialization and further, super-specialization. Technological advances helped in the diagnosis and management of many diseases. With such an advance, one would have expected a "cure" for many diseases resulting in satisfied patients and a healthier population. Has it happened?

In the past, when science had not yet developed, doctors cared though could not often cure, they showed empathy and concern for the patient and were responsible, accountable, and transparent. They followed moral principles, true to the Hippocratic oath and enhanced the image of the profession. Patients had faith in the doctors, respected doctors and were grateful to them, irrespective of the outcome.

The advancing science and technology were so attractive that medical practice became "high-tech" and soon traditional "high-touch" gave way to "no-touch". Humanity was blunted. Patients don't care to know how much doctors know but they want to know how much doctors care. They expect communication, counseling and time from doctors to answer their questions. Unfortunately, the traditional art of practice is lost in pursuit of advancing science. While science is dynamic with frequent changes and uncertainties, the traditional art of practice has stood the test of time for generations. Doctors must look beyond science and it is the need of the hour to serve the community better and salvage the image of the noble profession. It is possible only if the medicine is humanized.

Dr. Y. K. Amdekar

Part 1

Doctor, Look Beyond Science

1 Is Medicine A Science or Art?

Medicine is where science marries art

– Aldous Huxley

Medicine is a science of experience

– Samuel Hahnemann

Introduction

The medical mission – the calling of a doctor – is to feel connected with the purpose and value of the medical profession that is well represented by offering holistic care. A holistic approach needs the use of all faculties endowed by nature to all of us and they are body, heart, mind and soul. When translated into medical practice, the body refers to knowledge (**science**) while the heart as compassion, mind as commitment and soul as own conscience are all parts of **art**. Medical science without art remains short of a desired expected care.

Is Medicine a Science?

Science is an intelligent activity encompassed with a systematically organized study based on evidence to acquire knowledge capable of accurate prediction. Science is not the absolute truth but the search for the truth that may often elude us. Unlike physics or mathematics, medicine is a science of uncertainty and so at best considered to be a scientific study. Medical science is dynamic and ever-changing and its half-life of observed facts is short. Hence, we need to learn, unlearn and relearn all the time. The belief that medicine as science is further enhanced by the development of "evidence-based" medicine. However, there are limitations even to double-blind randomized control trials (RCTs) and a lack of evidence is not necessarily an absence of evidence. Moreover, evidence also has several grades and is often diverse in views. Consensus guidelines are at the best a summary of practical wisdom and not the evidence. Thus, there is a need for experience as well. In fact, evidence and experience are two sides of the same coin. Evidence and consensus guidelines are based on generalization while an experience fine-tunes to suit the individual patient thus overcoming grey areas of science. Of course, bias and prejudice are inherent with experience and one must have an open mind and honesty to accept when wrong.

Uncertainties in Spite of Medical Advances

There have been great strides in medicine helped by technological advances but most inventions that are supposed to result in a cure still fall short of the desired. In fact, management of most diseases can be categorized into 3 P's – placebo, palliative and plumbing. It is not only the uncertainty in the diagnosis of a disease because of the wide variation in presentation but also in its predictable outcome. This is because the **outcome of a disease depends on body, mind and genes** and hence the study of the body alone cannot predict the outcome. A genuine **"cure"** is rare but **care** is always possible. Medical practice based on science alone often fails because it cannot deliver "care". Bacterial infections and a few other infections can be cured but even then, the final outcome is not guaranteed for various reasons such as antibiotic resistance, host immune responses and genetic predisposition. Modern advances have improved our understanding, but a cure is still elusive in most diseases, besides the issues of accessibility and affordability. The present motto in medicine is thus **"cure, if possible, but care always"** and this is where the art of medical practice comes in to play a major role.

Medical Practice an Art-Based Scientific Study

Art involves skills developed by experience and observation in the application of science. The art of medicine has remained the same over generations and is the foundation of medical practice. It is permanent and evolved through centuries based on human values and intuition. Its thrust is to allay anxiety in the minds of patients. If you have human qualities of head and heart, they encourage the healing power of a patient. Healing of the damage is done by the human immune system, the stimulation for which comes from the mind of a sick person which in turn depends on the patient's confidence and faith in his doctor. It is an art of caring and comfort. There has to be an ideal art-science ratio though the pendulum has swung too far toward science ignoring art and hence a disaster. Early on, medical practice was art like other arts such as poetry and painting, practiced with love and passion. However, today it is based on science alone ignoring the art of medicine.

Must Integrate Art into the Science of Practice

Basic components of the art of medical practice include skilled planning, time management, communication and counseling. Besides, philosophy (patient hearing and offering honest opinion), ethics (do not harm, do good, privacy and justice) and culture (courteous behavior and empathy) form important constituents of the art of practice. Science treats the body, art comforts the mind and soul. One without the other is incomplete. Medicine and meditation both mean healing and are intended to offer "care" definitely, "cure" if possible.

The Emotional Side of Medicine

Beyond every illness is a human being. Sir William Osler said "it is most important to know what sort of a patient has the disease rather than what kind of disease the patient has", It represents a simple definition of empathy. Empathy is rooted in humility and in being humble and humane. Empathy is not an emotion but cognition; it means recognizing the suffering of others and it is a prerequisite to compassion. It is compassion that generates the desire to help others. The secret of "care" for a patient lies in caring for the patient and it needs a human connection that helps to heal. It is as important as medical science and physicians' competence. Especially, it comes to doctor's rescue in case of poor outcomes, complications or medical error. Empathy is the most under-appreciated human skill. It is present in every individual but further boosted by learning from role models. In medical practice, listening is the first step toward empathy. Detailed history-taking sets the tone for communication. Appropriate physical contact during physical examination boosts emotional connection. Counseling denotes compassion and generates faith. The physician must simply follow the art and offer help to patients without judgment.

Holistic Approach

Humans are endowed by nature with multiple qualities which include body, heart, mind and soul. When applied to medical practice, body means knowledge, heart the compassion, mind the commitment and soul our inner conscience. Knowledge is important and as medicine is dynamic and ever-changing science, we must keep up-to-date. But knowledge alone cannot deliver "care". We need to commit to doing the best for every patient with compassion. And finally, we are responsible to our own inner conscience. We must use the brain and heart together – the heart is referred to as "little brain" – it is innervated with large number of neurons. We must be honest, transparent, responsible and accountable. Thus, when every patient is treated in a holistic way with devotion (selfless dedication), it results in divine healing. It is easy to understand that healing is a natural process, mainly supported by the art of medical practice with rational use of science. Science alone fails.

Beyond the Art of Humanities

The art of medical practice also involves the art of clinical medicine. Analysis of detailed history should be based on "thought in action" which means each question has a specific purpose of inquiry and the answer to the question should lead to the next question. History should give a clue to probable differential diagnosis in most cases and this should be followed up with a focused physical examination that should be thorough and carried out the standard systematic way. The physician must learn to listen and not just hear, must observe and not just see and think not just collect information. Probable diagnosis must be based on Stutton's law to follow what is most common.

(When Mr Stutton - a bank robber was asked by the judge why he tried to rob the bank, Mr Stutton said that is because it is most common to find a large amount of money in the bank). Only after ruling out common conditions, one can think of an uncommon presentation of common problems and finally consider uncommon and rare problems, in that order. The patient is not an inanimate object that can be analyzed by technology and computers. Telemedicine has its own limitations though useful in providing access to medical facilities in remote areas. Patients expect physical contact besides time and conversation with the doctor. It is a rational approach to medical practice and constitutes an important part of the art of medicine.

Past and Present

A few decades ago, before modern science developed, physicians offered personal attention with compassion and concern for the patient that gave comfort, if not cure. Recent medical practice has thrust health care into an era of modernization with technological advances and computerization that allows physicians to access everything at their fingertips. However, there is indisputable depersonalization of patient care. In this fast-growing modern medicine, physicians treat diseases ignoring a human being in whose body, the disease resides but now, what is being treated is not the disease but test reports and numbers instead of a patient. This has resulted in patient dissatisfaction and disturbed patient-doctor relationships with its dire consequences including increasing the cost of health care.

Motivation Necessary to Reverse this Trend

Motivation is a psychological driving force that reinforces an action towards the desired goal. Intrinsic motivation should come from within, driven by enjoyment of work and pleasure without expecting a reward. Once intrinsic motivation gets started, habit sustains it. External motivation depends on reward/money or punishment/threat, it has a negative impact on life. Motivation determines what you do and attitude decides how well you do. Time management is the key along with communication, counseling and documentation. You must do to your patient what you would expect from your doctor if you were a patient. Mahatma Gandhi said, "recall the face of the poorest and weakest and ask yourself whether the step that you are contemplating to take would help him". If you apply this test, pride will be replaced by humility and dismay.

Personal Notes

During my entire medical education and especially during my post-graduate tenure, I was lucky to be exposed to the art of medicine from my teachers, besides learning the science of medicine from them. Though art was not taught in the curriculum, repeated exposure made a permanent impact. That was the time when I realized the art of medicine was as important as science or maybe even more relevant when science fell short of desired. I am aware that patients and parents of sick children facing serious or prolonged illness harbor fear, anxiety, frustration, and often self-pity or self-blame that also should be addressed by talking to them with empathy. Many times, I would spend more time talking to parents of sick children as compared to time spent over history taking and physical examination. I recall many instances when parents would express their gratitude just because I showed empathy and answered all their queries to their satisfaction. It also made me very happy. Once I was asked by a pediatrician couple to see their child who had a fever for more than a month without a diagnosis. I spent an hour discussing with them the probable diagnosis and management plan and they were satisfied and happy. Two weeks later, as the child was better, they came to thank me. Knowing that they see a large number of patients each day giving very little time to patients; I asked them whether their patients were satisfied. I was surprised when they said they were. I told them that their patients were not aware how much you owed them but you definitely knew it. And so, I suggested they change. But old habits die hard!

Take Home Message

We should not allow medical science to blunt humanity, ignore ethics and the need for empathy. High-tech medicine can do wonders only for a few but **high-touch** medicine can comfort all. Don't forget, doctors are criticized and manhandled due to a lack of art of practice and not because of poor knowledge of science.

2 Uncertainties in Medicine in Spite of Advances

Medicine is a science of uncertainty and art of probability

– William Osler

Must devote part of your mind to constantly processing uncertainty

– Scott Belsky

Introduction

Medicine unlike physics or mathematics is at best a scientific study rather than pure science. There have been rapid advances in medicine with the use of modern technology. However, as our understanding improves, it unfolds our increasing ignorance. "The more I learn, the more I realize how much I don't know," said Albert Einstein. Most of us experience the Dunning-Kruger effect that describes a hypothetical cognitive bias stating that people at a task overestimate their ability and confidence. The wisdom curve attains quickly a peak of stupidity followed by a valley of despair and then over time, the slope slowly moves upwards towards enlightenment.

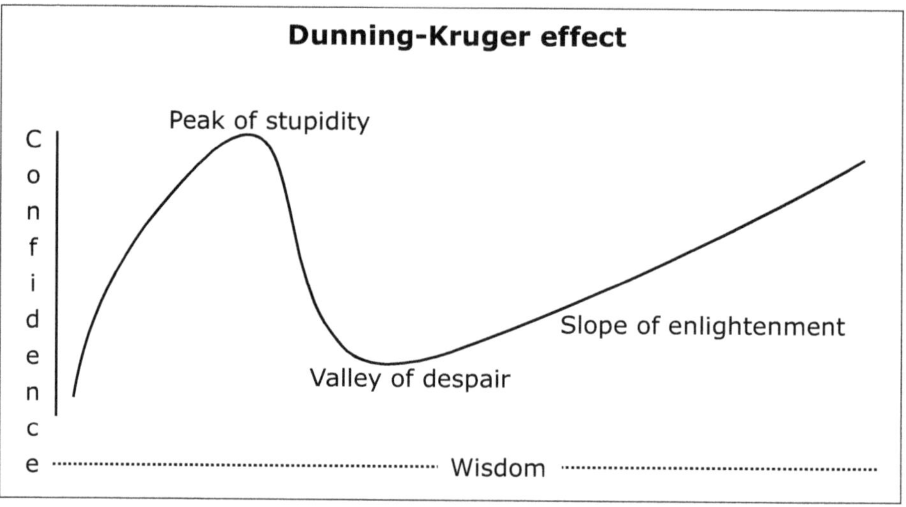

Over the last few decades, so-called advances in each decade have partly become obsolete by the next decade, exposing our stupidity and resulting despair. Hopefully, this leads to the beginning of enlightenment though the progress is very slow that takes a lifetime to realize what is right. Thus, uncertainty continues in medicine in spite of advances.

Disease Manifestation: a Result of a Tripartite Interaction

The presentation of a disease and its outcome depends on multiple variables and may not follow the standard pattern. The interplay of three major factors is involved in the manifestations of the disease and they include a primary triggering agent, a host and an environment. The **trigger** may exist in many different forms such as physical, chemical insult (poison, toxin or abnormal metabolite), infection being the most common besides many unknown forms. Detection of a primary agent has been increasingly possible with modern technological advances but for various reasons (technological limitations and human irrationality), proof of a primary agent often remains elusive. Even if the primary agent is detected, its characteristics are difficult to assess. For example, when infecting organism is detected, its severity or virulence is not known and so also in-vitro antibiotic sensitivity may not be the same as in-vivo efficacy. These are some of the technological limitations. The same is true about other primary triggering agents.

Host factors play an important role in the manifestations of diseases. **Human is 30% phenotype, 30% genotype and 40% mind.** It is not easy to anticipate phenotype, difficult to recognise genotype and impossible to assess the mind. Thus, we are mostly ignorant about the host except for few factors. Nutritional and immune status of the host can be evaluated to a certain extent but it may not translate into a predictable pattern or outcome in a disease. This is because even an immune-competent host may underperform to a specific challenge or overreact to a primary agent with its consequences (immuno-reactive disorders with organ damage, MIS - multisystem inflammatory syndrome). Science fails to preempt such possible immune aberrations and even after they occur, the cause of such reactions is a conjecture. Genetic predisposition is important but epigenetic factors decide the outcome. The role played by the "mind" in host response remains unclear. It is an irony that medical science has ignored the role of the mind in the causation of physical diseases though there is an attempt to correlate it with psychological problems. However, anatomy, physiology and pathology of the mind remain elusive but we know that communication and counseling with empathy do help the "mind" of the patient with resultant healing.

The **environment** also modifies disease manifestations. (Malaria in the hyperendemic zone may present without fever). Exposure to factors such as population density (overcrowding), state of general hygiene and seasonal variation may alter disease manifestations. Effects of drugs depend on pharmacodynamic and pharmacokinetic factors and vary with time of the day or night (circadian rhythm – steroids safe as a single dose in the morning), drug ingestion either on an empty or full stomach as well as the interaction between multiple drugs differ in their benefits as well as side effects. Such variables add to the complexity of medicine.

The Host Decides the Pathology and Hence the Outcome

Hosts of the same age with normal nutritional and immune status respond to the same infection with such a marked variation that no modern technology can predict. This is how it is mainly the individual host who decides the pathology (type of response) and its outcome that is unpredictable. Streptococcal pharyngitis is a classic example. There occurs a wide spectrum of host responses to streptococcal infection that may lead to markedly variable outcomes such as asymptomatic infection without disease, mild vague symptoms, standard presentation with cure with or without antibiotic, asymptomatic carrier state, recurrent disease, immune complications after curing of disease like rheumatic fever with its different manifestations, glomerulonephritis, PANDAS (neuro-psychiatric disorder) and also serious streptococcal skin-scalded syndrome or toxin-induced manifestations. All these patients look similar, to begin with, but they progress unpredictably in different ways. Modern science fails to preempt a specific pattern of response in a given individual and knows only after it occurs. Even then, treatment is not always helpful as management of immune complications is palliative and not curative and favorable outcomes cannot be guaranteed.

Tuberculosis is another example. Immune response to mycobacterial infection is T cell-dependent and it is the balance between hypersensitivity and immunity – two sides of host immune response. Depending on such a balance, manifestations vary from favorable response such as primary asymptomatic infection (requiring no treatment) to treatable pathology with good outcomes such as primary complex, progressive primary disease and pleural effusion, treatable pathology but with permanent damage such as chronic fibrocaceous cavitary disease and disseminated diseases such as miliary tuberculosis or meningitis. With such a different pathology, the outcome also varies from cure with or without permanent damage or even fatality. As mentioned earlier, drug-resistant tuberculosis is a challenge resulting from human irrationality (misuse by doctors and non-compliance by patients). It is clear that unpredictable responses and outcomes are a possibility in every disease. This is the reason that every disease may present with atypical or incomplete manifestations that pose a clinical challenge and the outcome is not certain in spite of early correct diagnosis and prompt compliant treatment.

Cause and Effect is often a Conjecture

Even when a cause of a disease is detected, one may not be sure whether the effect is related to the same. For example, isolation of a bacterium in a sample may not be the cause but simply a commensal or a contaminant. Similarly, in-vitro and in-vivo drug sensitivity may differ and the patient's response to a drug may not correlate with the test result. The normal test result does not necessarily rule out the disease as much as an abnormal test result in isolation is not the proof of a disease. Science does not know cause and effect in relation to congenital malformations. Though few risk factors are considered but it is not rare to find no risk factors to explain such problems and on the other hand, one does see an absence of any malformation in spite of the presence of risk factors. It is clear that we are still short of complete answers in spite of advances. There is no doubt that research should and will continue to find more answers but I fear our understanding will always lag behind in this race and this is how uncertainties will remain. That is how medical practice is based also on the art of probability.

Controversies due to Uncertainties Add Confusion

The recent pandemic of coronavirus is a classic example. It has left many unanswered questions and "experts" differ adding confusion. We are not sure about the origin of the pandemic. It took time for WHO to declare a pandemic. No government was sure of immediate action though most countries announced lockdown, few did not. No one was sure when to release restrictions. Several countries including India have faced multiple "waves". A balance between probable morbidity/mortality and economic losses was difficult to predict and there were controversies on every decision. The list of symptoms arising from covid infection kept on increasing to an extent that any symptom or even no symptom was considered possible to explain the disease.

There was confusion about different tests and their reliability besides affordability and accessibility. No test in medicine is 100% reliable, a false +ve and false - ve test results are inherent limitations. Treatment options were equally controversial with an initial favorable report about Hydroxychloroquine published in a reputable international journal that was soon confirmed to be wrong within the next few days. Several drugs have been tried with varying claims but not recommended and Remdesivir was the only approved drug. Even then, no one was sure about for whom and when to use this drug. The use of steroids, IVIG, monoclonal antibodies and plasma therapy have been tried with unpredictable varying success and so there were no clear recommendations.

Finally, it was felt that the only life-saving measures were steroids and adequate oxygenation. However, irrational use of steroids did result in Mucormycosis in a few patients. Similar controversies exist in the choice of vaccines and also the interval between two doses. The initial 4-week interval (based on the need to hurry through an immune response) was replaced by 6-8 weeks interval (for better immune response). Such uncertainties lead to confusion that is further promoted by different self-made experts. We are not sure whether present vaccines protect against various mutant strains. There is even a lobby against vaccination -imagine how evidence is elusive and the consensus is debatable. But what is universally accepted is the old traditional wisdom – social distancing, masking and sanitization.

Way forward in Spite of Uncertainties

Uncertainties in medicine are likely to be increasing as our knowledge improves with the unfolding of newer challenges. This is where experience and traditional wisdom come in along with scientific evidence. Experience is built over time with an open mind and willingness to accept mistakes and make necessary changes. Thus, we depend on consensus guidelines that at best represent a summary of the practical wisdom of experienced experts. Naturally, these guidelines need to be revised periodically as our knowledge (or ignorance) increases. It also underscores a fact that medical practitioners must continue to learn, unlearn and relearn forever.

Personal Notes

I was more confident about the diagnosis of a disease and its outcome when I started to practice with little knowledge (ignorance is a bliss). As I learned more, I developed a more cautious approach to being aware of a wide spectrum of presentations of a disease that may overlap with other possibilities. Similarly, I realized the outcome of correctly diagnosed and treated disease may not always progress in an expected pattern and hence there is always a need for constant monitoring. I have seen an unexpected recovery in a brain-damaged child and also met the worst outcome even when the disease was diagnosed early and treated in the best scientific way. It made me clear that there are other factors hitherto unknown.

Finally, I have realized that nature is so kind that most of our patients, but not all, improve in spite of uncertainties and we take the credit for the same. It should make us feel humbler not to take credit for success and be more watchful and try our best. I remember one of the pioneering cancer surgeons operated on a patient suffering from GI cancer and found an extensive spread that made him close the abdomen without any further resection and counseled relatives about the poor outcome. This happened in the early 70s and to his and everyone's surprise, the patient recovered completely. The surgeon considered his diagnosis of cancer was wrong but would not believe that cancer got cured by nature or any other measures followed by the patient. Such instances do occur though as mentioned before they are rare but make us aware of medical uncertainties. Such instances also remind us to look beyond modern medicine to other systems of medicine.

During the pandemic, medical experts were asked whether it was time to ease the lockdown – allergists were in favor of scratching it, dermatologists advised not to make a rash move, GI specialists had a gut feeling, neurologists felt the government had a lot of nerve, obstetricians felt everyone was laboring under a micro-conception, ophthalmologists thought the idea was short-sighted, pathologists could not opine without a post-mortem, pediatricians said 'oh, grow up", psychiatrists thought the whole idea was madness, radiologists could see through it, anesthetists thought the whole idea was gas, cardiologists did not have the heart to refute it, in the end, proctologists won leaving the entire decision up to the asshole.

Take Home Message

There is no doubt about rapidly advancing modern medicine has opened many opportunities for better health care. However, there exist too many variables in the causation and outcome of every disease and many of such factors are not yet clearly understood. Such uncertainties in medicine require watchful monitoring and empathetic counseling without instilling undue fear in the mind of a patient but at the same time not giving false hopes. Physicians must understand the limitations of science but continue learning also from experiences based on deliberate observation.

3 Changing Trends, A Challenge to the Already Trained

Is it not a bit unnerving what doctors call what they do is "practice"?

– George Courtin

It is astonishing with how little reading a doctor can practice but it is not astonishing how badly he does it

– Dr S. Venkatesan

Introduction

Medical science is dynamic and fast-changing so much that some of the prevalent trends a decade ago become obsolete by the next decade. The problem is we don't know which part of the knowledge would change to be invalid and so we need to keep learning, unlearning and relearning. Time may not be too far when what you read today was accurate when written, but may not be accurate when you read it today and what is used today may become obsolete tomorrow. However, the art of medical practice has been eternal over generations and so, once we learn the art of practice and perfect it, it is useful forever. With advancing modern science, art seems to be forgotten and this is a dangerous trend. It has resulted in patient dissatisfaction and led to loss of faith and image of the medical profession.

Changes in Disease Profile

Manifestation of a disease is a result of tripartite interaction between the host, environment and an offending agent. Over the last few decades, all three factors have shown changing trends. Changes in lifestyle have affected the nutritional and immune status of the host. Crowding, international travel, air pollution and many such factors have significantly contributed to changing trends in disease profiles. Offending agents, microbes, in particular, have been smarter than before and have successfully evaded host defense by mutation and acquiring drug resistance. Such changes have resulted in varied presentations of the same disease in different individuals and have been a challenge to the doctor. Unfortunately, neither of these three factors are easy to assess and hence evaluation of the interplay of these factors is getting more difficult. Standard presentation of the disease as described in a textbook is often not the way disease presents in actual life situations and such problems are a rule more than the exception. There are several such examples seen in day-to-day practice.

Changes Based on Host Factors

As malaria became endemic, it rarely presented as fever with rigors and may manifest with any type of fever including low-grade fever or at times even without fever. On the other hand, typhoid may present as fever with rigors. In fact, rigors represent a high rise in body temperature in a short time and would occur in any disease. Classical textbook presentation of tuberculosis is low-grade evening rise of fever. However, tuberculosis may present with any type of fever including a sudden high fever as seen in immune-mediated pleural effusion in a healthy child. This is because host response decides the type of pathology and its clinical presentation. Such changing trends have been observed in all diseases and pose a challenge in the diagnosis. Vaccines offer immunity that may not be fully protective and such a child manifests with a modified clinical presentation that is not easy to recognize. Similarly, a malnourished child presents in a non-classical atypical way. Even the outcome of therapy depends on the host's ability to respond appropriately and hence there could be a varied type of progress in a disease treated in the same way. At times, the immune system of the host mounts an inappropriate exaggerated immune response that is responsible for immune complications affecting multiple organs and it happens even after the infection is well controlled. Science does not know as yet how to modulate the appropriate immune response. This is a new challenge difficult to manage.

Changes Based on Environmental Factors

As the infective disease becomes endemic, the majority of persons including children in the community become infected and many of them develop immunity even without developing a disease. If infected again with the same offending agent, clinical manifestations are mild and often not recognizable. Similarly, exposure to tuberculosis infection that did not progress to disease leaves behind hypersensitivity and if reinfected, manifestations are different, take the form of destructive lesions as compared to first-time infection. Increasing air pollution has resulted in a higher prevalence of respiratory diseases including asthma and allergic rhinitis.

Changes Based on Offending Agent

Number of organisms and their virulence decide the severity of clinical presentation and drug resistance adds to the difference in the outcome. Clinical presentation is different in a child who has developed partial immunity as compared to a child who has no immunity at all against a particular infection. Misuse of antibiotics is universal that has resulted in antibiotic resistance with an increase in morbidity and mortality. Microbes keep on mutating and fooling our immune system. That is how the influenza viral vaccine has to be repeated every year. Lifelong immunity to natural infection is also likely to wane off necessitating vaccination even in adults and pertussis is a classic example.

Changes in Medical Practice

High Dependency on Laboratory Tests

There is a widening gap between traditional wisdom and modern science that has been further accelerated with the concept of evidence-based medicine. Availability and accessibility of modern tests have definitely made an impact though only in selected cases but it is unfortunate that is far more misused routinely even in non-affordable populations. Tests are offered without a provisional diagnosis and at times, there is a tendency to treat reports without clinical correlation rather than treating a disease or a person in whom the disease resides. Tests should ultimately benefit a patient and it is possible only when the test is able to define the cause of the disease for which specific treatment is available. Patients are dissatisfied when multiple tests do not result in final improvement. It is important to counsel about the need and benefit of test results before ordering tests so that patient and his relatives understand the implications of tests.

Evidence-Based Medicine

Evidence is of different degree, the lowest degree is an anecdotal experience. Evidence and experience both are two sides of the same coin. Evidence is based on averages and may not be a fit for all while experience is tailored to individual patients. Evidence depends on external research while experience on internal expertise. Both need to be judiciously used but there is a trend to consider the evidence without experience. With changing host factors, evidence may not be applicable to individual hosts.

Super Specialisation – Boon or Bane?

Superspecialist has to be excellent generalist to be rationally effective. It is ideal if a superspecialist spends 25% of his time with a generalist so that he does not overlook more common diseases with atypical presentation rather than trying to test for rarer ones. After all, several diseases affect multiple organs and it is not uncommon to see each superspecialist sees only through his biased angle.

Profession Tuned into Business!

Medicine is a profession and not a business. The business has a single motive of earning money while a doctor in the profession has a priority of providing holistic care to his patient while earning money. Business involves selling the goods irrespective of their worth whereas the profession involves giving the correct advice to the best of one's knowledge that is likely to benefit the patient. Unfortunately, there exists undisputable depersonalization of patient care with its consequences of patient dissatisfaction, legal suits or violence. It is a challenge to set clear goals of rational practice but it is very much possible with intrinsic motivation. It will bring more happiness in life than mere success. In fact, success lies in happiness.

Personal Notes

I witnessed changes in every aspect of life as so-called "development" had made life more complex and one had to adapt to such changes. Medicine is no exception. While it was difficult to keep updated in science, I was lucky to get opportunities to teach while in practice, after all, teaching is the best way of learning. It has taught me how to be careful at every step to avoid mistakes. And even then, mistakes did occur and I hope I learnt from them. I spent 4 hours a day attending my duties during my tenure as an Honorary teacher and many thought I had nothing better to do. However, it was much more challenging to refrain from unethical practices and conduct rational practice. I was aware when a few parents of my patients wondered why I spent so much time on detailed history and considered it as my inability to decipher the problem quickly. I remain motivated to adapt to changing trends, though I am aware it is difficult if not impossible. I have learnt to be vigilant to focus on my limitations and seek timely help from others. The community also has changed and so also their expectations from doctors as they have more faith in laboratory tests than in doctor's clinical diagnosis. I often meet parents who come with knowledge acquired from Google-God and challenge my opinion. In such situations, I end up with "you may be right but this is my honest opinion that is documented and it is to the best of my knowledge" and leave them without further argument. I have learned patient has a choice to follow your advice or not.

Take Home Message

Changing trends in medicine call for constant updating and the doctor has to be a life-time student. It is important to find time for continued education even in a busy practice. Changing trends in medical practice demand setting clear goals to achieve rationality and excellence and not fall prey to "rat race". Once you are motivated, habit sustains it to make life happy and worth living.

4 Diagnostic Process Often Reversed!

We need proper balance in medical approach

– Mark Twain

Before you examine the body of a patient, be patient to hear his story, once you learn his story, you will also come to know his body

– Suzy Kassem

Introduction

The process is nothing but a set of defined activities that have stood the test of time. It describes how a task should be performed and provides focus to make it better to ensure a successful outcome. The diagnostic process in medicine should follow the same principles. It is more important than a goal and the right process done in the right way leads to success.

Diagnostic Process in Medicine

The diagnostic process in medicine is complex but should follow the standard sequence. It should be a patient-centric activity of gathering information, information integration and interpretation (analysis of detailed history), complete and standard physical examination (with a focus on areas guided by history analysis) to form a working diagnosis. It is only after a provisional diagnosis is made that priority diagnostic testing is planned to confirm the final diagnosis. This is a process of diagnostic refinement followed by diagnostic verification. It brings in rationality, confidence, and consistency, enables planning, eliminates mistakes, improves outcome, avoids misuse of laboratory tests and drugs, saves time as well as cost and offers satisfaction to patients. Detailed history analysis contributes to more than 80% of provisional diagnosis and thus enough time should be spent on gathering the right information. History is not his story; the patient focuses on what bothers him the most and not what the physician would want to know. History should follow the principle of "thought in action". It means each question should be deliberate with a specific purpose, the answer to which should lead to the next relevant question. The thorough physical examination will further narrow down the differential diagnosis inferred from the analysis of detailed history. There exist increasing options for diagnostic testing, from which appropriate tests should be selected based on the provisional diagnosis. Epidemiology of common diseases should guide the priority of tests.

Reversed Diagnostic Process – A MISS Approach

Rising complexities of health care, ever-increasing advances, physician's time constraints and often cognitive limitations have been responsible for the reversed diagnostic process. **MISS** approach starts with **M**anagement first without consideration of probable diagnosis with polypharmacy and if it does not work, then the next step is to **I**nvestigate, again without any clue to a provisional diagnosis and hence multiple tests are ordered at random hoping to get a diagnosis from one of the several tests. Such a process results in confusion more than a diagnosis. However, such a diagnosis even when obtained may not correlate with clinical profile and so may be erroneous. Finally, when both management and investigations fail to provide a diagnosis, it is time to ask for **S**ymptoms and look for **S**igns on physical examination. These are shortcuts to the standard diagnostic process and such a reverse diagnostic process is prevalent in the modern era and is obviously a disaster.

Tests not for Diagnosis but for Confirmation

Diagnostic testing has become a critical feature of standard medical practice. Tests are expected to define anatomy, pathology and if possible, etiology and complement bedside medicine. The etiology of most diseases has been conjectural and remained elusive with an exception of infections. Limitations of tests must be kept in mind, sensitivity and specificity of tests need consideration. No test is 100% dependable as a negative test may not rule out disease and a positive test may not necessarily confirm the disease. For example, negative blood culture does not rule out bacterial infection and positive blood culture may be a contaminant or a commensal. Choosing appropriate tests need provisional diagnosis. Priority of ordering tests must be based on Sutton's law – common things first. It is said that when you hear hoofbeats, think horses, not zebras. Ordering multiple tests to rule out every possibility is an increasing trend that is not justified. It is irrational, not cost-effective and stressful to a patient. Unfortunately, patients demand tests as they consider tests superior to clinical diagnosis and doctors find it convenient to shortcut the diagnostic process. At times, you end up treating tests and not the patient.

Missing "High-Touch" Medicine

Interaction with the patient while history taking and physical examination in a standard diagnostic process help to build a rapport and a bond between the patient and a doctor. It demonstrates concern, honesty, responsibility, accountability and transparency on the part of a doctor and instills faith, confidence, satisfaction and compliance on the part of the patient. It in many ways leads to divine healing. "High-tech" medicine deprives all such benefits and treats a patient as an inanimate object. Thus, "high-tech" medicine should be judiciously used only after the "high-touch" process is followed.

Personal Notes

My teacher once told me that when he joined as a pediatric resident in UK, he had to undergo a routine health check before starting the post. A senior general physician examined him in detail including testing for the entire sensory system. My teacher was surprised as he thought this was a cursory requirement as young aspiring residents would be most healthy. He asked the physician why he had to examine in so much detail. To which, the physician asked whether it was not the way physicians conducted the clinical examination in India. My teacher understood the message and he became enlightened even before joining the post. It is common to find a junior colleague asking me for a second opinion because he has no clue to a diagnosis in spite of several investigations and trials with antibiotics. In one of such incidences, when I asked him what his provisional diagnosis had been, he quickly said he did not know and that was why he was requesting me to see his patient. This was a classical MISS approach.

I recall a bright undergraduate student who had learnt to take a detailed history including family history. He was taking a history of a lady who had fallen down from the 1st-floor gallery while putting clothes to dry and in thoroughness, he asked whether there was a history of any family member having fallen the similar way. He is today sincere rational doctor. The astute family physician observed mild puffiness of face, engorged neck veins and propped-up eyes in a person who had come for a minor illness and had no major complaints. The person was referred to a nephrologist, cardiologist and endocrinologist for an opinion on probable diagnosis but all tests were negative and each specialist vouched it was not the problem related to his specialty. The person confirmed from his family physician that he had the unusual disease, the fate of which was unknown. So, he decided to enjoy his life before he could worsen and so planned a world tour. He went to a store to buy branded shirts. The Attendant asked for his collar size and when is said 16, the attendant said if you wear such a tight collar, you would get puffiness of eyes, engorged neck veins and propped-up eyes. The person knew his diagnosis.

Take Home Message

The diagnostic process in medicine should be followed sequentially in each patient – to find anatomy first, followed by pathology. (Medical curriculum is in the same sequence – it starts with anatomy and physiology and then goes on to pathology (it is disturbed physiology). Anatomy and pathology can be reasonably assessed by history and physical examination while etiology is a guesswork based on critical thinking. It is only then that investigations should be ordered to confirm the probable diagnosis. Thus, tests are ordered as per the provisional diagnosis. It gives a thrill to a physician when minimum tests confirm the clinical diagnosis. Physicians must audit their clinical performance and it is the only way to be an accomplished doctor.

5 Super-Specialist – Boon or Bane

We have run into the law of diminishing returns in health care, where we are doing more and more, with higher and higher technology, at more and more cost and less and less benefit

– Richard Lamm

The whole imposing edifice of modern medicine is like a celebrated tower of Pisa – slightly off balance

– Prince Charles

Introduction

Super-specialist has a depth of knowledge in a small part of medical science at the sacrifice of breadth. He has a deep understanding of a narrow field that is vital in management of selective complex cases related to his specialty. It means there has to be a generalist who can detect such a case that needs the services of a super-specialist. If a patient visits a super-specialist directly, there is a greater chance of a doctor ruling out diseases related to his super-specialty with as many tests as possible and patient referred to a generalist. Generalist has a wider but superficial knowledge, breadth without depth and should have an ability to detect a problem that needs a referral to a super-specialist of relevant specialty. Super-specialties are well developed in adult medicine/surgery in India and are also developing over last 2-3 decades in Pediatrics with increasing speed, so also in most other branches of modern medicine.

Diseases do not Respect a Specialty

Apparently localized disease to a small area of the body also may affect structure or function of other systems and hence most diseases are general in that sense. It is therefore necessary that every patient must be thoroughly examined even when presented with localized disease and every doctor – generalist, specialist and super-specialist - must be knowledgeable and competent to do so. Moreover, few symptoms represent multiple systems. Surgical diseases often are first seen by physicians generalists and at times, medical problem may simulate a surgical issue and be seen by a surgeon. Is it not then necessary that irrespective of specialty, every doctor needs to be a basic generalist? Ideal superspecialist for the community at large is a wide-based generalist.

Making of a Super-Specialist

After completing basic graduation (MBBS), specialty training spans over three years (MD/MS). A specialist must continue to be an excellent basic generalist with deeper knowledge – increased depth in common problems but maintaining wider breadth and so should be able to handle atypical presentation or complications of common diseases in the community. However, during super-specialist training, the trainee focuses on a narrow part and loses the contact with general medicine/surgery. As time passes, he gets more detached from the generalist approach of basic medicine. As mentioned above, no disease respects the boundary of any system. Thus, super-specialist has to refer a patient to one or many specialists for even simple issues that are perceived to be beyond his domain. In such a situation, often there is no single doctor coordinating views of different specialties. It is nearly impossible for direct communication between different specialists and is often a cause of concern to a patient. In such a situation, a patient could be treated by doctors of different specialties without coordination between all of them.

Pros and Cons of a Super-Specialist

With deeper knowledge of a small part, super-specialist is able to diagnose common as well as uncommon presentation of rare diseases. He is able to keep up-to-date in his narrow specialty and thus knows the latest advances in his field. This is a boon for a patient suffering from such a rare disease. However, a super-specialist often tries to rule out every possible disease in every patient, forgetting Sutton's law "think common first" or as it is said "when you hear hoofbeats think horses, not zebras". (Suttan's law is named after Willie Sutton – a bank robber who when asked by the judge why he thought of robbing the bank, he said that is where most money lies). Thus, super-specialist does not consider common diseases as he has lost exposure to common problems and in turn depends heavily on multiple tests rather than clinical judgment. He does not consider provisional diagnosis to plan investigations as he considers possibility of every disease in each patient and so can opine only after all test results. All of us are aware of fallacies of test results. This assumes far more importance when resources are limited.

How to Ensure "Boon" and Avoid "Bane"?

There is no doubt, we need super-specialists and in future also super-super-specialists – one who would know everything about a smaller part of a super-specialty. Super-specialty is for the few and by the few. But to ensure rational benefits to the community, a super-specialist must be an excellent basic generalist. In order to be a sound generalist, super-specialist must spend 3 months of each year in general medicine/surgery throughout his career. If not, a super-specialist could become a bane. I recall having met the Chief Pediatric endocrinologist at Great Ormand Street Children's hospital in London who insisted that each faculty member in his department worked in general pediatrics for 3 months of each year. This was necessary because children referred for short stature to his department from all over Europe were often suffering from non-endocrinological problems such as celiac disease or chronic renal dysfunction. In absence of such a periodic exposure to general pediatrics, patients would be subjected to multiple investigations to rule out endocrine issues and then referred to a generalist. Super-specialist should not make a diagnosis on the basis of tests alone but must consider bedside provisional diagnosis thereby limiting tests to a minimum. While making a definitive diagnosis is a priority, rational practice demands minimum laboratory tests planned on the basis of provisional bedside diagnosis. Super-specialists often miss this approach and consider possibilities more than probabilities in every case. Then it becomes a bane. Let us not forget medicine is an art of probability.

Supply should be Commensurate with Demand

We need to estimate future demands of super-specialists and plan supply chain accordingly. India is close to achieve an ideal doctor-population ratio of 1:1000 though it is skewed in terms of geographical distribution and it includes generalist doctors (family physicians) and also specialists-generalists (MD/MS). As per Pareto principle, 80% problems are solved by 20% efforts and remaining 20% problems by 80% efforts. This applies well to medical practice. Thus, we definitely need more family physicians than specialists and more specialists than super-specialists. Of course, at all levels, doctors must practice preventive medicine promoting health rather than just being disease managers. Present generation of medical graduates are attracted to ever advancing medical technology to become super-specialists. If this trend continues, community may not be best served with shortage of generalists. Super-specialists are necessary for the few and should be few in numbers. Facilities for modern technologically advanced super-specialists such as transplant surgeons, immunologists and geneticists should be restricted to few centers so as to develop a large expertise rather than every small center dabbling into it. In USA, ratio of general pediatricians to pediatric super-specialists is 2:1. This is ideal only when vaccine and hygiene preventable diseases are extinct in the community. However, our epidemiology of diseases is different and as of now, we need far more generalists than super-specialists.

Personal Notes

It is not rare for the community to seek super-specialty opinion directly with a focus on one major symptom. I have seen a patient with vomiting directly meeting a super-specialist, GI specialist who rules out problems of his domain after several tests, surgeon ruling out intestinal obstruction, neurologist asking for neuroimaging to rule out brain tumor, nephrologist ordering renal function tests and metabolic specialist going through many tests. Highly accomplished doctors ask for all these tests so as not to miss any disease. Only if these super-specialists were excellent generalists, diagnosis could be achieved most rationally with minimum tests. As a senior generalist, patient often seeks my opinion after visiting few super-specialists, especially when symptoms are vague and overlapping such as prolonged fever or persistent vomiting. This is a reverse referral and speaks of compartmentalization of medical practice that becomes a bane. I recall when my father as a family physician would accompany a patient to a specialist that facilitated better monitoring of a patient and also a learning opportunity to a family physician. He could also question the specialist for clarification. Such a rapport between a referring doctor and a specialist is almost non-existent today. A cow was shown to an intern and asked to identify the animal. He instantly said it was cow and when asked whether he would investigate to confirm, he emphatically refused, he was sure. Same animal was shown to a specialist who also identified the animal right but wanted to confirm by tests "just to be sure". He had learnt "evidence-based medicine". He did not want to miss any other diagnosis. Finally, same animal was shown to a super-specialist. After a close intelligent look at the animal, he said there would be many possibilities such as hypertrophied goat or atrophied elephant that he would investigate to rule out. He also cited case reports in world literature in his support. And once all such possibilities were ruled out, he would consider it to be a cow. Finally, everyone got it right but intern was most rational, specialist cared for evidence-based diagnosis and super-specialist would not take any chance.

Take Home Message

Every doctor must be a competent generalist irrespective of his specialty or super-specialty. Success is achieved with wider experience achieved through formative years and sustained through periodic exposure to general approach. Thus, every doctor must try to be both – a generalist must know bit of specialty and specialist and super-specialist must know enough of basic general medicine. This alone will avoid perverse effects of super-specialisation and serve the community better.

6 Old and New – Make the Best of the Two

Old is gold but new may be a diamond but don't forget it is the gold that holds the diamond

– Igeenell Timmons

In modern medicine we have a name for everything but cure almost for nothing

– Charles Coleman

Introduction

Modern medical science is advancing rapidly and newer technology attracts everyone's attention. It has made a significant impact on health care but also is vulnerable to be misused. This is because majority patients in the community can be well treated by time-tested old methods of basic medicine and do not justify use of modern technology. Modern technology also has limitations and hence it should be used selectively only after proper counseling. Though it has widened our understanding of diseases, present knowledge lacks ability to offer significant advantage to majority patients. Level of clinical suspicion and probability of a given test result can be correlated, higher the degree of clinical suspicion, more likely the test result will confirm the diagnosis. Therefore, it is time that present generation of doctors must learn when to avoid use of modern technology, instead excel in use of basic medical approach of making a provisional diagnosis. At the same time, older generation of doctors must be continuously updated to know where modern technology can benefit the patient.

Old not Entirely Gold but all that Glitters is also not Gold

Science has changed but......

Over last six decades of my medical career, I have seen a drastic change in understanding of diseases and their management strategies. This has been possible only because of modern technology. I recall the days when simple chest X-ray was also not freely available and fluoroscopy was used routinely with its inherent dangers and subjective interpretations. Today we have many imaging modalities that depict not only structural but also functional changes. Infections can be diagnosed with precision and with the development of Immunology and genetics, it has been possible to get deeper insights into causation and progression of diseases. Invention of newer drugs and therapeutic interventions have revolutionised treatment strategies. Thus, "old" ignorance in science has been replaced by "new' understanding. Previous generation of doctors must keep updated and take help of technologically trained newer generation of doctors. It is important to realize that part of the present-day advanced knowledge will be obsolete by next decade as medicine is ever changing, hopefully for the better. It calls for continuous learning.

Science has changed but not art of medical management

Art of history taking and physical examination as well as art of communication and behavior with the patient has been time-tested and so remained the same over centuries. Ethics, empathy, concern for the patient, honesty, transparency, responsibility, accountability, communication and counseling made patients feel better, even when science had not much developed. Physicians always cared for the patients if not able to cure and patients showed gratitude and faith in doctors. Present generation of doctors have largely ignored this aspect of patient management in pursuit of modern science. It has made patients feel unhappy and lose faith in doctors. Thus, image of medical professions has been maligned. Present generation of doctors must reverse this trend and follow this part of "old" while using "new" selectively and rationally.

Limitations of Modern Technology

While taking history, an uninterrupted and patient listening to what the patient has to say is an exercise in developing a rapport between the doctor and a patient. It is a measure of doctor's empathy and concern about the patient and it makes the patient feel assured. Further, physical examination establishes a bond with appropriate human touch – "high-touch" technology. This sets the tone for developing faith in the doctor and helps in recovery of a patient. Misuse of modern technology lacks such opportunities and thus misses an important factor in the management of a patient. Diagnostic technology has also many inherent limitations. Peripheral blood smear is the most important part of blood investigations and modern technology is of no use as it needs an experienced and committed pathologist to examine the same. Similarly, treating physician has to correlate test results with his clinical judgment. In fact, every technology has inherent issues that come in the way of correct interpretation. Today, most laboratories perform CBC on automated counters that differentiate blood cells based on the size of cells, smallest size is a platelet and largest size is a leukocyte and size in between is an erythrocyte. If erythrocytes are of smaller size as happens in commonly prevalent iron deficiency anemia, automated counter includes them in platelets and platelet count goes higher than actual. If a child suffering from thrombocytopenia also has iron deficiency anemia, platelet count on automated counter may be normal and diagnosis can easily be missed. Besides the issue of interpretation, technical error in performing the test can give erroneous results as happens in case of a small blood clot while loading the sample. Commonly available counters can differentiate polymorphs and lymphocytes but not monocytes, eosinophils and basophils that are all clubbed together in one common category. So, in spite of automated counter, a pathologist must see the peripheral smear to assign relative value to these three types of cells included in another category. This means that a pathologist must have good basic knowledge.

Of course, now latest generation of counters are being invented to overcome such difficulties. Further, CBC results by themselves are not diagnostic of any disease and even a simple difference between an infective and non-infective disease or between viral and bacterial infection are also not possible. This brings in a point that basic knowledge of medicine is required for right interpretation in spite of modern technology. If it is true of a simple test, then it must be more problematic in complex tests such as genetic or immunological tests. Even in case of monogenic genetic defects (for example, cystic fibrosis), more than several hundred mutations are known and as all mutations cannot be tested, negative test does not rule out the disease. In such a situation, physician has to fall back on clinical approach and treat the patient. In case of oligogenic or polygenic defects, problems are further compounded even though newer tests such as microarray or gene sequencing are invented. Finally, positive genetic test has very little relevance to the index patient and theoretically may be useful for prenatal detection. Immunology plays an important part in causation, progression and outcome of diseases. However, such tests merely suggest the probability but are not diagnostic of autoimmune or infection induced immune disorders and need correlation with clinical profile. It is clear that modern technology cannot replace basic clinical approach and competence. Technology must be used as a servant (summon whenever required but ignore, if necessary) and not as a master (to dictate actions). Besides, the cost is a concern.

Rational use of Modern Technology

Diagnostic technology must be used judiciously with primary aim of offering direct benefit to the index patient. It is important to estimate pre-test probability of usefulness to a patient before ordering the test. It helps to decide whether to order a test or not. However, there could be indirect benefit of diagnostic tests to the family or community, even if not to the index patient and also could improve scientific understanding for doctors. For example, genetic tests in an index patient may be useful to predict recurrence of same defect in the next pregnancy and similarly RT-PCR test for covid helps monitoring epidemiology of the disease. In such a situation, patient and his relatives need to be well communicated and counselled before ordering the test so that they understand the advantages and limitations of these tests.

Therapeutic technological advances have been much more useful to patients. Interventional radiology and cardiac procedures, minimal invasive and robotic surgical techniques and organ/stem cell transplants have definitely benefited patients though often not affordable or accessible. In such situations, communication and counseling play very important role to explain risk-benefit ratio and long-term implications that are inherent with some of these advances.

Personal Notes

I have often seen patients complaining about doctors ordering multiple tests and interventions. This is true more when the results of tests are negative, suffering continues and diagnosis is at bay. When desirable outcome is achieved, even irrational use is mostly condoned. It is not wrong on the part of doctors to use modern technology only if its use is rational, can be justified, patients are adequately counselled and explanation is properly documented. Doctor should be accountable to his own conscience about rationality, justification and proper counseling. This is found lacking in many present generations of doctors. It is not rare for doctors to pursue final diagnosis even when final outcome is known to be poor and in absence of pre-test counseling, parents feel cheated in spite of doctor's good intensions to arrive at a final diagnosis. In such cases, patient must be given a choice of making a decision regarding further testing. What concerns the patient most is the individual benefit and not future of science. I saw a bird watcher focusing at a distance through his high-tech binoculars but the bird was sitting just behind him and it must be wondering whether to alert the bird-watcher to look behind. Many times, physician focusses at a distance but misses what is near.

Take Home Message

There is a need for intergenerational learning. Doctors of previous generation must at least be acquainted with newer developments and direct patients appropriately to seek better advice. They should therefore keep updated by attending CMEs and through interactions with the highly trained present generation. This alone will offer the advantage of modern science to patients. At the same time, present generation of doctors must attempt a provisional diagnosis before ordering tests and avoid misuse of modern technology by judicious selection. Art of medical practice is most essential part of patient management and will remain so irrespective of modern technology and this fact should be born in mind by present generation of doctors. This is the only way to make old and new work best together.

7 Doctor-Patient Relationship

Doctor is both a scientist and humanitarian, his most decisions lie in the field of patient relations

– David Allman

Doctor patient relationship is critical to the placebo effect

– Irving Kirsch

Introduction

Relationship refers the way both the parties behave with each other. Naturally, both are equally responsible for maintaining harmonious relation that is vital for successful outcome. For a doctor, professional success should be a long-term continuous process and depends on "word-of-mouth" publicity while for the patient, success is one time issue related to cure of his illness. Besides, sick patient is likely to be unrealistic in his expectations and pose a challenge. Hence, primarily it is doctor's responsibility to forge a harmonious relation with patients and must learn to handle situations that have potential to become a roadblock.

Foundation of Ideal Relationship

Contemporary medical ethics is the foundation of doctor-patient relationship. Medical ethics is a system of moral principles that apply value and judgment to medical practice. There are four pillars of medical ethics – beneficence (do best to the patient), non-maleficence (do no harm), justice (impact of decision) and autonomy (respect patient's rights). There are many more related important issues such as patient empowerment, confidentiality, informed consent, communication, counseling and documentation, don't run down peers, don't hide ignorance and equity (treat everyone as per the need). Ethics in medical practice is a measure of honesty, transparency, responsibility and accountability and is inseparable from medical competence. In addition, patient hearing and empathy result in quality care that builds mutual faith, respect and trust between doctor and patient. Patients don't care how much you know but definitely want to know how much you care.

Integrate art into Science of Medical Practice

While scientific knowledge and constant updating is essential, art of medical practice is as important as science to foster ideal doctor-patient relationship. Art includes, besides ethics, basic components such as skilled planning and time management, philosophy – patient hearing, honest opinion and explanation, culture – organized, disciplined, courteous and respectful behavior. Perfect combination of ethics with art and science offers "care always, cure if possible" in medical practice that builds mutual faith, respect and trust between doctor and patients.

Deteriorating Doctor-Patient Relationship

Both parties are responsible though as mentioned above, doctors are expected to be proactive in fostering good relation with patients. Current scenario is far from the ideal.

Deficiencies in doctors' behavior

There is an indisputable depersonalization in medical practice. Instead of making sensible decisions with basic clinical skills, there is a spurious outsourcing of common sense to modern technology. Doctors tend to treat tests rather than the disease and ignore the human being in whose body the disease resides. This has resulted in opportunity for exploitation and unethical medical practice, with profession turning into business. Rapid-fire investigations and gun-shot therapy is often based on external motivation either fear/punishment or incentives. Thus, affordable health care becomes an area of ethical conflict. Ethics, communication, counseling and documentation are often missing in pursuit of scientific outreach. Doctor-centered approach projects doctor as an expert and patient is expected to abide silently without asking questions. Conversational dominance and short time spent with the patient do not offer opportunity for discussion. Sadly, art and ethics of medical practice are not taught in medical schools and absence of role model teachers deprives medical students to learn this important aspect of medical practice. Further there is lack of control on quality of medical education and medical practice. All these deficiencies have eroded faith and image of medical profession and is the cause of deteriorating doctor-patient relationship. While every doctor would like to see his patient recover completely, his efforts must be made visible by repeated communication and counseling so that patient does not judge the doctor by the outcome. This is the only way to ensure ideal doctor-patient relationship.

Deficiencies in patients' behavior

It is patient's right to know about his disease and management plan. However, most patients expect "cure" of the disease and relate outcome to doctor's competence and efforts. They do not understand limitations of medical science and that of a doctor who cannot cure every disease even with best of competence and intentions. Earlier generation of patients had full faith in their doctors and they were satisfied with doctor's best efforts irrespective of the outcome. Lack of faith in doctors of present generation of patients is the cause of poor doctor-patient relationship for which I consider doctors equally responsible. Poor outcome of a disease is often beyond control of a doctor but patients in such circumstances behave with vengeance and unacceptable violence. Outcome in other professions does not decide level of competence of a professional. A lawyer is not blamed for a defeat in a law suit and teacher is not blamed if students fail. People understand multiple variable factors involved in final outcome. Same is true and even to a much larger extent in medical practice as outcome primarily depends on patient's ability to fight and not just on doctor's competence. Even when life and death is the question in medical practice, patients are not expected to behave irrationally. After all, humans are not immortal.

Consequences of Deteriorating Doctor-Patient Relationship

Unethical practices by doctors and unrealistic expectations leading to irrational behavior of patients have resulted in erosion of faith, trust and mutual respects for each other. Present generation of doctors practice defensive medicine that demands large number of tests and interventions with increase in cost of health care. It is a known fact that error of commission is more acceptable and condoned than error of omission that is punished. Doctors look at every patient as a potential litigant while patients look at the doctor as one who would cheat. This kind of behavior on the part of patients has led to increase in number of legal suits against the doctors and hence doctors justify defensive medicine. Besides doctors have to face danger to their own life and property. Hence, present generation of doctors have to spend for professional indemnity insurance against such possible events and such extra expenses are indirectly borne by patients. It has further vitiated doctor-patient relationship with disadvantage to both the parties. As such we are short of doctors in proportion to the population in India and present generation of doctors prefer their children to pursue any career other than medicine due to many adverse factors.

Can we Reverse this Trend?

It is possible if both the parties introspect their behavior pattern and change appropriately.

Doctors must change first

Time management is the key to better communication, counseling and documentation. Doctors are also required to keep updated constantly and find time for the same as medical science is dynamic and the only constant is the change. In busy practice also, doctor must find time without sacrificing quality of practice and it is possible only with group practice. This is necessary as doctor is not supposed to deny seeing a patient irrespective of time constraint and still is expected to offer best quality of service. Thus, group practice is ideal also for life of a doctor as he can find time for family and his own leisure, hobbies. Rational practice needs integration of art and science and doctors must acquire art of practice that involves ethics and empathy besides many other moral principles. Unfortunately, this is not taught in medical schools but it is left for individual doctors to follow art of practice by internal motivation that comes from within. It is the same motivation that should sensitise a doctor to keep updated in science. Once internal motivation gets started, it becomes a habit and is sustained forever. External motivation depends on fear/punishment or rewards, it is short lasting and often is a cause of stressful life.

Patients also must change their behavior

Patients must learn to be patient. They also have equal responsibility to facilitate ideal relationship with the doctor. They must have full faith and trust in their chosen doctor. They must understand limitations of medical science and not expect unrealistic outcomes. They must come prepared for doctor's visit that enables them to describe relevant details of their complaints. They must follow doctor's advice and instructions for follow-up. They must report back irrespective of improvement or otherwise. It is commonly seen that patients rarely report if they are better and it deprives the doctor of knowing his good results that boosts his confidence. Patients are expected to be transparent and honest. They should not hide any information that itself may prove to be a disadvantage to themselves such as other opinions. Lastly any bad outcome cannot justify vengeance and violence damaging doctor's life, property and image. There are better methods to challenge the outcome, if so desired.

Personal Notes

I am very happy when patient leaves my office with satisfaction and gratitude, my day is done! I recall few instances when patients were argumentative and I have learnt not to counteract even if patients are wrong. I remember an incidence when a child with fever was brought to me for second opinion and his mother asked me whether fever could be due to multiple myeloma. I was surprised to hear such a question. She informed me that she herself had similar fever that was finally diagnosed as multiple myeloma and her doctor had missed it completely for which she had decided to confront him and take him to the court. I knew the concerned doctor as most honest and competent physician and felt bad for him but avoided any further conversation. Few months later, when I met this mother, she herself narrated what happened when she went to fight with the doctor who had missed her diagnosis. When this doctor was shown final diagnosis made by another doctor, he banged his fists on the table and agreed that he had missed the diagnosis and it was his fault. This honest behavior of the doctor made this lady to decide against going to the court. Honesty is the best option and not the defensive argument to justify wrong action. I know of a very competent doctor when asked by his patient whether he was sure of his diagnosis, was upset and angrily said "do you know whom you are questioning, I talk only when, I am sure." This is ego and rudeness. Patient swore not to see him again in spite of his competence and commitment. We must mind our tongue!

Take Home Message

We must accept the fact that there is definite deterioration of doctor-patient relationship. Cordial relation plays such an important part in management of diseases. It is bipartite responsibility though doctors should be proactive in forging such a relationship. Time is the key factor for doctors and they must find ways to manage time for which group practice is an ideal solution. It also improves doctor's private life. Patients must be equally honest and transparent and must have full faith and trust in their chosen doctor. Unrealistic expectations and irrational behavior is not acceptable at any cost as there are better methods available for redressing their grievances.

8 Doctor-Doctor Relationship

What you do not want done to yourself,
do not do to others

– Confucius

Ultimate test of relationship is to disagree but
to maintain mutual respect

– Alexandra Penny

Introduction

Ayurveda – ancient science of life – had laid down code of conduct for physicians, to be righteous in every action. Aristotle – Greek philosopher – 384-322 BC advocated good conduct for physicians. American Medical Association formed a committee to formulate code of conduct for physicians in 1846. World Medical Association formed international code of conduct for physicians in 1947. In 1970, traditional medical ethics were found to be inadequate to deal with changing medical practices that led to widening scope of ethics. Besides four pillars of medical ethics – beneficence, non-maleficence, autonomy and justice, there are many other related issues that are very much part of medical ethics and one of them relate to doctor-doctor relationship. Medical council of India in its notification has elaborated on doctor-doctor relationship." I will treat my colleagues with all dignity and respect to maintain honor and noble traditions of medical profession". It adds "don't run down peers. Relation between doctors should be one of friendship and cooperation. However, physician should expose without fear or favor, incompetent or corrupt, dishonest or unethical conduct on the part of members of the profession."

How Important is Doctor-Doctor Relationship?

While doctor-patient relationship is at the core of holistic care, doctor-doctor relationship has clear importance and indirect contribution in boosting confidence of patients and thereby helping healing process. Unfortunately, this aspect is mostly neglected. Modern medical science has advanced with leaps and bounds to an extent that no physician can claim to know to treat every patient well enough, under his/her care. There is old Greek proverb "one man is no man". Owing to increasing complexities of modern medicine and technology, interdependence of doctors is assuming more importance with need for its close collaboration. Every doctor, be it a family physician or specialist, is likely to need advice or help from one of his/her colleagues. On the other hand, a doctor is called upon to help a colleague, either suggested by a treating doctor or requested by patient or his relatives. Such a consultation is intended to do more justice to the betterment of a patient without causing confusion, even in the face of difference of opinion. It is vital that both the concerned doctors "discuss" without "argument" and convey unified action to the patient. Discussion is to find out what is right while argument is to decide who is right. Responsibility of good conduct during such a consultation rest more on senior colleague whose help is sought by primary treating doctor. In such a consultation, no insincerity, rivalry or envy should be indulged. Doctor must behave with his colleagues the way he would expect his colleagues to behave with him. Doctor should consider it a privilege to help his colleague when asked for. In this relationship, every doctor must learn to make unambiguous statements with measured words to avoid any misunderstanding or misinterpretation. At times, same message delivered in different words sounds contradictory to each other that adds to confusion in the minds of patients. Ideally, such a consultation is usually "one time" help to a primary treating doctor who thereafter continues to treat his patient in the suggested direction. Doctor who provides help to a primary treating doctor should refrain from direct contact with the patient. Such a conduct between doctors not only boosts confidence of patients but also improves image of the profession. It has a direct benefit to the society and is a win-win situation for doctors and the community.

Introspection - Quo Vadis – Where are we Going?

Contemporary medical ethics is the very foundation of medical practice and is inseparable from medical science and doctor's competence. Unfortunately, art of medical practice is missing while there is scientific overreach with outsourcing common sense to modern technology that has increased cost of health care. Unfortunately, technology has de-humanised medicine. Patients consider medical profession as business and suspect every action irrespective of doctor's intentions that has maligned image of medical profession. Medical council of India has miserably failed to maintain high ethical standards that are required to promote moral values. Indian Medical Association has equally failed to control irrational methods of practice that has hurt general welfare of the community and has eroded faith in doctors. Negative professional criticism of another doctor, in the pursuit of money and prestige, damages reputation of the profession. May be an unintended (or was it intended?) casual remark such as "I wish I was called a bit early, it is already late" can spoil the situation. I know a doctor who would change the brand of a drug claiming better response as compared to a brand prescribed by primary doctor, making a patient doubt the very competence of his primary doctor. Such "one-upmanship" to take an advantage of a situation is a gross violation of code of conduct. I must admit that such an overt misconduct is rare today but one can always feel an undercurrent of occult attempts at such behavior between doctors in the present "rat race". After all, even if you win the race, don't forget you are a bloody rat.

Can Good Conduct be Taught?

I understand that Medical Council of India has now included "medical ethics" in undergraduate curriculum. However, art of medical practice is not learnt in classrooms but must be witnessed at the bedside of patients through a role model teacher. It should start from teacher-student relationship during undergraduate training period. I was lucky to have had teachers with high ethical values whom we tried to emulate. Present generation of medical students need such teachers. During my tenure as a post-graduate student, an intern was posted in our unit who was in a habit of expressing his views on every patient during ward round and we all thought his undue and untimely enthusiasm had to be curbed in order not to waste time on rounds. But Dr M.M. Wagle, my chief differed and said "it is good this boy is thinking even though he does not know enough. So, give him time to understand his limitations but don't stop him, he is after all learning". It was a lesson on how to behave with a student. I recall first day of my joining as an honorary assistant Prof in Pediatric Department at J. J. Hospital, Mumbai. Dr Wagle greeted me and asked me to conduct ward round when he and other senior faculty member would join me on rounds. It was a lesson to respect and promote a junior colleague. Such a behavior builds a close bond between one another. Dr Wagle addressed every human being as a gentleman, irrespective of status. It was only such role models that made it possible for us to learn art of interpersonal behavior in medical practice. I have tried to emulate my chief as much as I could throughout last 50 years of my professional career and I hope this legacy is passed on at least to few students.

What is appalling is lack of comradeship that starts right from training days. Five decades ago when I was a trainee, there was not only cordial relationship between students and resident doctors but also with faculty members who were our friends more than our teachers. Thus, we were closely knit. Over last one decade that I have experienced during my tenure as Medical Director of a teaching institution, that there is no comradeship between first, second and third-year residents as each junior addresses his one-year senior as "sir or madam". I feel it comes in the way of building relationship and thereby affects smooth working together.

Self-Regulation – Need of the Hour

There is no doubt about the role played by role model to promote good conduct. However, role model can't ensure good conduct unless one is motivated enough. Ethics is internally defined based on motivation while morals are externally imposed. Motivation is a psychological driving force that reinforces an action towards desired goal. Intrinsic motivation driven by enjoyment of work – pleasure without expecting reward – must come from within that has positive impact on life. Once intrinsic motivation gets started, habit sustains it. On the other hand, extrinsic motivation is driven by reward, money, threat or punishment and it has negative impact on life. While motivation leads the way, it is attitude that decides how well you behave. It is the attitude that takes you to altitude. Do you know – when each alphabet is assigned a numerical number in sequence (1 for A, 2 for B), word "attitude" totals 100!

Testing Time When Faced with Specific Situations

Few common situations occur in medical practice that really test individual behavior pattern in doctor-doctor relationship.

1. A doctor may be called to attend a patient whose regular doctor is not available. It is important to attend to problems that demand immediate attention, avoiding discussion and offering opinion on other problems for regular doctor to handle. It automatically takes care of difference of opinion, if any. Best way out is to reiterate that ideal advice comes from a regular doctor who knows the background health status of his patient. Such an explanation is reasonably acceptable.
2. Problem is tricky when senior doctor is called for second opinion that differs completely from the original. Even if senior doctor is convinced about need to change the diagnosis and/or management in favor of the patient's well-being, it is imperative to defend original doctor's opinion at the same time. It is easy to get away by making a statement "I would have done the same that your doctor did but now that it has failed, we need to change which we both doctors will discuss together and implement". It ensures the right change without damaging primary doctor's image and one could privately sensitise the doctor to correct his faults. This is very important as each doctor has faced similar situation, however experienced he may be and expects not to be fallen in the eyes of his patient. After all, medicine is science of uncertainty and art of probability and no doctor can claim to have made no mistakes.
3. It is not uncommon for patients to seek another doctor's opinion by themselves, without knowledge of primary treating doctor. Many of them may hide information about what was done by previous doctor. In addition, unhappy patient elaborates on how bad the previous doctor was. We should discourage such a dialogue and surely not comment on it lest it is considered as approval of patient's criticism about previous doctor or even an attempt to defend a professional colleague. It is best to move on with patient's physical problems, cutting short unnecessary gossip.
4. Cross-reference relates to an opinion asked for from one specialist to the other from allied branch of medicine. It may often pose a problem. It is duty of primary treating doctor to discuss with the patient and his relatives and justify need for a cross reference. It should be clear to everyone concerned whether it is "one time" consultation or "daily" review. It is often a bone of contention when it comes to

paying for it. It is much better to be transparent about it. It is ideal that in such a cross-reference consultation, both the doctors together convey unified opinion to the patient. However, if it is not possible for both the doctors to be present at the same time, primary doctor must explain the patient about joint discussion while other doctor should be very brief in talking to the patient and leave details to be discussed by primary doctor. This again would avoid any misinterpretation or misunderstanding on the part of the patient.

5. Biggest dilemma in doctor's mind is whether to protect a colleague in spite of unethical or negligent act or to expose him. Ethically, physician is expected to expose a corrupt, unethical or negligent colleague and it is also moral, social and professional responsibility. However, it may be construed as an act of vengeance by other colleagues. There is a room for constructive criticism. Positive criticism attempts to change medical practice for the better. It is right to criticize a colleague but face-to-face and only in strict confidence. Negative criticism amounts to fault-finding that serves no purpose than to damage someone's image. One should never malign a colleague. Honest comment offered in good faith is justified but how to do it is most important. Few years ago, one of my child patient's mother delivered another baby and wanted me to see her newborn at the maternity hospital to which I was not attached. I insisted that due permission should be obtained from treating obstetrician which was done. I went to see the baby by then 30 hours old. To my horror, I found imperforate anus though I was informed that baby had passed meconium. It was obvious a negligence. I had to inform parents about it and also need for urgent surgery and at the same time, I was obliged to protect the obstetrician. I was aware that rarely anal opening is seen as a dimple but there is a small membrane in the proximal part of anal canal that causes similar obstruction to passage of meconium. I explained the parents that as a pediatrician, I could diagnose such a condition but routinely it is not so easy to make out. Thus, I could save the doctor and also saved the baby. I also had to take the surgeon into confidence. I am sure my action is debatable but, in my mind, I acted right. Academic debates promote healthy criticism without naming a colleague, such as, one can present a real story of unethical act for audience reaction. It is likely the guilty colleague could be attending as well but without being recognized and in the process, he has learnt his mistake. I am sure every doctor wants to improve but without being made a villain.

Personal Notes

I started private practice in the year 1969 and ten years later, Dr Khare joined me. As another decade passed, we thought of adding another colleague in our group and Dr Chokhani joined around late 80's. By then we were three of us working as one unit, similar to unit system in teaching hospitals with three staff members. Subsequently Dr Pranjal Kale joined us and now we are four together. We share the place as well as patients though patients have a choice to select one of us as their primary pediatrician but are assured of help from others in the group whenever necessary. Interpersonal relations amongst us – all pediatricians - have been so good that only differences of opinion have been restricted to academic discussions and I give full credit to my colleagues. All of us have done reasonably well being together with many advantages of joint practice. This is just to make a point that doctors of same specialty can also work together as one unit, only with mutual trust and faith.

I recall when I met one of my senior colleagues soon after I had started joint practice, he wondered whether my decision was right as I would lose patients to my partner. I realized he had not understood that we were one unit.

Take Home Message

Basis of good relation between doctors lies in mutual respect and understanding. There are rules of good conduct for doctors – referred as medical etiquettes but they are never taught in medical curriculum. Anyway, they can't be taught in classroom but must be witnessed every day in live situations during training period to have a lasting effect. However, beyond an exposure to role model behavior, good conduct is self-regulated and all that one needs is motivation and attitude to follow it. Surely it brings joy and happiness in life. Of course, same is true about relationship between any two individuals that we need to learn from childhood through exposure in the family itself.

9 Building Blocks of Patient Care

Practice of medicine is an art, not a trade, a calling not a business, a calling in which your heart will be exercised equally with brain

– William Osler

What patient needs is more conversation

– Glenn Close

Introduction

"Care always, cure if possible" should be the motto of every doctor. In spite of advances in modern medicine, cure is not possible in many diseases. In the past much before modern science developed, physician could comfort patients only by quality of care they offered beyond prescribing medicines. Unfortunately, this aspect often is ignored by present-day doctors.

Attributes of Quality Care

Quality is an abstract and not a discrete entity. There are two dimensions of health care – provision of care (clinical standards) and experience of care (communication, counseling, empathy, ethics and emotional support). There is no doubt that clinical decisions must be based on science that include analysis of detailed history, focused physical examination, relevant minimum tests and rational therapy. However, there are other patient-centric aspects of quality care that relate to individual patient's needs, preferences and values, patient education and patient satisfaction. Therapy must be safe (no harm while trying to do good), effective - services provided based on scientific knowledge to all those who could benefit (avoiding underuse) and refraining from providing services to those who are unlikely to benefit (avoiding overuse), timely (reducing undue waits and harmful delays for both care-givers and receivers), equitable (providing same quality as per the need) and efficient (avoiding waste of drugs, equipment, tests, procedures, supplies, ideas and energy). Doctor should give adequate time as per the need and not just the standard time slot for every patient. Some patients may need extra time either for diagnosis or counseling and it is necessary for a doctor to manage time in such a way that quality of care is not sacrificed. Dignified and respectful approach is expected and success of quality care depends on patient empowerment that helps him to manage his own illness effectively.

Holistic Care Ensures Quality Care

We humans are endowed upon by nature few faculties that must be put to use in every act of ours to obtain best outcome. These include body, heart, mind and soul. When translated into medical practice, body means knowledge, heart the compassion, mind the commitment and soul the inner conscience. Compassion makes us understand the suffering of a patient which in turn would deliver quality care. Of course, we should not be too much attached to a patient lest we go astray in our clinical decisions. Commitment is necessary to do the best to the extent of our ability and should be the way you would expect other doctors to behave, if you were a patient. As medical science is dynamic and fast changing, we need to keep ourselves constantly updated. However, in spite of knowledge-based care delivered with compassion and commitment may not achieve desired results and it is where inner conscience plays a part. As outcome in a patient depends on many variables beyond our control, even at the end of poor outcome, we should be so clear in our conscience that we had left nothing undone. After all we are answerable to our own conscience.

Thin Line Between Great and Good Doctor

Good and great are both adjectives that superficially seem to be similar but are different. Great is an adjective that may be used for both good and bad behavior such as "he is a great crook" or "a great liar". But good as an adjective refers to only right behavior. There exists a thin line between great and good doctor. Great doctor is one whose performance is above average and so is admired while good doctor fulfills the expected or desired outcome including patient satisfaction and gratefulness and such a doctor commands respect. Average doctor treats symptoms, great doctor treats the disease while good doctor treats a patient and beyond.

Is Motivation Necessary?

Motivation is a psychological driving force that reinforces an action towards desired goal. Intrinsic motivation is driven by enjoyment of work, pleasure without expecting a reward and should come from within. In such a situation, even work load induces eustress – enjoyable stress that does produce positive impact on health and well-being. Once intrinsic motivation gets started, habit sustains it. As against, extrinsic motivation is driven by reward, money or threat, punishment and in which work load results in stress that has negative impact on life, results in life-style disorders. It is the intrinsic motivation that determines what you do but attitude decides how well you do. It is the attitude that takes you to altitudes. If you give a numerical value to each alphabet – 1 for A and 2 for B, then attitude is the word that totals 100. It is important to cultivate right kind of attitude to reach heights.

Personal Notes

I set up a joint practice so that quantity of practice could be shared with a motto to maintain good quality and I could give enough time to a patient with proper counseling and documentation. All my partners do the same. We are blessed by parents who appreciate care that we give and it brings us an immense joy. Of course, few patients want a quick fix and we are happy that such patients never come back to us. I have met patients who felt I talked more than prescribing drugs and so, they were not satisfied as they thought they wasted their time. Obviously, they don't care for "care" but only value the drug prescription. God bless them to find better doctor!

Take Home Message

Doctor is expected always to offer holistic care and cure, if possible. One must develop intrinsic motivation and right attitude that will help building right blocks of patient care. It will benefit both the patient and a doctor himself.

10 Nurturing Self

It's not selfish to love yourself, to take care of yourself and make happiness as a priority. It's necessary

– Mandy Hale

If your compassion does not include yourself, it is incomplete

– Jack Cornfield

Introduction

Nurturing is an act of encouraging, nourishing and caring for someone or something to promote ideal functioning. Nurturing self refers to continued care necessary to maintain good health that is totally in our own hands and for which we are solely responsible. Most of us are lucky to be born with good health but as we move along with our life, we often fail to maintain good health due to sheer neglect. Ironically this is more likely with doctors who look after health of others but are deficient in looking after their own health for various inexcusable reasons. Thus, they often miss out on good health. Good health is not a "divine" gift but needs ideal self-nurture, possible in older children and adults. Younger children require parents to nurture them and set the health in right direction, while older children may need supervision.

What is "Health"?

Health is complete state of physical, mental and spiritual well-being and not just absence of disease or infirmity. However, individuals vary in their potential to achieve total health and so one must understand that this definition relates to expected performance commensurate with age and prevalent cultural norms in the society.

Physical health

It is measured by common parameters such as weight, height and BMI – body mass index and should be within normal standard limits appropriate for age, ethnicity and family pattern. It is best assessed by functional competence in terms of energy to perform physical activities. Child during growing periods must maintain centiles on growth chart and an adult must maintain weight within small variations throughout life.

There are five important inputs necessary to maintain good physical health and they include balanced diet (plenty of vegetables and fruits with control on sugar and salt intake), ideal physical exercise (appropriately strenuous for an hour a day), adequate sleep (7-8 hours a day), proper hygiene (skin, teeth, genitalia) and time for leisure and hobbies that rejuvenate for better performance.

Mental health

It consists of emotional (empathy, coping up with stress, tolerant and remaining happy), philosophical (self-regulation, contented, satisfied, work with passion beyond rewards) and social health (socially accepted behavior, build stronger relationship and bonding). Mental health is nurtured during childhood by parents and other family members, further guided by role model teachers and thereafter fine-tuned and sustained with internal motivation by an adult.

Spiritual health

It has nothing to do with religion but consists of spreading love, avoiding jealousy and hatred, altruism, harmony, concerns about others and trying to help the needy. It is also nurtured in a similar way as mental health.

Happiness a Part of Good Health

Happiness is not included in the definition of health but I feel it is the **measure of maximum health.** Happiness is a state of mind and complete health can be nurtured only with harmonious relationship of body with mind. "Mens sana in corpore sano" – meaning healthy mind in a healthy body - is an emblem of Grant Medical College in Mumbai – my alma mater - third oldest medical college in India started in 1845 and this emblem is so apt to sensitise medical students starting their career. Meaningful life is be useful, helpful, compassionate and be blessed and daily acts of such kindness add up to happiness. Happiness is a spectrum of satisfaction, contentment, joy and bliss that results when you appreciate what you have. Happiness is different from pleasure that is transient and felt only by a single organ but happiness pervades through entire body and gives you long lasting experience. It is also different than success that is based on reward, recognition, position or power and is what is perceived by others. Both pleasure and success do not give happiness.

General obstacles to happiness are desire, anger, greed, ego, hatred and attachment. When translated into medical practice, causes of unhappiness include getting into "rat race", depersonalized approach to a patient, lack of holistic care resulting in patient's dissatisfaction, increasing stress to the doctor in addition to, poor life style and burnout. It is one's motivation that decides what one wants to do and the attitude to decide how well to do. Happiness resides in everyone, don't search outside but be motivated to find it.

Personal Notes

Most doctors tend to neglect their own health with an excuse of busy practice. My teacher always said that busy people had enough time because they knew how to manage time. Our joint practice has given me time for my own health. It takes just an hour to work out each day that is just 4% of daily time. Same is true about disciplined eating and sleeping time. It has made my life healthier and more enjoyable. I always took a break for 10 minutes after working for two hours in my clinic that rejuvenate me. Once a patient who had a next appointment started arguing with my attendant and barged in my room. When he saw me having coffee, he got angry and said "my child is sick and you are relaxing." I softly told him that I was having coffee to rejuvenate myself so that I could see his child in a better frame of mind and energy and requested him to wait for few more minutes. He obliged and when came in, I told him my break was for his child's benefit and he apologized.

Take Home Message

Every doctor must nurture himself and take care of his own life. Besides maintaining good life style that would ensure physical health, one must give equal importance to nurture mental and spiritual health. However, happiness should be the ultimate aim to boost complete health. Be always grateful for what you have, don't compare with others but compete with yourself to improve. Work hard with passion and share work with others to maintain quality of work. It will give you peace and leisure that makes life enjoyable and boosts health and happiness. Don't forget life has an expiry date. If you nurture yourself well, you will die young but as late as possible.

11 Balance in Life Beyond Bank Balance

Don't think money does everything or you are going to end up doing everything for money

– Voltaire

Everything in moderation is a perfect balance

– Ryan Robbins

Introduction

Balance ensures relative distribution to avoid fall. Balance in life is an act that demands attention to multiple activities in order to cope up with all of them in spite of conflicting factors. Life earlier was much easy with happiness and containment. Unfortunately, life has been increasingly complex, competitive and stressful, more so for the doctors. Bank balance provides financial security but does not ensure healthy and happy life. We work and earn only to enrich our life. Life has many components – physical (diet, exercise and sleep), mental (stimulation), psychological (success), emotional (happiness) and spiritual (empathy and harmony).

Concept of Work-Life Balance

This concept developed in the western world about 40 years ago and remains mostly ignored in India. Fierce competition, increasing aspirations and modern technology led to ignoring life. Consequences of imbalanced life affected both work and life. After all work is to enrich life and so all of us must define our goals in life clearly and time spent to achieve the same.

Balance in Life of a Doctor

Two major factors that need balance are related to **medical practice** and **personal lifestyle**, each of them consists of multiple components. Both factors are dynamic and changing but highly interdependent. Doctors in general ignore life in pursuit of medical practice and bank balance. Such an imbalance has its consequences affecting personal and family life as well as quality of medical practice resulting in increasing stress and unhappiness. Unfortunately, by the time one realizes effects of such an imbalance, it is often too late to change.

Balance Related to Medical Practice

Balance between art and science of practice

Medicine is a science of uncertainty and art of probability. Science refers to acquiring knowledge and clinical skills while art consists of ethics, communication, counseling, documentation, time management, dignified and respectful approach and patient empowerment. One without the other fails to provide holistic care. Every doctor must spend enough time with the patient and art of practice is equally or more important than medical competence and skills.

Balance between practice and updating

Medicine is a dynamic science and change is the only constant. So, we need to learn – unlearn - and relearn. Thus, constant updating is a need and one can learn by priority what is most applicable in practice. Interactive learning is ideal and one can form local groups to facilitate such learning. It is most important to keep updated so as to give the best to the patient and for which time spent is a good investment. It is possible but choice is yours. If you are not updated, check your pulse, you may be academically dead.

Balance between evidence and experience

Evidence and experience-based medicine is an imaginary divide as both are two sides of the same coin. Evidence guides decisions based on averages and not fit for all. Clinical judgment is the key component of evidence-based medicine. So, we need to keep balance between evidence that is based on external research and experience based on internal expertise, One without the other is not desirable.

Balance between traditional wisdom and modern science

Much before modern science developed, traditional wisdom helped to comfort patients. While modern science treats disease, traditional wisdom treats a patient in which resides the disease. Modern science offers a new test or a drug, traditional wisdom decides for whom to use and when to use. Thus, modern science must be guided by traditional wisdom and we need to use both.

Balance Related to Life

Balance between profession and personal health

Medical profession goes through three phases. First phase is one of aspiration and expectation, second phase of compulsion and greed for money and last phase of addiction to pursue the same. It is a “rat race”. We have time for patients but not for ourselves. We ignore our own health with irregular eating time, sleep deprivation and lack of exercise. We need to set our goal, regulate work pattern by group practice and create time for many other activities that keep us healthy, happy and still work with passion.

Balance between profession and family

Finding time for family during busy practice is a challenge but possible with adjusting work schedules. Group practice helps to achieve his balance. There are many benefits of spending time with the family such as bonding with family members, nurturing positive behavior, promoting healthy life, relieving stress, imparting good values and improving self-esteem of children.

Balance between time, money and energy

During initial days of practice, one has enough time and energy but no money, when practice flourishes, you have enough money and energy but no time and finally at the end of practice, you have enough money and time but no energy. So, one must enjoy life when you have money and energy and find time even in busy practice. Otherwise, you will collect money at the cost of health and later, spend all that accumulated money to regain health.

Balance between success and happiness

Success is you get what you want at any cost but happiness is you want what you get or what you need. Success lies in happiness. We must learn to "give" more than "take" because it gets back with more happiness. Success beyond limits "kills" but happiness takes care of your life so that you can die young as late as possible. Don't forget life has an expiry date that is not known.

Current Scenario of Medical Practice

Rational and ethical practice as well as academic updating is sacrificed in pursuit of money. Burnout leads to long term health problems such as obesity, hypertension, acidity, digestive complaints, depression, anxiety, sleep problems, chronic aches and pains. Quality of practice goes down with patient dissatisfaction and poor self-esteem. In turn, it increases stress worsening health problems and unhappiness. It is at the cost of personal health, family time and happiness. This trend must be reversed and it is possible best at the early phase of practice. However, it is never too late.

Personal Notes

I maintain friendly relations with my students. I recall when one of my ex-students and now a busy successful pediatrician told me that I always lacked ambition in life. I asked him why he felt so. He said if I had an ambition to become the most sought-after pediatrician, there would have been large crowd of patients in my waiting room at my office. I told him that my ambitions were different and I wanted to lead a balanced life with focus on happiness and passion and not just to build a large practice. I am convinced that person who excels in one area is considered most successful by others but he may not be happy because of imbalanced life. Priorities do change in life at different times but emphasis must be on a balance all the time.

Take Home Message

Set your goals to begin with and balance work and life. It is necessary to develop enough practice but far more important is to enjoy practice and life. It is possible only when you achieve an ideal balance. Final goal of life should be happiness and make life worth living.

12 Miles to Go ----- Before Teaching Becomes Learning

Education is not learning of facts but
training the mind to think

– Albert Einstein

Student, you don't study to pass the test but
study to prepare for the day when you are the
only one between the patient and his grave

– Mark Reid

Introduction

There is often a slip between cup and lip. Teaching is meant to learn but it may not happen. International program for students' assessment at the age of 15 years has been conducted every three years since year 2000. Results of this program in the year 2018 revealed that India ranked 72nd out of 73 participating countries. It is obvious that a gap exists between teaching and learning and we need to define this gap and take corrective measures. We must get inspired to make a change and we owe this to the next generation.

What is Teaching?

Teaching is a learning activity for students that includes learning for the teacher as well. It is an act of great optimism but it is incredibly complex. It should not be a mere source of information or knowledge that student can obtain even without a teacher. In fact, a teacher is expected to stimulate and equip students to think so they are able to seek, analyze and implement what is gathered. Purpose of teaching is to shape character, caliber and future of students. Quality of future doctors depend on our teaching today. "I can't teach anything to anyone, I only make them think," said Socrates.

What is Learning?

Learning is a process that starts at 32 weeks of gestation. It is the time when nervous system is primed to start learning. Learning is meant to acquire new information or modify and reinforce existing information. It is not a rote learning but meaningful learning. Understanding information is what is effective learning. Formal conventional learning often occurs through monologue that does not facilitate ideal learning. Informal interactive discussion between students and guided by a teacher is the best way to fulfill the very purpose of learning that is student-centered and not teacher-centered. Student initially is a dependent learner (depends on someone else to teach), if he becomes an interested learner and becomes involved in learning, he soon becomes a self-directed learner (he starts learning on his own).

Who is a Teacher?

Teacher is a person who creates a change that facilitates learning. In fact, one can learn from anyone who fits in the above definition irrespective of his professional status. In medicine, patients are the best teachers who suffer so that we can learn from their sufferings. Paramedical staff including nurses and ward boys as well as senior resident doctors can be good teachers and senior students can teach a junior student. In fact, formal designated teacher learns from students when they ask difficult questions. Even "dead" can teach as postmortem often reveals what was missed. I recall having learnt from a ward boy how to place the patient in the right position when performing a lumbar puncture and from a nurse how to give an enema. Thus, there are opportunities to learn all the time only if we wish to learn – age and time is no bar and this is the need for every doctor to keep learning as medicine is dynamic with change being the constant. Thus, doctor is always a student and it is true for every teacher as well.

Types of Teachers

Unfortunately, we call an individual a teacher only when he is designated or authorized or supposed to teach. Naturally every one of us must have met different types of "teachers" right from school, college and elsewhere. In general, there are three types of teachers. First type of teachers were those who "were in our school or college", second type were those who "taught us" but third type were those "from whom we learnt" I have a fond memory of third type of teachers and I am forever grateful to them. It is said that mediocre teacher tells, good teacher teaches, excellent teacher demonstrates but outstanding teacher inspires and motivates.

Quality of an Outstanding Teacher

A teacher must have good knowledge, competence and communication skills but equally important are factors like passion, perseverance, aptitude and attitude. He should be able to foster clinical thinking and cultivate curiosity, inspire hope, ignite imagination and instill love for learning. A teacher in medicine must deliver clinical facts (science) but also address human facts (art). It is a philosophical exercise besides biological one. He should develop sense of responsibility and ethical standards in students to fulfill Hippocrates oath. Of course, he has to be a good human being – honest, sincere, accountable, empathetic, and patient and above all a good listener.

How Does an Outstanding Teacher Teach?

He makes learning process interesting to engage attention of students. He does not simply impart factual knowledge but explains intricacies involved in a topic under discussion. He is able to make difficult problems simpler by giving examples in real life that students can easily grasp. He promotes interactive discussion among students so that every one learns. He scrutinizes own performance through a feed-back from students.

Is "Teacher" Born or Made?

I am not sure whether it is a "natural gift". However, even if one is gifted, it needs refining with continuous learning because "gift" may otherwise remain dormant. Australian professor John Hattie in his book "visible learning" says teaching is an art any one can learn for which one needs four psychological assets – interest, practice, purpose and hope – to achieve success. Interaction is the key and role model is an integral art. Practice makes one perfect but it has to be a deliberate practice that is effortful, mistakes-ridden and repetitive. What it means to a teacher is to observe own mistakes and employ special efforts to correct them. It leaves a question to ponder whether teachers need formal training.

Personal Notes

Besides excellent teachers from whom I learnt both art and science of medicine, I recall several others, though not designated as teachers, who taught me medicine and different aspects of life. As mentioned above, Rajaram was a wardboy who taught me first hands-on lesson in performing lumbar puncture in an infant. Our ward sister-in-charge showed me how to give an enema to a child. I have formed an organization called "clinical pediatrics" for teaching of medical students free of cost with the help of my colleagues who have taught me a lot as each one of them excel in one way or another. They are all practicing pediatricians and not formally designated teachers but teach with enthusiasm and passion. Finally, I continue to learn from my child patients and so I have dedicated all my books to "children who suffered so that we could learn". Of course, I owe to my parents and school teachers for inculcating good values in life.

I recall a school principal who told me that if teacher alone talks in the class, no one learns but if students talk in the class everyone learns. What he preached was learning through interactive discussion and not monologues. We have been following the same in our teaching sessions.

A doctor looked perplexed while viewing laboratory reports and so, patient asked whether there was anything serious. Doctor said "Not sure because I had left this part of study in option." Study of medicine continues through life and no portion can be optional.

One of my undergraduate students had asked me why they had to study many subjects but each subject was being taught by different teachers, why not from same teacher? He had a valid question. I explained to him that each specialist was able to explain intricacies better in his domain. I pondered with his question that also emphasizes that every teacher in medicine should possess basic knowledge.

Take Home Message

Teaching is a noble profession. We need to promote it. Focus on quality is a key factor and quality assessment tools must be in place so that teacher's performance is monitored. Students must assess teacher's performance as well. System must offer opportunities to passionate teachers wherever they may be even if they are not designated as teachers. It will benefit all. High performing educational systems in the world select best teachers and look after them well. They must be paid as per their performance. Only then best teachers will enter teaching profession.

13 Art of Communication and Counseling

He that won't be counseled can't be helped

– Benjamin Franklin

He was a patient with a diagnosis that he could not understand

– Maggie Stiefwater

Introduction

Communication and counseling are essential skills that every doctor must learn. It is a key to success as it instils confidence in the mind of a patient and improves compliance and thereby also recovery. Communication and counseling are not the same. Communication refers to meaningful information while counseling goes much beyond it. Good communication skills are a prerequisite for effective counseling. Counseling is not mere information but should provide professional help, assistance and guidance to resolve problems and difficulties that would make it easy for patients to face the situation.

Basics Revisited

Communication and counseling should be accurate, brief and clear, preferably documented, relevant to individual situation and needs, must avoid complexity by using simple language that lay person can understand, ideally by giving simple examples of day-to-day experiences. Courteous behavior and empathy are most essential components of counseling. It is important to read the mind of a patient and his relatives and address their concerns. Every patient would like to know about the disease – what is it, why did it happen, which tests are necessary, how would it be confirmed, how would it be treated, options available for treatment, safety of drugs and their side-effects, expected outcome, suffering and disability, time frame and cost of treatment. Communication offers relevant information and counseling takes care of hidden factors such as anxiety, worry, uncertainty, frustration, self-pity, self-blame etc by empathetic approach, giving support and confidence. Patient must feel that his doctor is with him to guide and help to face the situation.

Varied Situations Requiring Counseling

Every patient must be counselled relevant to his needs. However, physician is faced with many situations in practice that requires counseling at different levels. Rational practice during routine outpatient service, chronic diseases requiring good compliance, chronic functional disorders, disabilities with permanent handicaps, worsening conditions are some of the situations that need relevant counseling. But, most challenging situation for counseling is uncontrolled outbursts of anger and agitation by the relatives of patients that may lead to violence.

Counseling in Office Practice to Ensure Rationality

It is often not possible to arrive at a provisional diagnosis on first visit. Rationality demands that patient is advised to "wait and watch" without specific therapy till diagnosis evolves. It is necessary to ensure and convey safety of "wait and watch" by giving proper instructions to monitor danger symptoms and if observed, report immediately. We may have to explain dangers of empirical therapy and futility of ordering investigations at random. It is most important to document short summary of the problem along with advice given that ensures legal safety. Most appropriate action taken by a physician but if not documented, is not accepted as evidence in the court of justice.

Counseling for Chronic Conditions to Ensure Compliance

Many chronic diseases remain incurable but can be controlled to an extent to maintain reasonable quality of life. However, it is possible only with patient's compliance to follow advice given by the doctor and for which adequate counseling is required. Most patients default on advice once symptoms disappear, wrongly considering it as control of disease and fearing side effects of drugs. Besides, there are often "well-wishers" who advice to stop medications on feeling better. We need to emphasise on safety of long-term use of drugs and also dangers of non-compliance that may end up with worsening condition necessitating a greater number of drugs for longer duration. We must discuss periodic monitoring strategies and of course document the same.

Counseling for Chronic Functional Disorders

Functional disorders are on the rise even in children. It is important to realize that symptoms of such disorders are genuine even in absence of organic disease and are triggered by multiple factors such as home/school environment, stress and individual personality. The disorder presents with varied symptoms mediated through the mind. Abdominal pain is a common presentation of such a disorder as a result of gut-brain functional axis. We need special skills to convince the patient/parents of a child about the nature of the disease, lack of laboratory proof, diagnosis based on circumstantial evidence and management depending not much on drugs but participation from entire family and not the patient alone. Counseling should start with a discussion about organic disorders responsible for the symptoms and rule them out one by one before suggesting the role of mind over the body. We often meet denial to accept such a diagnosis from patients and parents and hence counseling in such situations becomes a challenge. We should be careful not to suggest malingering that is different than functional disorder. Patience and empathy are the key factors in counseling of such disorders and multiple counseling sessions may be necessary as improvement may be slow.

Counseling in Case of Permanent Handicap

Many chronic disorders end up with some permanent disability. Patient or parents often feel guilty, blame others or curse destiny. We need to remove such feelings and induce positive thinking to focus on retained functions with best of the efforts. Proper explanation of real situation is necessary but without undue hopes or despair. It is important to emphasise that every handicap can be overcome by compensatory mechanisms. For example, if a right-handed person loses his right hand, he can learn to work effectively with left hand and if one loses both the hands, there are persons who could learn to use toes as fingers. Such things are possible only with determination and best efforts by the handicapped individual under the guidance of an expert. We must encourage and support rehabilitative measures and not forget that for such individuals, we are the last hopes. We need to be empathetic to do our best.

Counseling When Faced with a Dying Patient

This is the most difficult part of counseling. We need to prepare the relatives for the inevitable but the process should be slow and smooth not to give them a sudden shock. They do sense the grave situation but still harbor a hope. We must inform them real situation of poor response to treatment but add that one has seen improvement even at such a worsening stage and assure them that everything possible is being done. It is ideal to allow within limits two or three close relatives in rotation to witness efforts being put in. We must communicate with relatives every half an hour and answer all questions that may be asked repeatedly. During counseling sessions, we must be careful to phrase statements in a way that they are not misinterpreted and it is best that only one person counsels them. Patience and empathy are the key factors for successful handling of such a crisis. It is best done by senior-most doctor in charge of the patient and not left to juniors.

Counseling When Faced with Angry and Agitating Relatives

This is a tricky situation that calls for remaining calm avoiding arguments and allowing the relatives to vent out their feelings without interruption. Patient hearing of their complaints is likely to reduce the tension a bit. We must not vehemently refute their allegations but must be tactful. We must say that we do understand their concern but explain them the correct view of the situation. We should not try to appear defensive but demonstrate confidence in handling the situation without instigating them. Don't forget, such a situation often results from lack of communication and counseling and should be mostly avoidable.

Personal Notes

I learnt the counseling skills during my training by observing how my teachers talked to patients and their relatives. I realize that it is possible to explain most complex disease in simple lay language. I give examples of real-life situations which are similar to their own medical problem. I was counseling the parent of a child with neurodegenerative disorder. I told them that as one gets older, many functions such as hearing, memory, body balance, speech etc. start getting impaired, this is called degeneration. It occurs in adults anytime from 60 years onwards but may also start occasionally bit early. However unfortunately, such degeneration started in their young child at an early age. But as degenerative impairment cannot be corrected with medicines, one has to adapt to such situations with relevant help from gadgets and supports. Explaining with such similarities, lay persons understand even the most complicated medical problem such as neurodegeneration. It is the art that each doctor must develop.

I recall mother of an infant who was instilling oral anti-cold medicine into nostrils. When she found it difficult, she phoned her doctor, who advised her to instill the same with dilution with water, to which she reported it was impossible. At that time, doctor realized that she was instilling oral medicine into nostrils. When reprimanded, doctor was blamed for unclear instructions as he had not mentioned it was for oral use. Even simple facts should not be taken for granted and clear instructions must be documented. Patients often make mistakes about formulation in drops and syrups as concentration is so different and may be harmful if one is mistaken for the other. I have known rectal suppository for constipation being swallowed orally. Other issue is poor handwriting of most of us. I know about a pharmacist giving Ascabiol (anti-scabies medicine for local application) instead of Ascoril (oral cough remedy). It may be ideal to write name of drugs in capitals or better is a digital print-out.

Take Home Message

Counseling is an art that is not taught in medical school but must be learnt by observing a role model and improved by experience. Communication and counseling are as important in practice as knowledge and competence. It is equally important to document every action that serves as evidence. Problems arise when we don't follow these norms.

14 How to Keep Updated in Busy Medical Practice

To improve is to change, to be perfect is to change often

– Winston Churchill

If change is constant then learning has to be continual

– Meir Liraz

Is there a Need to Keep Updated?

Medical science is dynamic and only constant is the change. Diseases caused by hitherto unknown organisms have come to light while well controlled older infections surface again. Large number of drugs are available and it is difficult to keep track of them. Vaccines were administered only to children but now they are also recommended for adults. Newer modalities of investigations are now in vogue and several new techniques of management are being practiced that include interventional procedures and organ transplants. Add to all these advances, we are now witnessing a surge in life style diseases with increasing incidence of obesity, diabetes, hypertension, coronary artery disease and strokes. So, the profile of disease pattern is changing fast and every doctor is going to meet these challenges, hence the need to keep updated.

How to Keep Undated?

It is impossible to learn everything that is new and it is also not necessary. One may have to be selective. We must make a note of problems that are more prevalent in our day-to-day practice and focus on updating in those areas. We must know recent advances in those areas so that we can offer the best to our patients. There are several sources of updating. Print or digital source of information is easily available. One may choose articles that are likely to be useful in your own practice and ignore other articles. This can be done at convenient time and it is possible if one plans it well. It is said that most busy persons have enough time as they plan their time well. Another source is attending CMEs. It is mandatory for every doctor to earn credit points by attending CMEs. One can again choose where to go and what to listen. It is not mere physical presence at such CMEs and you don't attend just to get credit points. During CMEs, it is important to make notes of information that you sensed useful in your practice. However best way to keep updated is to discuss a problem faced by you with someone who knows – such a doctor could be a specialist or your own senior colleague. It is ideal to form a voluntary group that meets periodically to discuss problems and try to solve them together.

When Practice is Flourishing, is there a Need to be Updated?

Patients will keep on coming to us not because we know best but because they have faith in us. They presume we would be doing our best and it is not possible to do best without being updated. It would amount to cheating if we don't do our best because of lack of latest knowledge. This is bitterly felt when one is called upon to treat our own relation. Of course, one can always get the best help from someone else for our own relation. But I am sure every patient of ours deserves the same from us and we are morally responsible for it. It is important to know what we know and also what we don't know but many times we don't know what we don't know. It is said that ignorance is a bliss but it is not true in medical profession as we deal with life.

Do You Need Motivation to Keep Updated?

It has to be an internal motivation that resides in your own self and you need to kindle it. You would get a thrill when you diagnose an uncommon condition and cure the patient. Such instances make routine practice satisfying and enjoyable. Once you are motivated, it becomes a habit that is sustained throughout life. It brings happiness in your life. So, start today if not done before. It is never too late. Read every day about the problem that you faced and I am sure there are problems every day. It may take just half an hour to know more about it. If you update in one problem a day, you would be the most updated doctor. If you don't keep updated, please check your pulse, you may be academically dead.

Personal Notes

During my residency in Pediatrics, I witnessed how Dr P.M. Udani would keep himself abreast with latest knowledge. He used to be a voracious reader and had large collection of books, vacant space on each page of his books was filled with his own notes. He could do it in spite of spending 8 hours a day at J.J. Hospital and 3-4 hours a day at his clinic. Teaching is the best way to learn and I was lucky to be appointed as honorary teacher in Grant Medical College. I used to spend four hours a week in college library and make relevant notes to be filed systematically for easy retrieval. Those days, we did not have computers or note pads. Over years it became easy to store notes electronically. Each time, I saw a difficult problem, I would search the answer in my notes or on other digital sites and then store newly acquired information on separate file. Updating is not only the need and it has also become easy now at the finger-click.

Take Home Message

Try to be selectively updated in areas that concern your practice the most. Invest just 2% of your daily life (half an hour a day) to keep updated. Be internally motivated to do your best, it brings happiness.

15 How to be Rational in Practice?

Rational man is guided by his thinking, by a process of reasoning, not by his feelings or desires

– Ayan Rand

Rational practice is to be taught not in a lecture hall but at the bedside of patients where it is applied

– Robert Owen

What is Rationality?

Rationality refers to judicious and well-reasoned sensible use of resources to offer quality service. Judicious use of resources in medical practice simply means minimal intervention (investigations and drugs) to get maximum benefit (cure, if possible, comfort always). Quality service in medical practice implies holistic care. Holistic care is possible with use of all modalities endowed upon humans by nature – namely body, heart, mind and soul. When translated into medical practice, body is knowledge, heart the compassion, mind the commitment and soul the conscience. If it is done with devotion – love and loyalty, it becomes divine - coming from supernatural powers and it is so sacred that helps ultimately the healing.

Medicine and Rationalism are Inseparable

Medicine is the most touching science of all – it involves healing, caring, soothing, reassuring, understanding and offering hope. Medical practice should be a perfect combination of science and art. Rationality of science involves detailed history, keen observation (it is well known that eyes don't see what mind does not know), focused physical examination, objective reasoning and analysis, introspection and learning from own mistakes. Rationality of art includes empathy, compassion, communication, counseling and documentation. It is only when judicious use of science and art is combined that rationality is served.

Universal Pitfalls in Medical Practice

There is not enough time spent on detailed history. Proper information is not sought because of lack of time – it is an excuse. Whatever information is obtained, it is not analyzed and interpreted due to lack of thinking. Once this habit is lost, thinking itself becomes a disuse atrophy. This leads to unfocused physical examination likely to miss abnormal findings. It sets in a vicious cycle of unnecessary tests, empirical therapy often with multiple drugs. It is obviously not conducive to communication, counseling or documentation. This is irrationality at its height. However, ironically, it may still work and gives false sense of competence to a doctor. Unfortunately, patient may not know about poor quality of service but the doctor should introspect.

How to Ensure Rational Practice?

Care always

For whatever complaint patient may come to you, offer advice on preventive health issues such as growth monitoring, developmental screening including vision and hearing, ideal diet, proper hygiene and life style.

Use clinical skills

Try to arrive at provisional diagnosis by analysis of detailed history and focused physical examination. Order investigations only after provisional diagnosis and that too, if necessary.

Be a good listener

Every parent of a child or child himself may give you a clue to a diagnosis only if you care to listen to them carefully and allow them to express what they wish to say. Most illiterate persons also know enough to express though one must have a skill to get relevant information and to filter out what is not relevant.

Test a test

Before you order a test, think what way such a test would help you to arrive at a diagnosis. Don't order a test because you don't know probable disease and if so, then you also don't know which tests to order. **There are no routine tests.**

Be a rational prescriber

If you don't have any provisional diagnosis, decide whether it is safe to wait for disease to evolve. Empirical therapy is justified only in serious situations and that too after ordering relevant tests. Prescribe minimum number of drugs. Symptomatic therapy is necessary only if symptoms are very discomforting to a patient and that too it should be employed only at the time of intolerable symptoms. This should be explained to the patient and left himself to decide when to use. Doctor should not advise the timing of such symptomatic therapy, though frequency has to be limited.

Communicate, counsel and document

Inform patient about his illness and therapy in simple words which improves compliance of treatment. Counseling is an art that guides the patient to go through his illness which instils confidence in a patient. Document in brief relevant facts that signifies transparency and accountability. It also helps to be legally safe.

Choose Your Own Way

You have to set your own goals in practice and pursue them. Let your goals be professional credibility, peer acceptance and social respect. To achieve this goal, be rational in practice and once you adhere to rationality, it becomes a habit that is sustained throughout life. It may take time to begin with but spending time for rationality is worth. It leads to happiness and promotes your own health.

Personal Notes

I formed a habit of documenting my provisional diagnosis with supporting facts that ensured rational drug prescription and advice. Even when I could not come to any provisional diagnosis, I would mention "no clue to any specific diagnosis" and add "it is safe to wait and observe any new symptoms and inform". I would end with "no specific medicines except symptomatic therapy". Such a commitment was accepted by most patients as it signified not only honesty but also confidence and it helped me to be rational in my approach. This is the best way to inculcate rationality. Unfortunately, most prescriptions contain only the drugs without any preceding justification and hence rationality is never monitored.

Once a parent of my patient requested me to see their neighbor's child for whom their pediatrician had prescribed an antibiotic. When I saw the child and confirmed the need for an antibiotic, child' s parents exclaimed saying "Oh, you also write an antibiotic" because I had never found the need to prescribe an antibiotic for their neighbor's child. They thought antibiotic use is irrational. Such beliefs must be countered and corrected. Rationality can't be stretched to irrational level.

One of my junior colleagues said that if everyone around him prescribed an antibiotic without reason, he could not afford to be rational. I told him a story. There was a vasectomy camp in a village where every eligible person underwent the procedure. When organisers were about to close down, an old man of 80 years came in and wanted to undergo vasectomy. He was told that he did not need it. He explained "if any lady got pregnant in the village, he would be blamed as all other men had undergone vasectomy" Old man had a valid point but it should not apply to medical practice. Hence practice rationally, it will give you happiness and community will recognize it eventually.

Take Home Message

Rational practice is possible if you set your goal to achieve it. It does not take time and with repeated practice, it becomes a habit. It offers satisfaction to a patient, happiness to a doctor and promotes good health in both.

16 How to Enjoy Medical Practice?

The best way to enjoy your job is
to imagine yourself without one

– Oscar Wilde

When you enjoy what you do,
work becomes a play

– Martin Yan

What Does the Word "Enjoy" Mean to You?

Enjoy means to receive joy while joy is a feeling of happiness and cheerfulness. In order to enjoy, one has to act before you experience joy. Thus, enjoy is an action, joy a feeling, an outcome of enjoy. Joy is a momentary but intense feeling of positive emotions. Such little moments experienced repeatedly lead to happiness. It is clear that joy is not dependent on external influences, it resides in your own mind that needs to be exposed and perceived by your own action. When mind is pure, joy follows like a shadow that never leaves, said Gautam Buddha. Joy is the emotional dimension of life that is well lived. Once you experience joy with your own action, in turn, whatever you do with joy will make you enjoy further. This cycle will continue and sustain as a habit. Joy has one characteristic – once you feel joy, you will strive for it again and again. Secret of joy is contained in one word – "excellence" and to know how to do well is simply to enjoy what you are doing.

Medical Practice is Stressful

Medicine is a science of uncertainty and hence doctors use art of probability to arrive at a diagnosis. Every individual reacts differently to same disease and even same individual responds differently at different times to a same disease. However, patient expects best outcome irrespective of several variables that are beyond control of a doctor. Stakes are high as minute error may result in major consequences. In no other profession, risk-outcome ratio is so screwed. Teacher is not expected to produce good results in every student and is not held responsible for failure of student. But doctor is expected to "cure" every disease, otherwise held accountable for the result. Every other professional can think over time and decide best possible action whereas medical practice demands "thought in action" – you think and act at the same time. Hence it is natural that medical practice is quite stressful.

What are the Compounding Factors to Stress?

Besides undue expectations from patients, burnout (60-80 hours a week with forever "on call") leading to physical and emotional exhaustion, alienation from personal life and peer pressure are other factors responsible for stress. However, we need to realize that stress is inappropriate or exaggerated response to situation that may be beyond your control but we need to modulate it to a tolerant level so that it has no negative impact on our work as well as life. It is possible with deliberate practice and meditation helps to destress. If unduly stressed, our performance goes down resulting in more stress. One can understand anxiety when you face serious situation – anxiety is the appropriate response and has a positive impact on outcome.

Can You Enjoy Medical Practice in Spite of Stress?

Don't forget that you have chosen to be a doctor and now let your life be well lived as a doctor. It is in your hands. No profession is all roses and even roses have thorns. So, we need to enjoy fragrance of our profession, coping up with thorns. There is a silver lining to our profession. Medicine is the most touching science as it involves caring, healing, soothing, reassuring, understanding and offering hopes with empathy, compassion, commitment, communication, counseling and documentation. This represents art of medical practice and is as important as science. One without the other falls short of desired outcome. Many of us have lost touch with this reality, ignoring how valuable it is and not cultivating it. Patients don't care about how much you know but they want to know how much you care. If you follow art of medical practice, care that you take becomes evident and even poor outcome is accepted as a part of destiny. As doctors, we are aware that disease heals not just because you chose the treatment right but also because patient responded correctly. It is not rare that correct diagnosis and ideal treatment fails to cure a disease. However, when we do our best and patient gets better, it brings joy to a doctor and much more so if difficult problem is solved rationally, it gives a thrill. Good deed is remembered by patients and as a doctor, every one of us have experienced it. So, if you do your work well, you will enjoy medical practice. It is possible.

How to Ensure You Enjoy Medical Practice?

"Care always, cure if possible" is our motto. Let us accept that perfection in medical science is impossible but it is possible in art of practice because it is entirely in your hand. Start practicing "holistic" care by using all the faculties endowed upon human beings by nature namely body, heart, mind and soul. When translated to medical practice, body refers to knowledge, heart to compassion, mind to commitment and soul to your own conscience. While knowledge is important, other three domains are most vital. Medical science is developing fast and one needs to keep updated. I have dealt with this issue in one of the articles. Try to see the problem from patient's perspectives and you will be compassionate. You must feel the pain that patient experiences though you should learn not to suffer from this pain. Commitment should be at the level when you are treating your own relative. And finally, whatever the outcome of treatment, you should be answerable to your own conscience that you did utmost whatever you could. Be humble, don't run down peers and follow ethics. Such behavior results in peer acceptance, respect in the profession and faith among patients. Once you follow these principles, there will be abundant joy in medical practice.

Balance Beyond Bank Balance

Besides art of medical practice, don't forget balance between profession and life to remain healthy and enjoy practice as well as life. Don't go after bank balance only because it may provide financial security but not ensure healthy and joyful life. Most doctors ignore health due to irregular eating time, lack of exercise, sleep deprivation and "rat race" in practice. Train yourself and your patients in such a way that you are able to look after your personal life. One ideal solution is to establish group practice so that you can modulate your work as well as personal life. You must find time for the family and take a break from practice. There can't be any excuse about busy practice as most busy people are never short of time because they manage time well. Develop some hobbies that can distract you from stress and makes life enjoyable. Finally learn to balance between time, money and energy. When you start practice, you have time and energy but no money, at the peak of your career, you have money and energy but no time and at the end, you have enough money and time but no energy. So, enjoy life as much as you enjoy practice. When you have money and energy, find time to enjoy life.

Personal Notes

One of my colleagues once told me that he had started enjoying practice ever since he started making and documenting a provisional diagnosis and to find that it was subsequently confirmed by relevant tests that gave him a thrill. He continued to do so in every patient that made him learn that every patient was different even when suffering from same disease. That is how he started enjoying his practice and looked forward to attend the clinic. It is the best way, otherwise practice becomes monotonous and stressful. I started a group practice as work load increased and every ten years, one colleague joined our group. We are now four in our group. It has given me and my colleagues time to enjoy life. Besides practice, we all spend time in voluntary teaching that is another source of joy and repeated joy brings happiness.

Take Home Message

Medical practice is stressful but turn this stress into an enjoyable stress –eustress. Follow the art of medical practice to ensure "care always, cure if possible". Avoid burnout and learn to balance between work and personal life. Manage time so that you can devote attention to your own health and family besides practice. You cannot enjoy practice without enjoying personal life. Manage time, energy and money well. If you follow this, you will look forward to work and life every day.

17 How to Find Time for the Family?

Time is free but it's priceless, you can't own it but can use it, you can't keep it but can spend it, once you lose it, you can't get it back

– Harvey Mackay

If you are too busy to enjoy time with your family then you need to evaluate your priorities

– Dave Willis

Family – Our First Responsibility

As a doctor, we owe a lot to our family. To begin with, we got higher education thanks to our parents who often struggled to make it happen for us. Besides education, we learnt culture in the family, value of sharing and "give and take", only because parents and extended family were available for guidance, support and encouragement. They were there in situations of despair and difficulties. Such a background stood good during subsequent life. After marriage, it was our spouses who made us comfortable and looked after our children even in our absence. Role and contribution of each doctor as parent is paramount for ideal growth and development of children, more so in nuclear families. It is our responsibility and it is our family's privilege. Hence there is a need to find time for the family in spite of busy practice.

Concept of Time Management

Time management is the key to efficient working. It is ability to use time more productively, more output in lesser time. It is the process of organizing and planning how to divide your time between specific activities, ensuring right time for right activities. It helps fulfill all responsibilities. One can achieve a lot, if time is managed well which in turn reduces stress and enhances our achievement. Everyone has 24 hours available each day but some can function effectively only because they manage time. Key is not spending time but investing time.

Work–Family Balance Beyond Bank Balance

Surely bank balance provides financial security but it does not translate into personal and family health and happiness. Both are equally important and so we must strike a balance. In initial days of medical practice, doctor has enough time as practice takes time to build and, in this phase, there is enough time to spend with family. It brings in happiness forgetting stress of waiting for patients. Problem surfaces when practice builds and with increasing work load, family is ignored. Not only family is ignored but personal health is also at risk because of burnout. This is also the time when children are in formative stage of development and they need proper grooming. We must decide how to strike a balance at this stage and it is possible. Once you miss this phase, habits die hard and as one gets senior, you are likely to continue the same way. However, it is never too late.

How to Find Time for the Family?

Every one including all professionals work as per "office time" with weekly holidays. But doctors work all the time that is most convenient to patients which happen to be most inconvenient time for their personal life. Besides they are available at any odd hours. If banks and post-offices work at the same time that students are in school and parents at their work, still people manage their banking or other needs and find time for the same. Well today in digital revolution, you can do banking from home but it was not so all these decades. If someone is not well, obviously he or she is likely to be at home and so can visit a doctor during "office time". In all western countries, doctors work at their own schedules and it is possible because they have developed "group practice". I feel it is the best way to practice that offers ideal work-family balance. I say this with confidence because I started group practice within first few years of solo practice. Today we are four pediatricians working together with ease and comfort of working without stress and time to look after our personal and family life. This is the best solution. What you lose by way of less income, you gain by far more happiness and sound health. Other solution is to restrict your work and direct it to your juniors so that juniors are happy and you are also happy. Many times, I hear that doctor feels his patients can't do without him but what is true is patients need to get better irrespective of who makes them better. Those patients who have faith in your competence will also find the same or even better with other doctors. You can recommend right doctor for them and patients will be grateful to you and so you will be happy with your family.

How to Spend Time with Family?

Spending time with the family should be investing in time for creative activities rather than only worldly pleasures. Doctor can make himself available at the time of dinner where all family members dine together. This is the time where everyone speaks about how the day went. Children can narrate what funny thing happened in school and you can tell them a story related to how patient behaved. It becomes interesting and children learn to think and speak. Most important, everyone looks forward to this event and time is not wasted to discuss how children misbehaved. This is an enjoyable time spent most effectively. Age-appropriate discussion during such time makes it more interesting and time well invested.

If such a thing is not possible every day, at least try to make it few days a week, surely on holidays. Of course, there would be other pleasures offered to children and family such as dining out or going for a movie but only selectively. In fact, I know few doctors who take off on one mid-week evenings in addition to weekends.

Hazards of not Spending Time with Family

In today's fast and wicked world, it may spell a disaster. Lack of communication leads to poor bonding. Children are left to themselves and remain unmonitored. You are most likely to offer them worldly pleasures that they would ever long for more and more. You do it as a guilt feeling of having not spent time with them. This sets them on a wrong path. They are likely to suffer because of such upbringing and it could be irreversible. I see increasing prevalence in psychological problems and obesity in children. Junk food, lack of physical exercise, addiction to electronic gadgets, sleep deprivation and often loneliness at home are spoiling children.

Personal Notes

During my earlier years of practice, I had to spend entire day out of home as I spent 4-5 hours a day at J.J. Hospital as an Honorary Professor and equal time for private practice. But once I settled in practice, I started a joint practice with one of my ex-students and every 8-10 years, one more Pediatrician joined our group. Over last 10 years, we four practice together as one unit and it gives all of us time for our family and to pursue other hobbies. In spite of initial struggle that kept me busy, I have been lucky not to miss a single occasion when my presence in the family was necessary. Every ten years, I started reducing my clinic hours to find more time with the family and it was possible only because of group practice. In fact, during formative years of our children, we need to spend time for them. It helps bonding that lasts forever.

Take Home Message

Don't give an excuse that you have no time because you can always find time only if you understand dangers of not doing so. Money can't buy health and happiness. While money and professional satisfaction are important, far more vital is personal and family's health and happiness. You did well because your parents spent time at home and at the same time, made available whatever was needed. Remember worldly pleasures can't replace time spent with the family.

18 How to be Legally Safe in Medical Practice?

Many doctors don't need laws to tell them to act responsibly, few others try to find the ways around the laws

– Plato

Only thing more dangerous than ignorance is arrogance

– Albert Einstein

Moral Duties of a Doctor

Hippocratic Oath developed 2500 years ago by Greek physician who laid down moral principles of conduct for doctors. WHO developed Geneva Declaration and Medical Council of India brought in an act that has been amended few times as per the need with changing medical practice scenarios. It has widened the scope of expected conduct of a doctor. Every doctor is bound by such rules to follow medical ethics. Its main pillars are beneficence (do good), non-maleficence (do no harm), autonomy (patient's right to make independent decisions), confidentiality (information communicated by patient is in confidence and should not be shared with others without patient's permission), justice (equality of rights, fairness and morality). Medical Council Registration is an agreement to follow these rules and so we are all bound by the same.

What is Expected of a Doctor?

Every doctor is expected to act with reasonable care and skill appropriate to the standards set up by professional bodies. Standard of care varies as per the qualifications, experience and environment in which doctor practices. Irrespective of these variables, each doctor is expected to offer "care always, cure if possible". Care involves action with empathy, concern for the patient, communication, counseling and documentation besides time management, good conduct, honesty, transparency, not to hide ignorance and not to run down peers.

Evolution of Legality in Medical Practice

Ethical standards are based on human principles of right and wrong while legal standards are based on written law. Moral principles were set up by the community and every doctor was expected to follow the same in order to offer the best to a patient. It was left to individual doctors to follow and generations of doctors followed the same, till recently.

However, with changing scenarios in medical practice, few doctors strayed away from moral principles that made the Government of India to bring in Consumer protection Act in the year 1986. According to this Act, dissatisfied patient may complain to consumer forum at local level and if not satisfied with outcome, may go to state or further national level. Indian Medical Association protested against such an Act but finally it was implemented. It became necessary only because of few doctors not following moral principles laid down by competent medical bodies. We ourselves are responsible to bring our services into legality. Unfortunately, every law is likely to be misused as well.

What Constitutes Medical Negligence?

Medical negligence is a breach of legal duty to care as per the expected standards that causes harm to the patient. It could be in the form of error of diagnosis, under or over investigations or treatment or deficiency in care. When doctor accepts a patient, it becomes an implied undertaking to offer standard care. It assumes that he has enough skills to handle such a patient. Every doctor is expected to act with reasonable care and skills. Error of judgment is considered as negligence only if other professionals in the same situation would not have done the same. Only because something went wrong is not considered negligence if professional experts opine that adequate care was exercised while treating a patient. No doctor is supposed to give warranty of perfection of their skills or guarantee of cure. If action of a doctor is appropriate to the standard laid down by professional body, error in diagnosis or outcome is not negligence.

How to be Legally Safe in Medical Practice?

Burden of proof of negligence is to be provided by a complainant. However, it is ideal that doctor can provide evidence of standard of care given to a patient. It is possible only if actions are not only communicated but also documented. Communication refers to offering relevant information about medical action while counseling is an act of guiding and supporting the patient to go through the illness in best possible way. Every doctor must follow these principles and document the same with attested signatures of both the parties. Documentation is the legal proof of having done it and without documentation, law considers it as not done. In serious situations where poor outcome is possible, it is best to record the counseling session on video. If doctor practices with principles of art and science of medicine, it builds good patient-doctor relationship with attendant mutual trust. It forms the core of avoiding legality in medical practice.

Personal Notes

I recall when medical practice was brought under consumer protection law, there was an objection raised by our Association. It was argued that medicine is a profession and not a business. However, I had openly differed because many doctors were not behaving as professionals and those who did adhere to professional standards had not to worry about consumer protection law. I formed a habit of writing short clinical notes and provisional diagnosis followed by drug prescription and general advice. It served dual purpose of ensuring rationality and also honesty. This habit of documentation along with proper counseling automatically takes care of legal safety and shows transparency and accountability. Law does not punish a doctor even if he fails to cure a patient provided, he has followed standard guidelines as expected. I am aware consumer protection Act may also be misused but such a risk is minimized by good behavior.

Take Home Message

We are now bound by law and not only by morality. However, if one follows moral principles, there is no worry about legality. Every law may be misused and so we must exercise utmost care. Documentation is all important that alone is considered as legal proof of your action. There is no need of defensive practice that itself may be questioned. Good doctor-patient relation with attendant mutual faith is the key to be legally safe.

19 How to Deal with Incurable Disease?

Never must the physician say disease is incurable, nature has hidden powers and mysteries

– Morris Fishbein

I don't have a choice about incurable disease but there are other choices in life to make

– Michael Fox

Concept of "Cure"

Word "cure" comes from Latin word "cura' meaning care, concern or attention. Rational medical practice includes care, concern and attention in the management of every disease. Thus, in literary sense, it should be possible for every doctor to "cure" every disease. However general expectation of "cure" refers to healing of damage caused by disease with complete functional recovery and regaining original state of health. But in medical parlance, "cure" is considered when there remains no evidence of active disease at the end of complete treatment irrespective of persistent functional disability.

What is Incurable Disease?

Medically speaking, disease is considered incurable when no more medical intervention is likely to help further recovery. However there exist non-pharmacological and non-surgical modalities of treatment other than medical interventions and doctor should not give up before trying them. For example, Down's syndrome cannot be cured but such a child can be helped in various other ways such as physiotherapy, occupational therapy and other rehabilitation measures and can lead a near normal life. Many diseases are controllable even if not curable and if well controlled, person can lead normal life with or without continued management. Diabetes and asthma are common examples of such controllable diseases. Many immunological disorders may get into remission by itself or by immune-suppressive drugs and remission may last even forever. It is important for all of us to realize that it is patient's immune system that cures the disease, albeit with the help of a doctor and his treatment modalities. However, if immune system does not act favorably, even completely "curable" infections such as Tuberculosis may be fatal due to immune-mediated complications. Thus, it is clear that incurable disease may still be treatable with the hope of natural control, if not cure. By convention, incurable disease suggests bad prognosis for life. However correctly speaking, it means science is unable to cure but proper management, immune system, nature or even luck or destiny may be able to control, if not cure. Finally, today's incurable disease may find cure tomorrow. Recently stem cell transplant or specific organ transplant has offered "cure" in increasing number of disorders.

Dealing with Incurable Disease

Once the disease is considered to be incurable, next step is to find out whether disease can be controlled or at least disease progression can be slowed down. In all such situations, aim is to make the patient as comfortable as possible with quality of life maintained to an extent feasible. This is done by nutritional support, hygienic measures, relief from pain, if any and psychological boosting provided by family and friends. All such measures can make a difference in ultimate outcome.

Counseling a Patient with Incurable Disease

Counseling refers to guiding and offering moral support to a patient so as to help him go through the ordeal. It is well known that **mind helps the body to recover**. Counseling is an art that is to be learnt by oneself. Unfortunately, it is not taught in medical schools. One should not consider helplessness even in incurable disease. Finally, "I treat and he cures" is the faith in our religions that most patients understand. Relatives must be informed fully about the incurable disease but not the patient directly. It is enough for the patient to know that you have not given up because you have seen many of such patients recover well. Once the patient knows that his doctor is with him, it gives him moral boost. We owe that much to our patients suffering from incurable diseases.

Personal Notes

Every doctor faces a challenge to deal with incurable diseases. In such situations, empathy plays major role. I recall an infant suffering from fatal neurological disease (spinal muscular atrophy) who would not see his first birthday. Even when diagnosis was certain, I subtly prepared parents over next few days to anticipate the inevitable outcome before announcing incurable disease. It is said that time heals. Within a week, parents asked me to ensure a painless death for their infant. In another incidence, a baby was born totally paralysed without myelin – the insulation cover to the nerves –another incurable fatal condition (congenital amyelinosis) and I knew that survival would depend on mechanical ventilation for life and hence impractical. It took some time to confirm the diagnosis and literature search revealed handful of such cases in the world and none had survived. But parents would not accept the diagnosis because their family astrologer opined that if life was maintained on a ventilator for a month, this baby would improve on its own. We did cooperate with their wish and ultimately, they accepted the inevitable. In this case, disconnecting a ventilator amounted to killing the child and we had to take legal advice before disconnecting the ventilator that also meant medical opinions from unrelated experts. But there are times when survival if at all, would be in a vegetative state and in such a case, relatives need to be counselled to consider signing DNR – "Do not resuscitate"

Take Home Message

Incurable disease is still treatable though may not be with specific curative drugs. There are other types of support such as nutrition, hygienic measures, pain relief, physiotherapy and psychological boost and they all help to offer comfort. Counseling a patient is an important part of management and knowing that doctor is around for any help makes the patient feel better.

20 How to Deal with Failure of Treatment?

Many medicines few cures

– Benjamin Franklin

Success is not final, failure is not fatal,
it is the courage to continue that counts

– Winston Churchill

Meaning of "Getting Well"

To a patient, it connotes total recovery back to original state of health. To a doctor, it refers to recovery to an extent possible depending upon multiple variables such as type of the disease (curable, controllable or incurable), stage of the disease (early or late diagnosed) and response to standard treatment (response also depends on individual patient's health and immunity). In other words, "getting well" is as per the expectation – patient expects total recovery and doctor expects what is best possible in a given situation.

Doctor Must Anticipate Progress

Once final diagnosis is achieved and standard protocol of treatment is defined, doctor must make time-wise anticipation of expected progress, considering variables related to disease and health status of the patient. Time to time assessment during treatment period would ensure that patient is progressing as per anticipation. In case of any deviation from expected course of events, doctor is timely warned about likely change in management that would again ensure necessary correction. Such anticipation is important as much as the correct diagnosis and treatment. For example, patient diagnosed to have acute bacterial pneumonia is expected to show improvement in tachypnea first, within 2-3 days, followed by reduction of fever over next few days and cough may worsen for a while at that stage before it resolves completely over next few days. Such an anticipation would not worry a doctor and in turn a patient, even if cough worsens as it was anticipated as a course of right direction of recovery. However, if temperature is normal but tachypnea persists, your antenna should go up to trace the cause, it may denote septic shock. Similarly, first symptom to improve in correctly treated typhoid fever is feeling of well-being and return of appetite and doctor finds feel of abdomen improving but fever continues to be high at that stage. So, for a patient who has sought treatment for fever feels he is no better but doctor knows that recovery is on the right path. Such is the importance of anticipation of course of events during treatment.

Need to Counsel and Document Anticipated Progress

It is not enough to know the diagnosis, treatment and prognosis or anticipated progress but equally important is to counsel the patient and document the same for records. Every doctor must develop skill of counseling and make a habit of documentation. It signifies honesty, transparency, accountability and responsibility. It instils faith and mutual trust that has a positive impact on outcome. As discussed above, patient must be informed about the best possible outcome which may change over period of treatment because of many variables. At times, patient may not be happy with the progress that may be short of his or her desired expectations, even when you are satisfied. In such a case, patient has a choice to take another opinion and one should suggest it upfront.

But When Patient Does Not Get Well as Expected

Problem arises when patient's progress does not keep up with what is expected and anticipated by a doctor. That is how time to time assessment of the course of events are important and should be informed to the patient or their relatives. Earliest deviation is spotted, not only patient is informed about change in the course of events but also there may be a change in outcome different than what was expected to begin with. It also needs to be freshly counselled and documented. Doctor must inform why in his view, course got deviated and how he is likely to correct the same. When things are not going the way they should, best way is to talk to the patient more often and try to answer patiently and calmly all doubts raised or at times even allegations made against the doctor. It is said that anger is demonstration of pseudo-strength of a weak person. One must not get defensive but inform the truth. It is important to let patient know that you have put in best of the efforts but they may not always equate to best of the outcome. Equally important is to let the patient see your best efforts and concern about the situation. Honesty pays and so if there are any mistakes inevitably occurred, it is best to own them instead of defending them. Always offer upfront a chance of getting second opinion and let the patient select his choice of second opinion. Most times, patients would ask a doctor whose second opinion they could seek and in such a case, suggest 2-3 alternatives so that they can still choose one of them. It proves your transparency. Once patient has developed faith and knows doctor is doing his best, invariably he would leave choice of second opinion to a doctor. It means half the battle is won. After all patients are not bothered about how much you know but they want to know how much you care. So not only care always but it also must be evident to a patient. Modesty and honesty are two virtues that come handy in difficult situations.

Personal Notes

During training days, responsibility is shared by seniors but in private practice, one is totally responsible for the outcome. Parents are not satisfied unless child completely recovers and at times, one has to face unrealistic expectations from parents. I recall a child suffering from typhoid fever who was improving well with regaining of appetite and energy but was not yet afebrile. Fever is the last symptom to disappear in typhoid. In spite of explaining these facts and assuring that fever would soon disappear, parents were upset. It took some time for me to learn by myself how not to argue with parents but suggest alternative opinion. I also learnt to anticipate "troublesome" parents and sought help in time from senior colleagues. It is ideal to convey a possibility of a rare exception of treatment failure due to patient's inability to respond to medicines. In such a situation, I assess the attitude of parents and suggest a second opinion.

Take Home Message

Medicine is a science of uncertainty and doctors act by probability supported by knowledge, experience and even an intuition. Naturally it is important to convey to a patient that best efforts are guaranteed but not equating to best outcome. However, it does not mean that you paint a gloomy picture each time to be defensive, it may fire back. But what is important is to anticipate, inform, counsel and document. Be honest and don't hide mistakes, to err is human. Be answerable to yourself and not blame others.

21 How to Communicate Need for Further Tests or Referral for Second Opinion?

If you can't measure it, you can't manage it

– Peter Drucker

If world thinks you are not good enough,
you know it's a lie but get a second opinion

– Nick Vujicic

Provisional Diagnosis a Must before Ordering Tests

Laboratory tests are specific to a disease and there are no "routine" tests. Thus, it is imperative that doctor thinks of provisional diagnosis based on analysis of detailed history and focused physical examination before considering specific laboratory tests to support bed-side diagnosis. It is likely that doctor may consider 2 or 3 probabilities and may like to exclude them all together at one time or by priority. Doctor should never consider all possibilities as there could be many. Of course, tests without any provisional diagnosis is irrational as test results have to be correlated with clinical diagnosis. No test result offers diagnosis and most laboratory reports end up with a statement "correlate clinically". It is ironical that laboratory person reminds a doctor to depend on clinical judgment for correct interpretation.

Not all Diseases Need Confirmation by Tests

Disease that is clinically evident and easy to monitor progress does not need any confirmative tests. Acute tonsillitis is a classic example. However, when a disease is not evident clinically such as urinary tract infection or when progress of disease is difficult to monitor as in case of meningitis, specific tests such as urine culture and CSF respectively are a must before starting treatment. Also, due to increasing drug resistance in diseases such as malaria, tuberculosis and typhoid, they must be confirmed before starting treatment.

Counseling a Patient Before Ordering Tests

After arriving at a probable clinical diagnosis, it is ideal to explain the patient why you feel the need for confirmation. It is important to preempt likely test results and how they would guide you further in proper management. Test results often mention insignificant abnormalities noted in a given test that may not be relevant as such findings may be seen in normal persons. For example, abdominal USG often reports small lymph nodes that are of no consequence but for patients it is an abnormality. In such expected situations, it is ideal to inform patients ahead of test results their insignificant relevance. It allays fears and doubts rather than defending results after they are received. Patients don't understand variation of test numbers nor its relevance. This commonly happens in CBC when patient is worried about numbers that don't tally with norms mentioned on test reports. This is more so when tests are done in infants or neonates in whom normal numbers are different than those of older children or adults and most laboratories have printed norms for adults and age-related norms are not mentioned. So when you order tests, inform patients why they are asked for and what could it mean if results are positive or negative. Such a discussion prior to getting test results is important. Unfortunately, most doctors depend on test results for their opinion as they have no clinical diagnosis. Don't forget test results are not reliable for final diagnosis without clinical correlation.

When First Set of Tests Provide no Clue

It is ideal to discuss interpretation of positive as well as negative test results and possible plan thereafter, right when you ask for first set of tests. It ensures that patient is not surprised and upset to know tests have not offered any clue to diagnosis. If first set of tests fail to diagnose the disease, obvious plan after negative test results would be to order second set of tests or consider second opinion. At this stage, you must discuss pros and cons of both the alternatives. I feel at this point, first choice should be second opinion. This is because second opinion invariably would end up with asking for more tests. However, if you order second set of tests without second opinion and if they also fail to diagnose the disease, second opinion will be followed by another set of tests. Drawing blood repeatedly is hated by patients and so also ordering more tests periodically. This is because it conveys to patients that doctor has no clue and he is searching for diagnosis without any specific direction. Besides, expenses mount up and all this may lead to dissatisfaction and even argument or allegation. It is best avoidable with second opinion that you must suggest at right time.

Personal Notes

I prefer to discuss every aspect of the disease with the parents to an extent that my medical assistants wonder whether I take a post-graduate teaching session with the parents. I also subtly inform them that outcome of treatment also depends on how patient is able to respond and follow it with what I would do in case of failure of treatment. If this is followed, parents don't question the need for some more tests or second opinion because they are preempted. Over years I have become more aware that I am liable to make mistakes and parents should be subtly warned about such a possibility. Though as I become senior, parents disbelieve that I could be wrong. Well, it is a bonus to seniority but I never depend on it.

Take Home Message

Communication and counseling are key factors in treating a patient. Relevant information about the tests being ordered and need of carrying out these tests must be conveyed to patients and so also possibility of positive and negative test results. This is the way patients must be involved in disease management that in turn leads to faith and mutual trust between doctor and patient. Once this relation is established, I am sure patients would be ready to follow advice thereafter, be it additional tests or second opinion.

22 How to Respond to Inappropriate Patient Requests?

Do not let behavior of others destroy your inner peace

– Dalai Lama

Most bad behavior comes from insecurity

– Debra Winger

What is Meant by Inappropriate Patient Requests?

What is considered to be inappropriate by doctors may be felt most appropriate by patients. So we need to be unbiased when considering patient request as inappropriate. In other words, we need to get into patient's shoes to be most fair and empathetic. It is doctor's duty to spend enough time, communicate and counsel properly and answer all questions however silly they may be. This should be the appropriate behavior of a doctor and if not, patients may demand, then it is not inappropriate. Only when we consider request as inappropriate, we must respond appropriately and not argue. Response comes from cerebral cortex while argument is only a knee jerk from spinal level. Response is a result of thought process that spells what is right while argument is meant to decide who is right in which case it becomes an ego issue.

Common Requests from Patients that are Inappropriate

1. Medical practice is the only profession where patients (clients) expect service at any time of their convenience, even in absence of emergency situation.
2. Many times, advice is sought on the phone including at any odd hours and is expected to be delivered without seeing a patient, irrespective of its feasibility and of course free of charge.
3. Cell phones have made it possible to speak to the doctor directly anytime and doctor is supposed to respond to each call, irrespective of being busy with a serious patient.
4. Every patient expects to be attended in a short time even if he has come later than his scheduled appointment time. After all there are enough excuses to offer for being late.
5. Majority patients have faith in medicines and tests so they insist to get them irrespective of whether they are required or not. Test results are believed more than doctor's clinical judgment that may be often questioned.

6. Test results are sent on WhatsApp for interpretation, instead of patient or his relative bringing them to a doctor and detailed discussion is expected to be delivered on phone.
7. At times, patient expects a doctor to Interpret results of tests ordered by another doctor or advice on medicines prescribed by another doctor. They expect a free second opinion without seeing the patient.
8. Every concerned relative or friend of a patient expects latest information about the disease and progress on one-to-one basis and feels it is doctor's duty to satisfy their queries, as patient is near and dear to them.
9. Finally, patient may expect concession in doctor's fees as no hospital, laboratories or pharmacies offer any concession.

How to Respond to Inappropriate Requests?

Most important "mantra" is not to lose temper but still make a point. For example, patient arrives when you are about to leave the clinic, inform him that you are going to attend an emergency and so you would offer him first aid and ask him to report next day. Don't spend much time or discuss any details. It conveys to a patient clearly that he did not get full advice but at the same time you have attended him and not sent him back without seeing. Wise patient learns not to repeat the same mistake.

In modern era of easy communication through cell phone, insist on messages and not calls on cell phone. Cell phone must be used only for emergency situations. However, every patient claims an emergency and so best way is to suggest urgent hospitalization to be on safe side, if they really think is an emergency. Most parents then have said that it is not that urgent. Encourage calls on land-line that can be attended by your assistants and answered accordingly. Assistant can be trained to reply to common queries. Automatically, calls on land-line come during working hours. Remember, **Supreme Court expects doctors not to offer advice on phone without seeing the patient.** Otherwise, doctor is held responsible for the outcome. I have been giving advice on phone all these years but now I add to say this is first aid advice and it is better that patient is seen. So, you are legally safe and at the same time you wish to help patients.

If patients insist on laboratory tests or X-rays, best way is to say that in your opinion they are unlikely to help though patient can get them done, if they wish. It takes care of occasional time when such a test proves to be useful though with inconclusive reports, patient knows that he has spent money for nothing. However, if patient asks for specific drugs like antibiotics that are not required, one must be firm not to prescribe. Many patients ask for tonics and I inform them that it would be useless so I won't prescribe but as it is harmless, they can decide to take it. If they insist, prescribe it. After all, manufacturer and chemist also must earn and everybody will be happy thereafter. If I am asked to opine on prescriptions or test results ordered by another doctor, I inform the patient that correct interpretation is possible only with correlation with physical examination. Most doctors don't document their physical examination findings and so it is not fair for you to offer advice merely on test results. In serious situations, every close and not so close relative and friend wishes to get first-hand information from treating doctor. Best way is to request immediate guardians to take care and if they wish, you should be ready to talk to all of them at one time.

Personal Notes

Our joint practice helps patients to contact one of us almost through 14 hours of working day from 8 am to 10 pm. This saves us from untimely requests from the patients. If occasional parent insists on unnecessary tests, I document my advice and leave it to them to undergo the test. There is no point in making an issue of it. However, demand for an unjustified antibiotic is not accepted and opinion to that effect is documented. At times, parents have objected to accept prescription of steroids even when scientifically indicated and in such case, I would document my advice and its justification but leave it for parents to follow or not. After all patients have autonomy but if they don't follow your advice, you are not responsible for the outcome. Once a VIP parent wanted me to see their child at odd hours even when there was no emergency and so I refused. It upset them and they never came back to me. I consider it as their loss and not mine.

Take Home Message

Consider patient request with due allowance to their fear or concern about the disease or treatment. So, within limits, what is inappropriate to a doctor may be most appropriate to a patient. Inappropriate requests must be handled with care, calmness and diplomatic way to avoid bitterness and arguments. At the same time, show gentle firmness in your opinion. Remember patient has a right to his own views and so we should leave it to him to decide whether to follow your advice or not. So be flexible to a large extent especially when patient's demands are harmless though may also be useless.

23 How to Communicate Risks Involved in Management?

As the world becomes more digital place, we cannot forget about the human connection

– Albert Einstein

Effective communication depends on trust and trust depends on trustworthiness

– Steven Covey

Concept of "Risk"

Risk refers to a chance of unacceptable outcome of any action. Life itself is a series of taking risks as every step has a margin of risk, however small it may be. No outcome is 100% certain or safe and so there is always a fear of uncertainty. In fact, medicine is a science of uncertainty and doctors have to depend on art of probability. Therefore, it always involves some risk. Moreover, outcome of medical treatment depends on many variables, of which most unpredictable variable is individual patient's response to treatment. Doctor has no control over patient's response as much as teacher has no control over student's response and therefore outcome is not in the hands of a doctor. Even the best of the treatment may not guarantee best outcome.

Risk Management

It is a process of identifying, monitoring and managing potential risk situation in order to minimize negative impact. As every act has a potential risk, doctor must evaluate risk-benefit ratio. One has to weigh pros and cons. First consider what may happen naturally if no action is taken. After all no action may be apparently safer than any action as in case of minor trauma that heals by itself or a viral infection that is self-limiting. However, in a curable bacterial infection, antibiotic should not be withheld just because there is a possibility of side effects of an antibiotic. In such a situation, side effects of antibiotic are so minor as compared to benefit of cure of bacterial infection which otherwise may endanger life. So clearly benefit outweighs risk and so such a risk is worth taking. In such a situation, it is best not to talk upfront about side effects. When asked by the patient, one should highlight safety of the drug with rarely minimum and inconsequential temporary side effect. Many patients are well informed through "google-doctor" and have read more about side effects than effects. Let patients know that you are responsible for correct information and google-God information is not necessarily applicable to everyone. To a very inquisitive patient who talks only about side effects, I often give them an example that makes them understand a point. I ask them whether it is safe to sit in my clinic under a roof that may collapse anytime. Well, there is always a possibility of collapse to a pessimist but optimist never thinks about it and he is mostly right. Every day one hears about fatal accidents on road and even then, no one stops travelling, simply because risk is negligible. However, situation where in chance of risk and benefit are equal decision is difficult and should be taken together with the patient. For example, treatment of some cancers may be equally dangerous to life as cancer itself. Besides, side effects of treatment may be unbearable requiring repeated hospitalization as against natural sinking that may be less painful. It is an individual patient's mindset that should decide best possible action. But there is always a hope for improvement and so many may be ready to take a risk. Calculated risk is a need to achieve a goal but the final decision must come from the patient.

Use Communication Skills

Communication refers to giving relevant information to the patient. Relevance must be appropriate to the situation. Information not only should be truthful but at the same time it should not discourage the patient to lose hopes of improvement. One needs to be tactful. Most important is the fact that patient should not feel doctor is hiding some information. Such a suspicion leads to despair. So best is to explain to relatives in front of a patient. Always emphasise on positives first. Even in a dire situation that holds significant risk, once you decide that risk is worth taking, talk to the patient about negative impact of not taking a risk. It may amount to a definite disaster while taking a risk may have equal chances of success. It is a good idea to describe your own experience about similar patients who have done well. At times such stories could be fictitious but bring in hopes. Mind plays a significant role in recovery. Doctor must imbibe confidence in a patient that success is always a possibility and so risk is worth taking.

Finally, universal faith on almighty is embedded in our culture, especially in high-risk situations. So, it is appropriate to convince a patient that you will leave nothing undone and put-up best efforts. After all outcome depends on luck and luck favors the brave. So, patient must pray and keep mind cool while you as a doctor do your best.

Personal Notes

I recall an incidence when a child was admitted with acute appendicitis for whom I suggested urgent surgery. Parents took few hours to decide and meanwhile child's abdominal pain disappeared but patient had started deteriorating. This child had developed gangrene (meaning appendix became dead due to loss of blood supply and so pain disappeared but child deteriorated). I explained in details to make them aware that child's life was in danger but they would not agree. In that situation, I asked them to sign a document that they had chosen to disregard my advice and so would be responsible for the outcome. At that stage, parents agreed and child was saved after surgery. I have faced similar situation when a child suffering from pneumonia was breathing faster and required hospitalization but parents refused as their doctor had opined against. I refused to treat this child and left them to decide what suited them.

Take Home Message

Risk is involved in every step of life. A drug that has an effect also has a side effect, there is no drug without a side effect. It is always right to take a risk when benefit clearly outweighs risk. Even in such a favorable situation, there exists a risk that should be downplayed. Doctor has to be tactful to communicate when risk is high but must be taken for hopeful outcome as against not taking a risk that is a sure disaster. It should be communicated in a way to offer hope. Your experience about stories of success in similar situations helps to boost morale of the patient. It has a positive impact that improves chance of success.

24 How to Prepare Yourself to Survive Violent Patient Encounter?

Most violent element in society is ignorance

– Emma Goldman

Aggression is the first step on the slippery slope of selfishness and chaos

– Anne Campbell

What Constitutes Violence?

WHO defines it as intentional use of force or power, threatened or actual, against oneself, individual, group or organization which results in or has high chance of resulting in hurt, damage, destruction or even death. It is an emotional outburst of destructive nature, an intentional use of physical force, an act of power of one person over another.

Changing Scenario of Medical Practice

Physicians of yester years commanded respect from the community to an extent that doctor's views were sought not only for health issues but also in every other family matters. Community had faith in their doctors as they witnessed how much doctors cared for them and community did not care about how much doctors knew. Doctors showed concern with empathy as they communicated, counselled and stood by their patients in times of stress. Patients felt confident and had tremendous belief in their doctors. Things changed for the worse with rapid deterioration in doctor-patient relationship. It is a great irony that medicine, the epitome of healing profession is now often exposed to violence. It is a paradox.

Genesis of this Change

Both doctors and community have changed. There is a brutal dimension to medicine in that what is intended to heal may cause pain, damage or even death. Doctors often succeed but at times fail in their goal. Physicians don't get pleasure in causing pain to their patients but their brains react to viewing pain less strongly than what patients feel. In fact, it is an adaptive response to be able to function effectively in the face of patient's suffering. This may blunt their response to patient's pain. This may lead to confrontation as doctors use harsh words, show rudeness, authoritarian approach and often intimidating behavior. On the other hand, community believes and expects that doctors should cure all problems and save every life. If outcome is short of desired, it is seen as carelessness, negligence and incompetence of doctors. With such a dichotomy of what doctors can deliver and what community expects, irrational behavior of few members of the community sets up a trouble that may escalate to any level with mob mentality.

How to Avoid Situation that May Lead to Violence?

When patient under your care does not progress the expected way, you must suggest to shift the patient to a better facility at optimum time. Doctor must anticipate poor outcome at the time when things are not looking so bad. One major problem arises when patient is shifted too late and hospital where he is shifted, doctor may loosely make a comment that patient should have been shifted much before. In the hospital setting, doctors should be cautious to explain real situation in a manner that seriousness is subtly conveyed. It is best to say that outcome depends on how patient responds and that will be known over next few days. In other words, patient's relatives understand the seriousness and are sensitized to an inevitable outcome. At such a point, relatives start losing cool and try to find mistakes including most trivial issues such as they were not allowed to enter the hospital and security person was rude. You must maintain calm, be empathetic to their problems but at the same time, justify the action that is in the interest of the patient. You must allow relatives to vent their frustration and anger, listen to them without interrupting and finally counsel them tactfully. It is the arrogance of a doctor that often sets up a problem and so learn to remain calm and confident. Another important fact is to allow relatives to witness care being taken, within limits and spend time talking to them periodically. It often avoids trouble. Finally let one doctor remain in communication as a spokesman so that there is no confusion created by different ways of expressing same message. It is at times conceived as opposing views and becomes bone of contention.

Personal Notes

In a general hospital, child was brought in a state of septic shock and attending doctors had appraised relatives about seriousness and danger to life. However, the next day when child was sinking, mob appeared in the hospital and started fighting with doctors and threatening them. Attending doctors anticipated bigger problem and summoned me as a senior doctor. First step I took was to make all of them sit in a room and told them that I would listen to their complaints and find a solution. I allowed them to talk as much as they wanted. They wanted to know why child was not improving in spite of correct diagnosis and proper treatment and so in their views, doctors were negligent and incompetent. As a lay person I thought they had a valid question. Before answering their question, I asked them whether any of them was a teacher in school and luckily for me one of them was. I asked this teacher whether every student in his class scores good marks and passed. He said not all pass, to which I told him that he is responsible for bad teaching. He immediately said that it was not correct because he did his job well but few children did not study or understand and so he was not responsible. I explained to him same thing has happened in this child. Treatment is correct but child fails to respond. He understood my point and I requested him to explain to others. I waited as mob became quiet. This teacher told me that I should try my best and I assured him that it was already being done. Other doctors were surprised how I could douse the fire within this mob so easily.

Take Home Message

One must anticipate trouble and act in time to share responsibilities. Doctors must learn to avoid harsh words and rudeness that always fires back. We have to remain cool and not shout but explain in a way that relatives cool down. Force of any kind and authoritarian attitude leads to trouble. We must not forget that failing situation results in inappropriate behavior of relatives and they need support rather than arguments. Doctors must follow what previous generation of doctors did. They were good listeners, empathetic and caring. If one follows this rule, trouble would be avoided. Of course, there has to be deterrent by law for such violence against doctors.

25 Doctor, Are You Happy in Life?

Purpose of our life is to be happy

– Dalai Lama

It is impossible to build happiness on someone else's unhappiness

– Dalsaku Ikeda

Life is a Journey and not a Destination

Each journey begins with a dream. Some of us may have dreamt to be a doctor while others became doctors by default. However, when a journey as a doctor begins, one definitely dreams of future life. This is the time to know what you want to achieve out of doctor's life, very purpose of life. You need to set priorities, decide what toad to take to reach there and assess whether it is reachable. After all, life is what we perceive! Life is best for those who are happy and so enjoy, difficult for those who analyze and so unhappy and worst for those who criticize and so frustrated. Life lived for others is a life lived well.

Purpose of Life as a Doctor

Fact that one exists does not make life worth! What is the measure of worth? Is it success or happiness or both? Both may not always go together in equal proportion. Success is you get by any means what you desire while happiness is you want what you need and you want what you get. Success is what others think about you while happiness is what you perceive yourself. Robin Sharma in his novel "monk who sold his Ferrari" defines success as an unintended side effect of an act done for anyone other than yourself. Such a success is most difficult and but possible to achieve in life. However, success lies in happiness and happiness in turn promotes success. Happy person is not the one who has everything but one who makes the best out of whatever he has. So, appreciate what you have and be happy, try to improve without competing with others – otherwise pursuit of happiness itself becomes the cause of unhappiness.

Life Journey has Three Phases

Generally, life journey evolves and creates new challenges from early age through middle and old age. During early age we dream, middle age we try to achieve our dreams and old age we introspect what better could have been done that we lost precious time and opportunities. During early age, we have time and energy but no money, in middle age we have energy and money but no time and in old age we have time and money but no energy. It is clear we need to strike a balance in life. When young and successful, you lose our health to collect wealth and then in old age, you lose wealth to regain health. Money is required but it also often brings in problems and hence make journey of life with minimal luggage that brings happiness more than success.

Phases of Medical Practice

To begin with it is the **phase of aspiration**. Initially there is wishful thinking of scientific, ethical and rational practice but waiting for patients makes one get restless and stressed. Slowly there is a drift from **aspiration to compulsion** leading to monetary pursuit that brings in wealth with increasing volume of practice. It appears to be end of stressful life with happiness forever. Soon life revolves around practice and money with increasing greed. It results in burning-out with deteriorating quality of practice, health and family – all at a time. It results in work-life imbalance with attendant cost to health. This is the **phase of success without happiness**. But habits die hard and so life continues the same way thereafter as it is too late to change. But as you entered third phase in which other colleagues start shining more and one becomes insecure about losing patients to other colleagues. By now if you have not developed any other hobbies, you remain frustrated and depressed. So, this is the **phase of eternal unhappiness.** This is how many end up without attaining happiness in life.

Be Responsible for Happiness in Your Own Life

Purpose of life is happiness more than mere success. Road to life twists and turns and so we need to turn rejection into an opportunity.

Stanford University in USA was born out of such rejection. Mr and Mrs Stanford were on vacation to Boston in their old age and suddenly thought of donating all their assets to his alma-mater – Harvard University. It was their last day in Boston and still decided to see the Dean if possible. They had no appointment but were ready to wait through the day in case Dean would have time to see them. Dean's secretary informed the Dean about old couple ready to wait till evening and go away if Dean had no time. So, Dean decided to see them when they offered all their assets to the institution. Looking at the old couple in informal vacation attire, Dean thought they would probably offer few dollars and so thanked them without accepting their offer. Mr Stanford was dejected and as they walked out, his wife said to him "why should we not start a university ourselves and compete with Harvard" and that is how today Stanford University stands as one of the most prestigious universities in the world. Life should be like a tennis game – you serve well, then return well but don't forget game starts with love-all. Life is like a piano where melodies arise from use of both black and white keys. Similarly, life also has ups and downs and we need to brave through to make ourselves happy. But don't forget life is like a bicycle – if you stand still, you fall. So, we must try to move forward in life.

Avoid one letter word "I", instead use two letter word "WE", overcome three letter word "EGO" because its outer edge cuts popularity and inner edge purity, instead use four letter word "LOVE".

Learn to "give" more than "take" – it comes back to you in plenty. So, we must give and forgive but often we get and forget.

Patience and silence are two great energies in life. Patience makes you mentally strong, silence emotionally strong.

How to Achieve Happiness?

Finale to perfection in life is to be happy. Happiness resides in you – search for it. Be grateful for what you have, it will make you happy. Motivate yourself to work with passion and joy – you will enjoy it. Once you are motivated, habits will sustain your happiness. You must develop an attitude to achieve happiness, after all attitude takes you to altitude. Share your happiness with others, spread happiness wherever you go and not whenever you go. Some people make you happy when they come, others when they leave. Happiness promotes health so that you can enjoy life.

Personal Notes

During final year of postgraduate training, I started teaching my juniors and also undergraduate medical students to help me learn the subject better. Teaching is the best way to learn. After completion of education, as I was appointed as honorary teacher in Grant Medial College, teaching for learning became a passion. It continues till today and it gives me tremendous happiness besides keeping me updated. Before starting practice, I went to get blessings from one of the first pediatricians of India – Dr Raghunandan Sanzgiri. On knowing that I was appointed at J.J. Hospital, he told me that I would be happy if I sincerely served the poor and teach medical students. He ended by saying that such daily acts of goodness bring happiness in life. Since then, I never missed attending J.J. Hospital for 30 years and I enjoyed my tenure. I believe in destiny – pre-determined course of events and I was never short of anything in life nor had anything in excess – a perfect balance. Thus, I could spend more time of my life in teaching rather than earning money and it has made me rich in happiness index. And even then, money did come, more than what I needed.

Take Home Message

Strive hard to be excellent and rational in your practice – passion and joy in practice makes it possible that in turn bring happiness. You must enjoy life – don't forget life has an expiry date. Growing old is natural but growing up is optional. Aging is the only way to live longer – don't worry about old age – it does not last long. Tragedy of life is not death but what you did not do when alive. Life is a long journey from human being to be humane. Finally, take care of your own life so that you can die young as late as possible.

26 Doctor, are you healthy? Mens Sana in Corpore Sano - Healthy Mind in Healthy Body

Health is not valued till illness comes

– Thomas Fuller

You have power over your mind, not on outside events. Realize this and you will find strength

– Marcus Aurelius

Introduction

Health was considered as "divine gift" till Hippocrates pioneered the move away from these notions of health and encouraged a focus on acquiring knowledge about health. He believed that sound health was the result of balance between various body fluids such as blood, bile and phlegm. Since then, concept of health has much widened. WHO defines health as "complete state of physical, mental and social well- being and not merely absence of disease or infirmity". Such a definition does not take into account changing concepts of health related to age and culture. For practical purposes, health of children refers to well-being in terms of acquiring destined growth (physical increase in size), development (maturity of function enabling acquiring new skills), activities and energy that facilitates the child to perform to his/her maximum potential and behavior commensurate with social expectations (emotional, social and spiritual). It is well known that body and mind are interdependent and together decide final health status of an individual. It must be nurtured by everyone of us right from childhood but it is never too late. As doctors, we should act as "health guides" rather than "disease managers".

General Health-Promoting Factors

Energy intake (calories consumed through food) and energy expenditure (physical exercise besides calories burnt for basal metabolism) must be well balanced to maintain sound health. Hence diet and physical exercise are important in promoting good health.

Diet – exclusive breast feeding for first 6 months followed by complementary feeding (from family pot) while continuing breast feeds as long as possible in first two years lays the foundation of good health. Vegetables and fruits are important components of diet along with dairy products, cereals and pulses in both vegetarian and non-vegetarian diet. Vegetarian diet is considered better for health, only if one consumes all groups of food items. It is equally important to eat happily, together with the family members.

Communication and bonding between all family members also help nurture sound mental development. Physical exercise – Parents must inculcate sports activities in children right from early age and avoid use of electronic gadgets. Age-appropriate physical exercise can be chosen as per the child's preference and continued regularly. Once a habit is formed, it is sustained for life.

Besides diet and physical exercise, body needs rest to rejuvenate after day's hard work and hence sleep is important. Similarly, mental health helps to ease stress and remain happy that adds to better health.

Sleep – Age-appropriate duration and timing of sleep is vital for sound health. Older child and adults need 6-8 hours of sleep while younger ones need longer duration. Ideal sleep time is between 10 pm and 6 am. One should avoid exposure to electronic gadgets at least one hour before bed-time and it is a good idea to meditate for half an hour prior to sleeping. Meditation refers to concentration over a fixed thought (it could be as simple as following one's breath) that takes away stray thoughts from mind. It helps to get sound sleep and one gets up fresh in the morning. It is ideal to ensure suitable environment conducive to sleep. Unfortunately, most children and adults do not follow ideal sleep hygiene.

Mental health – It includes emotional, psychological and social health. It relates to how we think, feel and act that in turn determines how we handle stress, relate to others and make choices. Mental health is facilitated by nurturing ideal culture of behavior inculcated during upbringing in the family by spending time with family members and friends. One must learn to express feelings and discuss with elders that helps coping up with stress. We need to avoid arguments but solve differences with discussion – arguments are to find out who is right but discussion to find out what is right. Spiritual behavior teaches us how to love and not to hate anyone that in turn promotes harmony. Healthy mind in healthy body is the ultimate health.

Many diseases can be prevented by nurturing health supported by good hygiene.

Hygiene – Poor hygiene is a common cause of diseases. Dental hygiene is often ignored but it is important to look after teeth and gums that otherwise become a source of infection, bad odor and poor health. Hand and genital hygiene are as important. Hands often carry infection from one to another. Food hygiene avoids infections transmitted by contaminated food.

Special Care for Health of Every Organ

Besides maintaining general health, it is desirable that extra efforts be undertaken to look after health of every organ in the body. It adds to better health through efficient working of all organs during entire life.

Lung health

Ideal breathing technique includes deep inhalation, ability to hold breath and relaxed exhalation ending with forceful expulsion of air. It helps in maximum breathing using all segments of lungs. Besides active sports, age-appropriate jogging or brisk walking and breathing exercises (as recommended by yoga or art of living) are ideal. Playing breath-driven musical instruments is a good breathing exercise and so also inflating balloons. One should be regular in carrying out such exercises. It is important to avoid smoking and minimise exposure to home pollution.

Intestinal health

Traditional wisdom knew importance of intestinal health. Castor oil was given to everyone once a week to drive away the toxins produced in the intestines. Methods have changed though principle has remained the same. Eat high-fibre diet – both soluble (oats, nuts, seeds, legume-pulses that is seed of legume) and insoluble (wheat bran, vegetables, whole grains). Avoid spicy and oily food, maintain regular eating schedules – eat slowly, drink adequate amount of water. Bowel habits are important to be inculcated to prevent constipation and its bad effects.

Cardiac health

Heart is a muscle and it keeps strong and fit with exercise, as do other muscles in the body. It is important to avoid smoking, overeating, obesity (monitor waist-hip ratio) and stress. Restriction of excess of salt (processed food is a rich source) and caffeine helps to maintain normal blood pressure.

Brain health

Brain develops fast from second trimester of pregnancy up to second year of life and development is complete by the age of five years. Thus, this is the most crucial period of brain development. Fetus can start hearing by second trimester. Talking and reading to a fetus helps in development of fetal brain. As brain development is nearly over by the age of two years, infants and toddlers must be mentally challenged and stimulated as per their age. Parents must encourage infant to learn new skills by providing opportunity. Talking to infants during wakeful periods develops communication skills. It is important to encourage exploration for young child and best way of learning is with interaction and not memorisation. After all, learning should continue throughout life, it keeps brain active and healthy.

Renal health

Functional maturity of kidneys starts around last trimester of pregnancy and is complete by 18 months of postnatal age. However, nephrons increase in number almost up to third decade and thereafter, there is gradual involution. To maintain renal health, one must remain active, drink plenty of water, control blood pressure and blood sugar, weight and diet control, avoid processed food that contains excess of sodium and phosphorus, take care of constipation, pelvic floor exercises, don't hold urine. Excess of protein intake is bad, avoid reno-toxic drugs such as NSAIDs and damage due to dehydration, electrolyte imbalance and infection. Special care in early life includes timely diagnosis of infection if any and its prompt management. eGFR (estimated GFR) must be monitored periodically and is good screening test. It is roughly calculated as follows. 0.5 X (height in cms divided by serum creatinine in mg%). Normal GFR is 80-100 ml/min. Serum creatinine rises only when GFR goes down to <30 ml/min and thus it is a late determinant of disturbed renal function.

Bone health

Bones store calcium-phosphorus to make them strong and also release them when needed for other organs. High calcium containing food, vitamin D (exposure to sunlight for at least 30 minutes between 11 am and 1 pm with minimum clothes is ideal) and adequate physical exercise maintain bone health. Risk of osteoporosis is increased by sedentary life style.

Hepatic health

Toxins from pesticides, chemicals, additives and unknown sources, hepatotoxic drugs such as anti-TB and anti-convulsants (must be monitored during therapy) and alcohol are likely to damage the liver and so best avoided as far as possible. Unsafe sex and contaminated needles are risk factors for hepatitis B and C viral infections which damage liver. Such infections may also be transmitted from infected mother to neonate. Hepatitis B vaccines protect liver from such infection while Hepatitis A vaccine prevents infection from contaminated food. Liver is also damaged due to accumulation of excess of fat in an obese person.

Healthy mind

Healthy mind is the best asset for the body as it promotes health through stimulating immune system as well as functioning of major organs. On the other hand, unhealthy mind is the worst enemy. Mind is the virtual entity and resides in grey matter of the entire cortex that functions through neural network and chemical and hormonal systems of the brain. Mind exists naturally as it is not the clean slate at birth but can be further enhanced by proper nurture. Mind plays an important role in healing of the disease. It is known that treatment is most effective when patient expects it to work and is optimistic. That is also how placebo works. To maintain healthy mind, we must remain physically active, keep learning, develop and pursue hobbies, meditate to avoid negative thoughts and keep positive attitude, connect with friends and family to remain socially active, be happy and enjoy peaceful life. It is not possible unless one tries proactively to achieve healthy mind. As a doctor, we must also look after mind of the patient besides the body. Application of science treats the body and traditional art of medical practice nurtures the mind of the patient. It is possible only when a doctor knows importance of healthy mind in a healthy body.

Personal Notes

I was lucky to be born to parents who taught the value of what we got rather than craving for more. They inculcated ideal virtues such as discipline, honesty and empathy. This helped me to develop total health as much as possible that includes besides physical and mental health, emotional, social and spiritual health. Subsequently during my postgraduate training, I was influenced by my mentor Dr Wagle who emphasised importance of being humane, respecting every person equally. He defined clearly difference between discussion and argument, discussion is to find out what is right and an argument to find who is right. After completing postgraduation, I was appointed as honorary assistant professor at Grant Medical College when I went to take blessings from one of the pediatricians of first generation – Dr Raghunandan Sanzgiri. He told me to serve the poor sincerely so that one of them would send me a rich patient in my clinic. I wondered how a poor patient in a government general hospital would refer a rich patient but soon it was clear to me how valuable are the blessings of people whom we serve well. All such influences and many more during formative years helped me to develop healthy mind in a healthy body. I continued to remain happy with what I got.

Take Home Message

Remain healthy, eat lightly, breathe deeply, exercise regularly, live moderately, cultivate cheerfulness and maintain interest in life. If you don't have time for wellness, you will have to make time for sickness. Aging process is normal for all the organs but can be delayed with proper life style, so that you remain healthy as long as possible.

PREFACE TO PART 2

History taking is the most important part of a diagnostic process to which it contributes to more than 80%. However, it is possible only if a physician has acquired the art of history taking. History is not merely a reproduction of the patient's narrative but it is much more. This is where the skill lies to gather information in a manner that would lead to a probable diagnosis. It requires "thought in action" where the brain constantly interprets every bit of information as it is gathered, leading to the next relevant question. Thus, patient's reply to a question should lead to the next appropriate question. This is how entire history would be able to unfold the probable diagnosis. Even a classic symptom pertaining to a particular system may also arise from other systems. For example, cough is a symptom of a primary respiratory system but it also may be secondary to cardiac, upper GI, neurological system or even may be psychogenic in origin. Therefore, physicians should be conversant with basic concepts related to each symptom. Collected information if analyzed properly can anticipate likely abnormal physical findings. When physical signs on clinical examination tally with what is expected on analysis of history, one is almost sure of the diagnosis. It can then be confirmed by relevant laboratory tests if necessary.

This book emphasises the need for every physician to develop adequate skills in history taking. It is important to follow simple rules and standard ways of history taking so as not to miss out any vital information. However, the relevant information is possible to gather only if a physician has clear concepts of the genesis of each symptom and understands what such a symptom conveys, then only, subsequent questions can be framed to obtain the best possible information. Correlation with other accompanying symptoms helps to define the anatomy and pathology of the disease, while etiology is guesswork based on rational thinking.

This book emphasises the importance of history taking, helps to understand the genesis of individual symptoms and demonstrates how such knowledge can be implemented to arrive at bedside diagnosis in routine cases seen in office practice. Each chapter ends with MCQ for a short revision contribution.

Dr. Y. K. Amdekar

Part 2

History is Not His Story, But Much More Analysis of Symptoms with Case-Based Discussion

Section 1
General View

27 Art of History Taking

The diagnostic process in medicine is complex but should follow the standard sequence. It should be a patient-centric activity of gathering facts through patient hearing, integration of collected information and interpretation (analysis of detailed history) that helps to guide a focused physical examination. It is the way to arrive at a bedside provisional diagnosis. This is a process of diagnostic refinement followed by diagnostic verification by appropriate tests, if necessary. It brings in rationality, confidence, and consistency, enables planning further management, eliminates mistakes, improves outcome, avoids misuse of laboratory tests and drugs, saves time as well as cost, offers satisfaction to patients and fulfillment to doctors. As detailed history analysis contributes to more than 80% of provisional diagnosis, enough time should be spent on gathering the right information.

History is not **his story;** the patient focuses on what bothers him the most and does not necessarily report what the physician would want to know. History should follow the principle of "thought in action". It means each question should be deliberate with a specific purpose, the answer to which should lead to the next relevant question. History should reveal not only anatomical diagnosis (site of the disease) but even microanatomical site (it is not enough to know the affection of the respiratory system but history must also suggest which part of the respiratory system may be involved, is it airways, lung parenchyma, interstitium or pleura).

Once the history suggests the microanatomical site of the disease, further questions should try to unfold probable pathology (inflammation, infarction, infiltration or tumor, degeneration). Etiology is guesswork based on using adjectives (acute, subacute or chronic, static or progressive, continuous or recurrent, worsening or improving). Thus, "thought in action" can arrive at a probable diagnosis. Every mother, however uneducated or illiterate, is observant about her child's symptoms and physicians must develop skills to ask relevant questions to get the right information. Patient listening is important and time spent on history-taking is always worth it.

28 Simple Rules of History Taking

In the Case of a Single Symptom

One may have to ask for other relevant symptoms, if present. Such other symptoms may not be reported upfront as the patient may feel they are not important and highlight only a single symptom that bothers him most. For example, a patient suffering from fever may not mention mild running nose or cough that may denote an oncoming respiratory infection. Similarly, a patient complaining of general weakness has no other symptoms but on direct questioning, one may come to know other hidden symptoms such as polyuria, polydipsia and polyphagia that may suggest diabetes mellitus.

In Case of Multiple Symptoms

Ask for a **chief complaint**. It is not rare for a patient to describe many symptoms such as fever, cold, cough, occasional vomit and one loose stool, headache and body ache, loss of appetite and disturbed sleep etc. But one should inquire about a chief complaint (it is the most prominent complaint). If it is fever, one can understand all other symptoms are related to fever and so fever should be a leading point to ask relevant history. Similarly, when the patient complains of abdominal pain, vomiting and fever, if the chief complaint is abdominal pain, it is likely to be acute appendicitis, in which vomiting and fever are secondary symptoms; if the chief complaint is vomiting, viral A hepatitis is a probability. Thus, chief complaint offers a clue to a probable diagnosis and guide to a focused physical examination and relevant tests. But at times, the patient may consider all symptoms to be equally severe – means no single chief complaint. In such a case, inquire about the **sequence of symptoms** appearance and disappearance, if any. For example: If a patient presents with fever followed the next day with a cold and then cough, it is likely to be a viral infection but if a patient presents with cold and cough first and two days later presents with mild fever, it is not an infection but allergy. Similarly, the sequence of the disappearance of symptoms is also important to note. For example, in a patient suffering from typhoid fever, fever is the last symptom to disappear but much before fever subsides, the patient shows improvement in appetite, general well-being and abdominal fullness. However, if the patient becomes afebrile before other symptoms disappear, one considers it to be a complication, such as septic shock. Thus, the sequence of appearance and disappearance of symptoms is also an important part of the inquiry.

29 Standard Method of History-Taking and its Relevance

General Information

Patient should be addressed by the first name which sets in a good rapport. Age is important to know as some diseases are more prevalent in particular age groups. The exact age in weeks or months is relevant to monitor growth in infants.

History Should Start with the First Question

Was the patient completely well prior to the onset of the present illness? Often, the patient refers to the onset of the major symptom as the starting point of illness. However, when probed further, milder symptoms could be existing prior to the onset of the present illness. "Apparently" normal patient may not really be normal prior to reported illness. This is important as milder symptoms are not voluntarily reported as the patient feels they are not important. For example, low-grade fever for a few days prior to the onset of high fever may not be mentioned. Missing such minor symptoms can lead the physician in the wrong direction. Similarly, acute onset of new symptoms in a previously healthy individual has a different interpretation than one presenting in a malnourished individual. A hidden disease, even without observed symptoms, does affect the general well-being of the patient and it is reflected by disturbed appetite, sleep, activity or energy level and behavior as well as change in bowel pattern or urination. Such minor changes are often not reported unless asked for. Thus, every effort must be made to make sure that the onset of the problem as reported is correct.

Chief Complaint

It refers to the main complaint or reason for which a patient presents to a doctor. It may not always be the first symptom noticed by the patient. For example, the patient starts with a running nose followed the next day with a high fever. In such a situation, fever is the chief complaint, though not the first symptom perceived by the patient but the first symptom that offers a clue to the respiratory system as the anatomical localization.

Onset, Duration and Progress

Hyperacute (in seconds) onset suggests mechanical cause such as trauma, inhaled foreign body, pulmonary embolism or pneumothorax, onset within minutes or few hours is often due to allergy or a vascular etiology such as thrombosis and onset over 2-3 days would suggest a probable infection. Thus, onset helps to consider probable etiology.

It is important to note the *duration* of symptoms. The short duration of fever may represent acute viral infection while fever presenting for two weeks or longer may be due to tuberculosis or non-infective inflammatory disease. Abdominal pain lasting for months without any disturbance in health may be due to a functional disorder. It is important to note that the duration of a symptom may not coincide with the duration of the disease. Mild symptoms may persist well after the disease is cured but on the other hand, symptoms may disappear completely but the disease may still remain active as happens in tuberculosis or malignancy.

Progress as noted in history helps to decide the type of disease. Symptoms may start improving as in common viral infection (recovering disease) or remain to the same extent for few days as in typhoid or tuberculosis (static disease, neither improving or deteriorating) or increase in severity or new symptoms may come up as in case of empyema following pneumonia or capillary leak syndrome following dengue fever (worsening disease). Viral infection may present with biphasic fever – recurrence of fever after the afebrile period in which the second phase of fever is mild and short, it settles down by itself. However, if in an infection, the second phase of fever is severe and prolonged, it suggests immune complications as happens in leptospirosis. However, if the interval between two phases of fever is longer, say a few days, it is likely to be the same infection with a variable pattern of fever as happens in tuberculosis (fever off and on) and in such a situation, the patient remains sick during the afebrile period. On the other hand, the patient remains normal in case of recurrent fever due to recurrent infection.

Past History

Cough is a common recurring symptom in routine practice and the presence of past history of similar cough indicates a probable hyper-reactive airway disease as in the case of asthma. Thus, past history of *similar disease* (not merely similar symptoms) is important. For example, a child with nocturnal episodic cough in the past, presents this time, with progressively worsening cough with a whoop, obviously, the disease is different (pertussis) but has a similar symptom of cough. Similarly, recurrent episodes of fever may be due to different causes each time. Thus, past history of similar symptoms is different from that of a similar disease. It is also important to ask for past history of *major illnesses*. For example, if a patient presents with acute bacterial pneumonia but has a past history of meningitis and osteomyelitis at different times within the last one year, it suggests underlying immune deficiency disorder. However, if a patient presents with recurrent pneumonia in the same lobe, it is likely to be due to congenital malformation in that lobe that predisposes to recurrent infection at the same site.

Family History

Few diseases may be *genetically determined* and hence recur in subsequent generations. Depending on the type of genetic inheritance (autosomal or sex-linked, dominant or recessive), one may get some clues to a diagnosis. For example. Hemophilia due to factor 8 deficiency is a sex-linked recessive disorder that means it occurs only in males but is transmitted by females. However, many disorders are autosomal recessive and hence occur in both males and females but both the parents are heterozygous – which means they harbor abnormal gene but are asymptomatic or minimally symptomatic which is often not noticed. Highly infectious diseases such as whooping cough often spread easily to other members in contact and hence, one may note the positive family history of a similar disease. Tuberculosis is another classic example. Thus, family history may also refer to a *history of contact* in the family.

Personal History

It refers to factors of general well-being as noted by the level of activity or energy, appetite, sleep, behavior, bowel movements, urination and weight record, if available. Subtle or hidden illness may be present prior to the onset of the main complaint and it may be reflected in items of abnormal personal history as mentioned above. For example, polyuria may not be mentioned unless asked for and so one may miss diabetes mellitus or renal tubular disorder. As noted at the beginning of this chapter, personal history indicates how well the patient was before reporting the present illness.

Drug History

Patient may be taking some drugs that may alter the presentation of his present disease as happens often in a febrile patient already on antibiotic therapy. Patients on any chronic drug therapy may present with symptoms of either excess of drug or due to missing a dose of a drug as may happen in case of diabetes. History of a drug allergy may be important to guide the further selection of drugs.

Diet History

Diet recall over a few days may bring about information of adequacy or inadequacy of nutritional intake. It would help in the management but also may offer a clue to the diagnosis. For example, a patient complaining of flatulence and gaseous abdominal distension may be consuming too much of sugar-containing foods including milk or change in bowel pattern may be related to consumption of wheat as in celiac disease.

Socio-economic History

Knowing the socio-economic status of the patient defines the risk of some of the diseases as well as affordability of therapy, based on which a physician must modify the diagnostic and therapeutic approaches to suit the needs of the patient. Of course, it has to be done without sacrificing the benefits of rational diagnostic and therapeutic measures. It is important to realize that the majority of problems in routine practice can be taken care of by clinical bedside medicine (analysis of detailed history and focused physical examination) using minimum laboratory tests and/or drugs. (Essential drug list as suggested by the Government is sufficient for the treatment of 90% of patients in routine practice). There are scales available to assess the socio-economic status of patients. (Kuppuswami scale is commonly used).

Growth and Development History

This part of history is important in children during growing and developing years. Primary malnutrition due to poor intake of food or secondary malnutrition due to severe or chronic disease affects growth (weight is affected first and if the problem continues then the height is also affected and hence growth is measured by both weight and height). Even In absence of weight and height measurements, parents are able to inform growth patterns only if asked for. Many times, parents complain that younger sibling looks bigger than the elder or clothes don't require to change in size indicating poor growth. Similarly, inquiry about milestones offers clues to neurological or behavioral problems such as autism spectrum disorder or learning disorder. It should always be a practice to call an infant of about 10 months of age and see whether he responds to your calling his name. If he does not, one may suspect either hearing impairment, intellectual defect or autism spectrum disorder. It is thus possible to pick up such defects early enough for a better outcome.

Section 2

Analysis of Common Symptoms with Case-Based Discussion

Analysis of Individual Symptoms

It is necessary to understand the basic concepts of the genesis of individual symptoms, nature's purpose behind such a response and how we should interpret the same and manage. A symptom may be common to any of the multiple systems in the body. Even an apparently specific symptom such as cough may primarily arise from the cardiac, neurological or upper GI system, though finally mediated through the respiratory system.

Similarly, vomiting may be due to stimulation of chemoreceptor trigger zone in the brain as a result of a variety of causes or even induced by severe cough and not necessarily only due to affection of GI system. A symptom may be so non-specific such as fever or generalized weakness that one needs to ask several leading questions for the right interpretation. Thus, knowledge of basic concepts should guide to asking relevant questions to seek desired information. It is equally important to realize that the symptom of the disease not only offers a clue to anatomical diagnosis (site of the disease) but also it is nature's intended way to protect the body. Nature is kind not to hurt but when faced with a disease, finds it necessary to present a symptom that not only protects but also alerts the patient and his doctor. It is well known that "fever is a friend and not a foe" and also pain is meant to protect the injured part from further damage.

In subsequent chapters of this section, you will find a detailed discussion of basic concepts related to individual symptoms, followed by clinical application based on live case scenarios experienced in office practice and also a few MCQs for revision at the end of a chapter.

30 Fever a Friend or a Foe?

Back to Basics – Understanding Fever

Why Does Body Temperature Rise?

Fever is the body's immune response to the entry of organisms or tissue damage that may result from either an infection or non-infective inflammation due to autoimmune disorders, malignancy, allergy or trauma. Rarely, fever may result from failure of temperature regulating system as in case of hypothalamic disorder, autonomic disturbances or heat fever and also due to increased metabolism as in case of hyperthyroidism. At times, a drug may cause fever, though the diagnosis of drug fever depends on the exclusion of other possibilities and by the withdrawal of the offending drug. Rarely, fever may be a fictitious symptom. It is clear that fever does not equate to infection but there are many other causes of fever. However, infection is the most common cause of fever but not necessarily a bacterial infection. Viral infections are more common, especially in healthy young children. Thus, antibiotics should not be used in the treatment of every fever.

How Does Body Temperature Rise?

Body's immune response is mediated through cytokines – chemicals produced by immune cells of the body such as monocytes/macrophages and neutrophils. These cytokines send signals to the hypothalamus that functions as a thermostat to raise body temperature to the desired set point. Hypothalamus acts through the autonomic nervous system and regulates body temperature. If the body needs to increase the temperature to a moderate degree, it is achieved by preventing heat loss by peripheral vasoconstriction that manifests as chill in the patient and cold periphery as compared to the warm central part of the body. However, when the body needs to increase the temperature to a much higher degree, it does so by increasing heat production by excessive muscular contractions that manifest as rigors. Once the desired temperature is achieved, the thermostat shuts down and fever starts coming down either naturally or induced by the antipyretic drug. Cooling is facilitated by sweating, especially in case of high fever. One can understand that chills or rigors are not specific to any disease but simply correlate with the degree and speed of rising temperature. So, malaria may not present with rigors if the parasitic load is low but typhoid fever may present with rigors if the infection is more virulent. The degree of fever depends on the virulence of the organism and the immune status of the host. Neonate or severely malnourished child may not present with fever in spite of a serious infection. Similarly, the child may not present with a high fever to infection against which he is partially immunised. A child staying in a highly endemic area for malaria may not present with high fever due to partial immunity derived from repeated exposure to malarial parasites. It is also true that the absence of fever may not rule out infection.

Is Fever Beneficial for the Body?

Fever is a friend and not a foe as it tries to prevent the multiplication of organisms. Raised body temperature leads to the increased blood supply to the damaged site that in turn brings in immune cells and antibodies at the site of damage. It helps to contain the damage and promotes the healing process. Hence, fever is always helpful though when such a response crosses the intended limit, it could also harm the body as happens in hyperthermia, fortunately, it is very rare. Fever being an immune response is an indirect marker of good immunity or fighting power denoting nature's attempt at healing and hence fever is a desirable response, provided it is appropriate to the given situation. Much before science developed, it was known that serious patients with high fever often got better than those with low fever, who often succumbed. Hence in the olden days, doctors tried to induce fever hoping for better outcome. Of course, it is no longer tenable.

If Fever is Helpful to the Body, Should it be Controlled?

Fever should be controlled only if it causes significant discomfort to the child in terms of extreme irritability or lethargy. Generally, discomfort caused by fever correlates with the peak of fever and it is the right time to use paracetamol. So, if a child's behavior is nearly normal in spite of fever, there is no need to bring down fever. Thus, we need to treat discomfort caused by fever and not fever itself. It is a myth and unfortunately a general belief, though wrong, that fever is harmful and so must be suppressed at any cost. It is important to dispel this myth with proper communication and counselling. Mild to moderate fever rarely produce significant discomfort and hence it need not be suppressed. Many children continue to be reasonably playful in spite of moderate fever. It is important to note that discomfort may be caused by factors other than fever that also need to be addressed. Fever in a seriously ill patient in ICU may increase the energy demands of the heart and lungs in particular and so should be suppressed, even if fever is moderate.

What About Risk of Febrile Convulsion?

Simple febrile convulsion occurs in 5% of normal children and it cannot be predicted. There is often a positive family history. Convulsion is short-lasting for less than a minute and self-limiting without risk to life or brain damage. It typically occurs within the first 24 hours of the onset of fever and rarely recurs in the same episode of fever. The first episode generally occurs in infancy or before the age of two years. However, recurrence in subsequent episodes of fever is likely up to the age of six years and can be prevented by a prophylactic drug – Clobazam that should be reserved for frequent recurrence. It is worth a note that control of fever does not necessarily prevent simple febrile convulsion though it is rational to administer paracetamol in case of high fever. In fact, many a time, parents notice fever only after the child develops a convulsion. Hence there is no need to worry about febrile convulsion though recurrence can be prevented. Convulsion in a brain-damaged child should not be considered as simple febrile convulsion and so also in a child with late-onset of the first episode and one occurring beyond the age of six years. Simple febrile convulsion does not increase the risk of subsequent epilepsy.

Which is an Ideal Antipyretic?

Paracetamol is the ideal drug that controls discomfort without undue reduction of fever. It helps in diagnosis as fever pattern due to the natural progression of the disease is not altered. Earlier generations of doctors categorized fever patterns as persistent, intermittent or remittent which was useful in diagnosing the cause of fever. Attempt to reduce fever by "strong" drugs, fever pattern is lost and is no longer useful for clinical diagnosis. If fever is suppressed unduly with a higher dose or more powerful antipyretic, it may lead to a false sense of disease control and one may miss worsening condition. Besides, it may also cause side effects. Paracetamol has an advantage over other antipyretic drugs in that it has a wide margin of safety and is devoid of gastric and renal side effects. Paracetamol is an ideal drug that relieves discomfort caused by high fever without disturbing the body's helpful immune response. Thereby it helps to diagnose the cause of fever. Besides, it is the safest antipyretic.

What if Paracetamol Fails to Control Fever?

If paracetamol is administered much before fever attains the desired peak, the fever will rise in spite of the drug. This is true for every other antipyretic because once the thermostat is set at a particular point, fever has to rise till that point is reached. So antipyretic is effective only when administered at the peak of fever which often coincides with significant discomfort. This fact is often ignored resulting in irrational therapy. Children are innocent and so they are often comfortable even at a moderate degree of fever. Discomfort is a subjective feeling and should be judged on an individual basis. However, if paracetamol fails to achieve desired comfort in spite of mild reduction of fever or otherwise, it in fact suggests probable serious infection that calls for judicious action. Thus, it helps to diagnose serious disease in initial stages. Another condition in which every antipyretic would fail is "central" fever – fever caused by hypothalamic dysfunction. It is a rare condition but can be suspected with total failure of response to any antipyretic. Paracetamol rarely fails as ideal response is to relieve discomfort and not to control fever and it does achieve desired action. No antipyretic helps if administered too early in the course of rising fever. However, in case of genuine failure, one should rule out serious infection and consider Ibuprofen as the next alternative. Tepid water sponging is another temporary measure that is effective and safe. Cold compress over forehead is useless.

How Does Tepid Water Sponge Reduce Body Temperature?

Temperature of tepid water should be around 25 degrees centigrade while body temperature in case of high fever may be around 40 degrees centigrade. When towel dipped in tepid water and squeezed is applied to skin surface and rubbed gently, heat from the skin surface is transferred smoothly to the towel due to physics principle of convection. It reduces temperature of that skin surface to which towel is applied. This process is repeated one by one on all four limbs, chest, abdomen, back and head. Temperature comes down by 2 degrees centigrade with two rounds of sponging the entire skin surface of the body. This method is useful when paracetamol fails to provide comfort or fever returns after paracetamol within a period of four hours. It is important to note that one should not use cold water. Application of cold water leads to vasoconstriction and in fact heat from the body is not allowed to dissipate. Further, child with high fever cannot tolerate cold water application and becomes more uncomfortable. Tepid water sponge is effective in reducing body temperature only when it is done in an ideal way. Though normally it should be reserved when paracetamol does not produce desired action. While sponging, child should not be exposed to wind and skin should be dried well at the end of sponging.

When is Urgent Control of Fever Necessary?

It is only in case of hyperpyrexia – temperature > 105F that quick control of fever is necessary. Heat fever is one such condition in which entire body – central as well as peripheral parts of the body are equally hot. In every other condition of high fever, peripheral parts of the body are cold. In case of hyperpyrexia, physical methods are quicker than drugs and include ice-water enema or tepid water sponging. In addition, parenteral antipyretic may be used. Fortunately, hyperpyrexia is a rare event, endangering life and it needs diagnosis of cause of fever as well as proper treatment. Such a patient is ideally treated in intensive care facility.

Take Home Message

Fever is body's protective response and in fact it helps the patient to recover from illness. It is rarely harmful. Fever pattern and its progress helps physician to diagnose cause of fever, provided it is not suppressed by irrational therapy.

Next article deals with clinical application of basic facts highlighted in this article with discussion on live case scenarios, representing day-to-day problems faced by practitioners.

MCQs

1. Which of the following statement is right - Fever may be caused

A) By infection
B) Without infection
C) Due to inflammation
D) By all of the above

2. Which of the following statement is wrong? Causes of non-infective fever include

A) Malignancy
B) Collagen vascular disease
C) Toxoplasmosis
D) Drugs

3. Which of the following statements are correct – non-inflammatory causes of fever include

A) Heat fever
B) Hyperthyroidism
C) Central fever
D) All of the above

4. Which of the following statement is right? Fever does not respond to any antipyretic in

A) Acute bacterial infection
B) Malignancy
C) Central fever
D) Collagen vascular disease

5. Which of the following statement is wrong? Body temperature rises because of

A) Production of cytokines as a result of tissue damage
B) Temperature regulation system defect
C) Increased metabolism
D) None of the above

Answers to MCQs

Correct answers as follows:

Q1 D	Q2 C	Q3 D	Q4 C	Q5 D

31 Can You Believe? History Leads to a Probable Cause of Fever

Clinical Application of Basic Concepts of Fever

Cytokines mediate the rise in body temperature and so the degree of fever depends on the number of cytokines produced. A large number of cytokines are produced in localized severe acute bacterial infection, wide-spread acute viral infection and non-infective inflammation such as collagen vascular disorder or malignancy such as acute leukemia. Hence these diseases present with a high fever at the onset. The sudden release of malarial parasites in blood also results in high fever at the onset. Low-grade fever at onset suggests low-grade infection or chronic infection. A moderate degree of fever at the onset that increases to a higher degree over the next 3-4 days – step-ladder pattern – suggests acute bacteremic bacterial infection in which initial bacteraemia results in a moderate degree of fever that worsens when infection localizes in a particular organ. Generally, acute bacterial infection responds poorly to paracetamol with persistent sick feeling even if fever is partially reduced while fever in acute viral infection responds better to paracetamol with the child feeling better even with minimal control of fever. Fever is often rhythmic in most infections except in the case of typical malaria. Fever in acute viral infections mostly settles by day 3-4 without any specific therapy, fever in untreated acute bacterial infection worsens by D3-4 while there is no change in fever pattern by D3-4 in case of malaria or non-infective inflammatory diseases. Accompanying symptoms if any help early localization of the disease.

Following questions help in arriving at a provisional diagnosis in case of fever, even as early as by D 2-3.

1. Degree of fever at onset (within first 24 hours)
2. Response to paracetamol (in terms of discomfort)
3. Behavior during inter-febrile period (even with a small change in the reduction of fever)
4. Rhythm of fever (regular every 4-6 hours or irregular)
5. Progress by Day 3-4 (without specific antibiotic therapy)
6. Any accompanying symptoms (often cold, cough or other)

Case-Based Study

Case 1

Two year old child presented with fever for a day. Fever was high at the onset, it responded fairly to paracetamol, child felt better during inter-febrile period, fever was rhythmic coming up every 4-6 hours. Physical examination did not reveal any abnormality. High fever at onset – four possibilities – acute bacterial infection at the site of entry (tonsillitis, bacillary dysentery, UTI), acute viral infection, non-infective inflammatory disease (collagen vascular disease, malignancy) and malaria. Fair response to paracetamol and better during inter-febrile period rule out acute bacterial infection. Rhythmic fever is unlikely to be malaria. So, at this juncture, fever is likely to be due to either viral infection or non-infective causes. One has to wait to see further progress.

On day 2, child developed cold and cough. It suggests localization to respiratory tract. Physical examination revealed fairly comfortable child, coryza, chest clear, no other abnormality. At this stage, you have already diagnosed it as acute viral respiratory infection.

One can anticipate quick recovery over next 2-3 days. Fever continued for another 2 days and then abated. However, cough continued for next few days.

Thus, it is **acute viral respiratory infection.** There is no need for antibiotic. It is anticipated that cough in acute viral infection may continue for few more days and it does not call for change in diagnosis or treatment.

Viral infection is most common cause of fever in healthy young children and it could also be frequent – few times a year. In spite of recurrence, as such episodes are self-limiting and do not affect well-being and growth, parental counselling is necessary to allay their anxiety and refrain from unnecessary investigations and drugs.

Case 2

Two years old child presented with fever for a day. Fever was high at the onset, poor response to paracetamol with child remaining sick during inter-febrile period. Fever would rise every 4 hours. Physical examination revealed no abnormality. Poor response to paracetamol with continued disturbed behavior during inter-febrile period would have warned of **oncoming acute bacterial infection** even before localization. Commonly acute bacterial infection may localize to upper respiratory tract (tonsillitis, otitis media), lower respiratory tract (pneumonia), central nervous system (meningitis), intestinal system (dysentery) or less commonly to other sites such as cervical lymphnode or bone/joint. So, one has to observe development of any localizing symptoms.

On day 2, he developed abdominal pain and loose stools with blood and mucous. He was diagnosed as acute bacillary dysentery. He was treated with an antibiotic and got better. Bacillary dysentery is caused by gram negative bacteria and antibiotic of choice could be cotrimoxazole or cefixime. Amoxicillin would work but may be reserved for gram positive bacterial infection such as pneumonia. It is possible that acute bacterial infection may be suspected even on first day of fever. However, one has to wait for localization before starting an antibiotic.

It is because infection at different sites vary in choice of antibiotic and also its dosage. There is no single antibiotic that will treat effectively every bacterial infection. As a general rule, acute bacterial infections occurring in organs above the diaphragm are due to gram positive organisms while those below the diaphragm are caused by gram negative organisms. Deep-seated or serious infections such as meningitis, endocarditis or osteomyelitis must be treated with intravenous antibiotics and so also all bacterial infections in neonates, young infants and immunocompromised patients.

Case 3

Five years old child presented with fever for a day. Fever was low to moderate at onset, fair response to paracetamol with normal inter-febrile period and rhythmic pattern. As this child's fever was not high at onset, those four possibilities (acute bacterial infection at the site of entry, acute viral infection, non-infective inflammatory disease and malaria) are less likely though acute bacterial or viral infection of low virulence would still be possible. In such a case, we would have to wait and observe further course. Fever increased to high degree on day 4 with poor response now to paracetamol and child looking sicker during inter-febrile period. So, at this stage it looks like acute bacterial infection. Increasing trend of fever during first 3-4 days – moderate fever rising to higher degree - a step-ladder pattern - suggests bacteremic bacterial infection. This child did not develop any significant localizing symptoms such as breathlessness (pneumonia) or headache, vomiting (meningitis), though did complain of vague abdominal pain. Physical examination showed mild abdominal distension and sick child on D 4. **Typhoid fever** was suspected and blood culture sent for confirmation. In such a typical presentation, one may start antibiotic after sending out blood culture and not wait for results. This is because typhoid is a serious disease and early institution of antibiotic is ideal. Blood culture proved diagnosis of typhoid fever. Antibiotic of choice depends on local epidemiology but third generation cephalosporin is preferred and macrolide may also be used.

During bacteremic stage, child develops fever that increases once infection localizes to some site. Three common localization sites include lung (pneumonia), brain (meningitis) and intestine (typhoid). Though, lung can be infected also directly through droplet infection reaching through airways. One has to observe localizing symptoms. Acute pyelonephritis is another bacterial infection without obvious localization. However, it starts with high fever unlike a typical typhoid fever with step ladder pattern.

Provisional diagnosis may not be possible in first 3-4 days in bacteremic bacterial infections. One has to wait for symptoms of localization that may be observed on D2-3 such as vomiting in meningitis or mild tachypnea in pneumonia. Typhoid fever may not present with any localizing symptom except vague abdominal pain. One should not start an antibiotic unless there is reasonable clue to diagnosis, which is mostly observed by D3-4. If situation demands to start an antibiotic, one must order relevant tests before starting an antibiotic.

Case 4

Five year old child presented with high fever at onset with fair response to paracetamol and better during inter-febrile period. This would rule out acute bacterial infection. Fever was rhythmic and so malaria is unlikely. That leaves only two possibilities - acute viral infection or non-infective inflammatory disease. Physical examination did not reveal any abnormality. Fever continued for next 4 days without any change. Acute viral infection would have some accompanying symptoms and would have settled down by D4. Besides, fever in this child would rise every 12 hours and not every 4-6 hours as often happens in acute viral infection. Typically effect of paracetamol wanes off within 4-6 hours. At this stage, acute viral infection is also ruled out and hence it is most likely a non-infective inflammatory disease. Physical examination on D 4 did not reveal any abnormality. One may not be able to guess further course that may evolve over another few days to sometimes even weeks. But it is clear that it is not an infective disease and so investigations and therapy should not be addressed to infections. Here again, one must wait and observe for evolution of disease. In such a case, one must watch for joint involvement, skin rash, mouth ulcers (all suggestive of collagen vascular disease), lymphadenopathy, pallor, purpura and bony tenderness (all suggestive of probable hematological malignancy). This child developed evanescent skin rash (rash appearing at the height of fever and disappearing when fever is controlled). It is a pointer to systemic inflammatory disease. Two weeks later, he developed joint swelling and pain suggesting the diagnosis of **systemic onset of Juvenile idiopathic arthritis.** Non-infective inflammatory disease can be suspected as early as 4th or 5th day though diagnosis is not known till disease evolves in a recognizable pattern. However, there is no need to start empirical antibiotic therapy just because fever continues longer.

Anti-inflammatory drug such as Naproxen is the drug of choice. Steroids are reserved only in selective cases, especially non-responders. Systemic onset inflammatory disorders simulate acute bacterial infection with high fever and neutrophilic leukocytosis. However, normal inter-febrile period and lack of localization to any organ would suggest noninfective disorder. Unfortunately, diagnosis of systemic onset inflammatory disease is made only after antibiotics fail to improve the patient.

Case 5

Five year old child presented with high fever at onset (four possibilities) with erratic rhythm irrespective of paracetamol (mostly malaria) and normal during inter-febrile period. Physical examination on D 2 did not reveal any abnormality. Fever continued without any change or any other symptoms. In a typical situation, malaria may be considered at the end of first day of fever. Diagnosis of **malaria** due to plasmodium vivax infection was confirmed on peripheral blood smear. Chloroquine is the drug of choice in uncomplicated vivax malaria. Ideal dosage schedule should be adhered to. Early in the course of malaria, there are no positive findings on clinical examination as pallor and splenomegaly come up later and are more prominent in recurrent malaria. However, history if well analyzed can suspect malaria. It is equally important to keep in mind that malaria can present with atypical findings. Confirmation with peripheral blood smear is a must before starting anti-malarial therapy to avoid drug resistance. Rapid antigen tests have limitations though easy to implement and hence thin and thick peripheral blood smear continues to be the gold standard for diagnosis of malaria. It also defines parasitic index denoting severity. Malaria being an endemic infection in India, it may present with wide variation of fever pattern. Hence, one may not expect each time fever with rigors but erratic fever pattern and normal inter-febrile period is a clue to diagnosis of malaria. Spleen may not be palpable in first attack of malaria. Epidemiology of infections must be taken into consideration for the etiological diagnosis of infections.

Case 6

Five year old child presented with low grade fever at onset. Low grade fever suggests infection with low virulence. Acute bacterial infection generally presents with high fever at onset but subacute or chronic bacterial infection may present with low grade fever as happens in tuberculosis. Acute viral infection may also present with low grade fever because host may be partially immune to such an infection either due to previous natural exposure to same virus or prior vaccination against same virus. Similarly, malaria may also present with low grade fever if host has had earlier exposure to malarial parasites. Systemic inflammatory diseases present with high fever at onset. So, in this child acute bacterial infection and non-infective inflammatory diseases are ruled out. Physical examination at this stage did not reveal any abnormality. So, one must wait before considering any antibiotic or laboratory investigations. This is because one does not know which antibiotic and which test to order. Moreover, this child is not seriously ill.

This child continued to run low grade fever for next one week without any other symptoms or signs. At this stage, viral infection as well as malaria are mostly ruled out. So, one starts thinking about subacute or chronic bacterial infections such as tuberculosis. Surely antibiotic is not necessary in this child as acute bacterial infection has been ruled out. Further tests may have to be addressed to rule out tuberculosis. This child showed pneumonia on chest X-ray and **tuberculosis** was confirmed by subsequent tests. Tuberculosis may also present with acute onset of high fever as seen in acute pleural effusion in a healthy person. This is because such a manifestation is immune mediated and hence acute presentation. Tuberculosis must always be treated with four drugs for first two months, followed by three drugs for next 4 months, irrespective of type and site of disease. However, therapy may have to be prolonged beyond 6 months, as in case of TB meningitis or disseminated TB. Empirical anti-TB therapy is irrational and it has resulted in drug-resistant TB. Thus, It is important to confirm diagnosis of tuberculosis by bacteriological tests such as sputum culture (in young children, gastric aspiration can replace sputum for culture as sputum is often swallowed by children and AFB can be picked up in gastric aspiration) or molecular tests such as GeneXpert that is available freely. It is also true that TB in a child is usually paucibacillary (a smaller number of bacteria) and so confirmation is not always possible. However, every attempt must be made to confirm the diagnosis. Contact screening of family members is an important tool in the diagnosis of TB in an infant. It is worth a note that there are enough facilities provided by the government for free diagnosis and treatment. Counselling a patient to ensure compliance of treatment is major responsibility of a doctor.

Tuberculosis presents with varied pattern of fever depending on the pathology of the disease. Acute onset pleural effusion due to Tuberculosis presents with short duration high fever, while typical primary complex presents with low grade fever without localization to lungs even in an apparently healthy child. Typical presentation with low grade fever, loss of appetite and weight are classic but not always seen and are also not specific to tuberculosis.

Case 7

Two year old child presented with high fever at onset with poor response to paracetamol and continued to be sick during inter-febrile period. This would suggest acute bacterial infection. So, one may carefully look for localization. (tonsillitis, otitis media, cervical lymphadenitis, UTI or bacillary dysentery). He did not develop any localization over next 24 hours. Physical examination showed no abnormal signs. So, this rules out above-mentioned conditions except urinary tract infection that often has no specific localizing symptoms and for which one should order routine urinalysis and culture, so as not to miss UTI. Routine urinalysis showed large number of pus cells and urine culture confirmed diagnosis of **Urinary tract infection.** This child was treated with antibiotics covering gram negative infections such as cotrimoxazole or norfloxacin and thereafter subjected to further tests to rule out congenital defects in urinary system.

It is true that localization of acute bacterial infection at the site of entry may get delayed beyond 2-3 days. However. non-localized fever in suspected acute bacterial infection in younger child demands ruling out UTI as early as possible. UTI is a serious disease in young children because it is likely to be due to congenital defects in urinary system and so, if not treated properly would damage kidneys due to recurrent episodes of infections. Chronic renal failure in children is often due to irrationally treated UTI and is a preventable disease with rational approach to fever. In older girls in particular, local unhygienic condition is the cause of recurrent UTI but it involves mainly lower urinary tract and hence less likely to damage the kidneys. It often presents without fever with local symptoms such as frequency of urination and burning or pain while passing urine.

Case 8

Five year old child presented with high fever at onset accompanied with headache. There was fair response to paracetamol and he appeared well during inter-febrile period. So, at this stage acute bacterial infection is unlikely. Does headache justify considering it as meningitis? Meningitis is bacteremic bacterial infection as infection cannot reach meninges without going through blood stream. In such a case, localization of infection occurs 2-3 days after the onset of fever. As headache appeared at onset, it is not likely to be meningitis. This child's headache was due to high fever itself as headache would go down as soon as fever was controlled. Child recovered within next 3 days and was diagnosed as viral infection. This child was treated without any specific therapy and was not subjected to any tests to rule out meningitis.

Headache is a non-specific symptom that accompanies any febrile disease. When such a symptom appears early in the course of disease, detailed history would reveal that headache disappears temporarily when fever is controlled by paracetamol. In meningitis, headache and vomiting continue irrespective of temporary control of fever. History of sequence of appearance and disappearance of symptoms gives a clue to such a problem and avoid undue tension.

Take Home Message

Analysis of detailed history of fever helps to arrive at a group diagnosis (bacterial or viral infection, malaria and non-infective inflammatory disorders (collagen vascular diseases and malignancy) within first 2-3 days of fever and at times even at the end of first day of fever. Until cause of fever is known, all that one needs to be sure is to rule out any serious problem. If child's behavior is reasonably normal especially when fever is temporarily controlled with paracetamol, urine output is within normal limits and pulse/respiration are not disproportionately fast, one can be confident to rule out seriousness. Once serious illness is ruled out, it is safe to wait for evolution of symptoms before an antibiotic is prescribed unless bacterial infection is suspected and preferably confirmed. Occasionally, localizing symptoms in acute bacterial infection may evolve over a week (typhoid fever, leptospirosis, brucellosis and endocarditis) and also in acute viral infection (EB and CMV). Symptoms of non-infective inflammatory diseases may evolve over several weeks. In all such cases, counselling and documentation play important role in rational practice. Misuse of antibiotics is universal in the world and has posed a danger to life and increasing cost of health care due to development of antibiotic resistant organisms. This is an emergency and time is running out.

MCQs

1. Which of the following statement about acute viral infection is wrong?

A) It affects all parts of a system or multiple systems
B) It usually settles down by D 3-4
C) Child is sick during inter-febrile period
D) Often family history is positive

2. How early can one clinically suspect acute bacterial infection in most patients?

A) Day 3-4 after onset of fever
B) Only when localizing symptoms appear
C) Within first two days of fever
D) When signs appear

3. Which bacterial infection may not have any localizing symptoms?

A) Acute pyelonephritis
B) Typhoid fever
C) Tuberculosis
D) All of above

4. Which one of the following features strongly suggest malaria?

A) Fever with rigors
B) Erratic rhythm of fever
C) Sick during inter-febrile period
D) None of the above

5. Which are the diseases in which fever may persist for more than a week without any specific treatment?

A) Viral infection
B) Collagen vascular disease
C) Malignancy
D) All of the above

Answers to MCQs

Correct answers as follows:

Q1 C	Q2 A	Q3 D	Q4 B	Q5 D

32 Cough – Distress to Patient, Challenge to Physician

Back to Basics – Understanding Cough

"Cold and cough" – these terms are used by lay persons as per their perception and are often misinterpreted. Physician must confirm whether "cold" refers to nasal discharge or blocked nose and whether "cough" is a sound produced by an attempt at forceful expulsion during expiration. It is not surprising to find there may not be either cold or cough, even when complained. Another loose term used by lay people is congestion in chest. This term may simply refer to noisy breathing that may or may not be accompanied with cold or cough. Similarly, congestion in throat is another misrepresented term. After all, congestion is a physical sign and not a symptom and so, patient will not perceive congestion, it is just presumed. Hence, it is necessary for physician to confirm the intended meaning the patient wishes to convey. Without such clarification, physician may be misled in interpretation of such symptoms.

Do "Cold And Cough" Go Together?

They are often together because most common cause of this combination symptoms is either a viral infection or allergy. Viral infection presents with fever followed by cold and cough while allergy starts with cold and cough but without significant fever (low grade fever is possible). In fact, sequence of events guides the doctor to diagnose the disease. Bacterial infection is mostly localized and does not present with cold and cough. However, allergy leading to cold and cough may be secondarily infected with bacteria and so may present as dual disease.

What is Cough?

Cough is a sound produced by sudden, forceful and often repetitive attempt at expulsion during expiration. It is a protective reflex that is expected to expel any irritant, secretions or foreign particles from larger airways – upper airways (pharynx, larynx and trachea) and lower airways (proximal or larger bronchi). Affection of other areas in respiratory tract such as nose, bronchioles, lung parenchyma, pleura and interstitium present with minimal or no cough. Cough arising from upper airways is dry while that from lower large airways is wet. Infants and young children may not be able to expectorate and wet cough at this age presents with noise produced by air moving in and out through increased secretions. However noisy chest may also present without cough.

How is Cough Generated?

Cough starts with initial deep inspiration that is followed by brief powerful expiratory effort with closed glottis resulting in generation of pressure in the airways and then sudden opening of glottis with closure of nasopharynx and vigorous expiration through mouth. It produces sound and it all happens reflexly. It is clear that cough due to affection of bronchioles, lung parenchyma or interstitium cannot be effective because low luminal airflow and velocity at these sites fail to generate enough pressure and hence do not present with significant cough or often without cough. However, if child cannot initiate deep inspiration or powerful expiration as may happen in case of severely obstructed airways or respiratory muscle paralysis, he/she may not be able to cough even in presence of irritant or secretions in larger airways. Neonates and younger infants are not able to cough effectively and it is obvious that child on mechanical ventilation would not be able to cough. Thus, absence of cough may not rule out large airway disease.

How is Cough Mediated?

Cough is mediated exclusively via vagus nerve. It is worth noting that pharynx is not supplied by vagus and hence isolate affection of pharynx does not cause cough unless irritant or secretions trickle down to larynx. This has a clinical relevance in that isolated pharyngeal disease as in bacterial pharyngitis would not present with cough and so cough in pharyngeal disease suggests extension of disease beyond pharynx as happens in viral infection. Airways extending from larynx to larger or proximal bronchi contain rapidly adapting pulmonary stretch receptors that quickly adapt to persistent stimulus thereby interrupting bout of cough transiently, facilitating normal breathing in between bouts of cough. This is important as cough must be interrupted at least for few seconds to facilitate act of breathing. If single bout of cough continues for more than few seconds, it may lead to cessation of breathing – apnea and may also be fatal as occasionally happens in young infant suffering from pertussis – whooping cough. Thus, pertussis is a serious disease in very young infant. However repeated bouts of cough cannot be prevented as nerve endings in mucosal epithelium sense the irritant or inflammatory secretions and produce cough. Finally vagal fibers enter brainstem from where cough reflex is generated via second order neurons. It also has clinical relevance as unconscious patient due to brainstem affection is not able to cough.

Factors in Airways Leading to Cough

There are several factors in airways that can stimulate cough receptors to produce cough. These receptors are sensitive to mechanical factors such as inhaled foreign body or compression pressure on airways as in case of mediastinal tumor and these receptors also are sensitive to acid or isomolar solutions such as water. This explains cough due to gastro-esophageal reflux (GERD) or aspiration of water or food particles into the airways.

Similarly, other events such as smooth muscle contraction as in asthma, vasodilatation and edema as in cardiac conditions, mucous secretions as in bronchitis and reduced lung compliance as in pneumonia are responsible to produce cough. Inflammation commonly due to infection or non-infective causes are responsible for cough in routine practice. Drugs such as angiotensin converting enzyme inhibitors (ACE inhibitors) and non-steroidal anti-infammatory drugs (ibuprofen) are known to trigger cough, though exact mechanism is not known. Similarly psychogenic factors, especially in children, present with cough referred to as "habit cough".

Why Drugs Often Fail to Relieve Cough?

There are several components such as neurogenic and mechanical factors that are involved in producing cough. Besides, most of the irritants or inflammatory products in airways are not easy to get rid of as consistency of mucous and efficiency of ciliary function determine ease of expulsion and so cough continues in spite of trial with different drugs. Even mere symptomatic relief is also difficult to achieve as there is no drug known to science that can control all these variable factors. That is why most cough remedies are cocktails of cough-sedative, expectorant, mucolytics and antihistamines with the hope that one of the constituents may work. But it does not do so. Temporary relief may be possible with inhaled bronchodilator in case of bronchospasm. Transient relief may occur with hydration of airways as is done with steam inhalation or sips of warm water or chewable item in mouth secreting more saliva (dryness of airways increases cough). Reclining with head high position offers bit of relief and so also adequate ventilation and comfortable room temperature. Of course, removal of inhaled foreign body can "cure" cough.

If Symptomatic Therapy Does Not Work, What Next?

Significant cough though distressing to a patient, has a purpose of expelling the irritant. So, unless irritant is expelled, cough would never stop. Hence attempt should be made to offer comfort to a child rather than suppressing cough. During day time, most children remain reasonably comfortable in spite of cough, simply because they are too busy with play and other activities that they ignore cough. However, cough disturbs them during sleeping time and hence attempt must be made to ensure proper sleep within limits. One can use with discretion an antihistamine (first generation like chlorphenamine) containing cough suppressant in a single dose at night. Codeine is a powerful cough suppressant but is addictive besides it also causes constipation and hence best avoided. Pholcodiene may be an alternative. Mucolytics may be tried in wet cough but often are not beneficial. If cough suggests bronchospasm, inhaled bronchodilator would offer relief better than oral medicine. There is no reason to use symptomatic drugs through the day and should only be administered when discomfort is intolerable. None of these modalities "cure" cough and this is the reason why treating cough is a big challenge to physician. Provisional diagnosis of the disease presenting with cough is vital, without which relief of cough may not be possible. Though luckily some of the causes of cough may be self-limiting but unfortunately, they are often recurrent.

Take Home Message

Cough is a reflex intended to expel the irritant in airways. Severe cough suggests affection of large airways (dry cough in upper and wet cough in lower airways) while mild cough arises from smaller airways and beyond (bronchioles, alveoli, interstitium and pleura). Pain is a symptom of pleural disease and may be present also in pneumonia (it is pleuro-pneumonia). Cough may also be a symptom of cardiac disease (left to right shunt or cardiac failure), upper GI system (GERD or aspiration syndromes), neurogenic (from ear drum or autonomic system) and psychogenic (habit cough). Drugs are not very useful to suppress cough except inhaled bronchodilator for spasmodic cough but cough suppressant with first generation antihistamine may be considered on SOS basis to relieve discomfort. Traditional home remedies are as good and must be tried.

Next article deals with clinical application of basic facts highlighted in this article with discussion on live case scenarios, representing day-to-day problems faced by practitioners.

MCQs

1. Which of the following statement is wrong? Mild cough is a feature of

A) Bronchiolitis
B) Pneumonia
C) Bronchitis
D) Pleural disease

2. Cough is generated with

A) Deep inspiration
B) Expiration with closed glottis
C) Forceful expiration with open glottis
D) All of the above

3. Which of the following statement is wrong? Cough may result from

A) Cardiac disease
B) Neurological disease
C) GI abnormality
D) None of the above

4. Which of the following statement is right? Cough may be absent if

A) Airways are affected

B) Airways are not affected

C) Heart is affected

D) All of the above

5. Which of the following statement is wrong? Cough is difficult to treat because

A) Correct diagnosis is often elusive

B) There are multiple mechanisms leading to cough

C) Irritant is not easy to expel

D) Cough receptors are not well developed

Answers to MCQs

Correct answers as follows:

Q1 C	Q2 D	Q3 D	Q4 D	Q5 D

33 Cough Should not be a Challenge any More

Clinical Application of Basic Concepts of Cough

Cough is a localizing symptom, unlike fever. It is often a primary respiratory disease though may be secondary to cardiac, GI or neurological disorder. Hence one must start with anatomical diagnosis – which system is involved and further which part of the system is affected – it is microanatomy of the disease. Significant cough localizes disease to larynx, trachea or bronchi. In other areas of affection in respiratory tract, cough is mild and often accompanied with other symptoms such as chest pain in pleural disease, acute breathlessness in pneumonia or bronchiolitis. Palpitation and breathlessness suggest cardiac disease while chocking episode denotes probable gastro-esophageal reflux or neurological disorder. Of course, if one fails to localize anatomy of the disease, it may be psychogenic. Unless microanatomy is known, one can't proceed to pathology. Most common pathological processes involved in production of cough are inflammation and allergy. Acute inflammation is characterized by fever while chronic inflammation presents with worsening systemic symptoms such as loss of weight and appetite. Allergy presents with sudden onset of cough that may also disappear suddenly but often would recur. Besides, there is often personal or family history of allergy. Respiratory allergy affects entire system so also in case of viral infection while bacterial infection is mostly localized to a part of the system and not generalized. Thus, probable etiology also can be guessed.

Following questions help in arriving at probable diagnosis in case of cough.

1. Is cough a major symptom?
2. If so, is there past history of similar illness?
3. Is cough worse at night as compared to day time?
4. Is there personal or family history of allergy?
5. Onset, duration and progress of cough
6. Are there other symptoms such as fever, cold or breathlessness?
7. Sequence of appearance of such symptoms

Case-Based Study

Case 1

Two year old child presented with fever followed next day with cold and wet cough. Cough was severe with watery discharge from nose. There was no past history of similar disease. Physical examination revealed febrile child with coryza but not looking very sick.

Chest was clear. Fever suggests infection and cough denotes airway disease along with involvement of nose as well. So this is generalized involvement of airways. This is typical of **viral infection** and so does not need any antibiotic or laboratory tests. Fever settled down within 3 days with paracetamol. Cold and cough also got better over next 2 days. In case of watery nasal secretions, one needs to wipe them and in case of nose block, instil normal saline drops in the nostrils. It helps to unblock the nose. Cough syrups are of no much use. Viral infection is often a generalized infection affecting entire system (cold and cough – upper and lower airways) and also at times multiple systems (cold, cough as well as diarrhea) and also self-limiting within 3-4 days. Besides, viral infections spread fast and hence similar illness in other family members or prevailing in the community would offer a clue to probable viral infection.

Case 2

Two year old child presented with fever followed next day with cold and wet cough. Cough was severe with watery discharge from nose. There was past history of recurrent episodes of cough often without fever. However, there was no history of allergy in the family. Physical examination did not reveal any localizing signs.

Onset of disease with fever suggests infection with generalized involvement of airways affecting nose down to bronchi. So, this is similar to previous case. However, in this child, fever subsided on its own within next 2 days but cough worsened and continued for next two weeks. Physical examination during this period continued to show no other signs. As fever had disappeared, infection was definitely controlled. If so, why did cough continue for such a long time? This is referred to as hyper-reactive airway disease. It is known as **WALRI – wheeze associated lower respiratory infection.** It means this child is susceptible to recurrent episodes of cough that could be triggered by either viral infection or allergy. It is evident in history itself as this child had recurrent episodes of cough in the past. Cough did settle down by itself though it lasted too long. Here is the need for proper counselling rather than trying some medicines. Of course, there is no question of antibiotic in this child nor does this child deserve laboratory tests or chest X-ray. Inhaled bronchodilators help.

Generally, cold and cough in a respiratory viral infection settles soon after fever subsides. However, when cough in particular continues for few weeks well after fever subsides, one suspects inherent susceptibility of host to suffer from recurrent cough triggered by viral infection and also by multiple triggers other than infection.

Case 3

Six year old child presented with high fever, thick yellow nasal secretions and cough for last two days. Past history revealed repeated episodes of cold and cough since the age of

2 year, at times accompanied with high fever, treated with antibiotics. There was history of allergy in the family. Physical examination showed highly febrile child, looking sick, adenoid facies, (open mouth suggesting chronic obstruction to breathing through nostrils due to enlarged adenoids), ears normal and no localizing findings in chest. High fever in a sick child favors probable bacterial infection. However, in the background is hyper-reactive airways disease that is allergic as evident by family history of allergy in a child with repeated episodes of cold and cough. So, this child is suffering from **acute bacterial rhinosinusitis in the background of allergy.** It needs to be treated with antibiotic for the present but once infection is controlled, he should be treated for allergic rhinosinusitis. Amoxicillin with or without clavulanate is the drug of choice for respiratory infections.

Secondary bacterial infection is a result of retained secretions (as in rhinosinusitis, bronchiectasis, pyelonephritis or cholangitis) and significant immune suppression following measles or varicella infection, chemotherapy and immune deficiency disorders. While treating bacterial infection with appropriate antibiotic, primary background cause must be evaluated and managed well to prevent recurrences.

Case 4

Four year old child presented with high fever and mild cough. Fever was high at onset with mild response to paracetamol and high fever would recur every 4-5 hours as effect of paracetamol would wear off. Child always remained sick during interfebrile period. Cough was mild and not disturbing the child. Physical examination did not reveal any abnormality except sick looking child. At this juncture, one is expecting bacterial infection to localize mostly in lung parenchyma as suggested by mild cough. Mild cough is also a feature of bronchiolitis, pleural or interstitial disease. Acute bronchiolitis presents with upper respiratory symptoms and often with mild fever followed by breathlessness while acute interstitial infection is often viral and so involves entire respiratory system with significant cough and so, both these diseases are unlikely in this child. Absence of chest pain rules out pleural disease. Though at times pleura may be involved in case of pneumonia and such a child may present with chest pain. Hence, even on day 2 of illness, **bacterial pneumonia** is most likely and one must watch carefully for further progress. A day later, he developed mild breathlessness and now diagnosis of pneumonia is confirmed by chest X-ray and CBC showing neutrophilic leukocytosis. Amoxicillin with clavulanate was started and child started responding with relief from breathlessness and fever was also in control. Though cough worsened by this time. Does it suggest complication or drug resistant infection? Neither of the two. In fact, as pneumonia starts improving, cough often worsens as inflammatory exudate liquefies and has to be expelled through airways. It results in temporary worsening of cough. It is nature's attempt to get rid of exudate to ensure complete healing. There was no need to change medicines and antibiotic was continued for 7 days with full recovery. There was no need of cough syrup as well. Recovering infection may worsen one of the original symptoms because of natural course of the disease (cough worsening in recovering pneumonia or diarrhea continuing in recovering rota viral infection). In such a case, it is ideal to communicate such an expected course of events ahead of its occurrence so that it allays anxiety on the part of patients.

Case 5

Eight year old child presented with mild fever and cough for 2 days. Physical examination did not reveal any abnormality. At this stage, there is no clue to diagnosis, but acute infection seems unlikely due to onset with low grade fever and it is best to watch further progress without any tests or medicines. It is safe to wait as child is not sick looking. Child continued to run mild fever for next 10 days but cough was worsening. So, this is subacute infection of respiratory tract with gradual worsening. Physical examination at this stage showed localized crepitations on right side of chest and child had lost one kg of weight. Diagnosis of **tuberculosis** was possible and was proved with chest X-ray and confirmed with GeneXpert. This child was treated with four drug treatment (HRZE) for two months and HRE for next four months. Child showed improvement within 2-3 weeks, though treatment must be completed for 6 months.

Low grade fever may suggest acute viral infection of low virulence or one occurring in partially immune host. However, if low grade fever continues beyond 3-4 days, one should consider chronic low-grade infection such as Tuberculosis or fungal infection. Systemic fungal infection is seen in immune compromised host and not in normal person.

Case 6

Four year old child presented with mild fever and dry cough for two days but over next five days, cough started worsening though fever disappeared. Physical examination at this stage did not reveal any abnormality. It is clear that this is upper respiratory tract infection as evident by dry cough but further progress suggests worsening local condition in upper airways without deterioration of systemic symptoms such as fever. On direct questioning, two other family members were reported to be suffering from similar cough for last one month. So, this is highly infectious disease and diagnosis of **pertussis – whooping cough** was made. He was treated with Macrolide. It took another week before he got well. In absence of family history, pertussis can be suspected with worsening bouts of cough in severity and duration, especially in absence of past history of recurrent cough. It is treated with macrolide but antibiotic is effective only if started early in the course of the disease. Even if pertussis is diagnosed late in the course of the disease, it is rational to start an antibiotic as even it does not help the patient, it would prevent spread of infection to other members of the family. Progression of severe cough is a result of uncontrolled infection such as pertussis or gradual compression of airways as in case of mediastinal lymphoma.

Both conditions may not present with any abnormal physical signs in the chest and must be suspected with consideration of other clues. Even chest X-ray is normal in pertussis but usually not in mediastinal lymphoma, though occasionally lymphnode may be hidden behind the heart and hence missed. Careful assessment can visualize compression of large airways in such a case.

Case 7

Two year old child presented with severe cough for last 2 days. There were no other complaints. There was no past or family history of allergy. Physical examination did not reveal any obvious abnormality. Acute onset of severe cough without fever rules out infection and suggests either mechanical problem or allergy. As there is no history suggestive of allergy, it is likely to be mechanical problem. On direct questioning, parents recalled that cough started all of a sudden in a minute while he was eating. It gave away the diagnosis of **inhaled foreign body.** It was a piece of groundnut that was removed through bronchoscope. Inhaled foreign body may not be picked-up by clinical examination, especially if it is lodged in smaller bronchial segment and also missed by chest X-ray as vegetable foreign body is not visible on X-ray. However, one may pick-up localized signs of either atelectasis or emphysema due to complete or partial obstruction of a bronchial segment respectively on physical or radiological examination.

Basic rule to inquire about onset of the disease is so important in case of cough. Inhaled foreign body is missed for several weeks simply because a doctor had not asked for an onset. There is no other diagnosis in case of sudden onset of cough other than inhalation of foreign body. Inhalation of other material as in case of GERD presents with chocking episodes with recurrent cough.

Case 8

Eight year old child was seen for cough going on for last 6 months. There were no other symptoms. Physical examination did not show any abnormality. Several tests and trials with medicines including antibiotics, cough syrups and inhalers had failed to control cough. Finally, he was advised to undergo bronchoscopy that he refused. What was missing? On detailed questioning, it was clear that he was never disturbed by cough during sleep and play activities. Besides he was eating well and had gained weight during last 6 months. So, diagnosis was **habit cough**. Such a child often would oblige by controlling cough, if you insist that he should not cough while you examine him so that you would be able to diagnose his problem. It is due to emotional stress and one must go into depth to find out what bothers this child. Generally, both parents and the child refuse presence of any stress. Empathetic counselling with confidence of the diagnosis is the need and at times, one may have to take help of a psychologist.

Every chronic symptom is likely to affect well-being as evident by changes in weight, appetite, sleep, play activity or behavior. Such symptoms appear early in the course of the disease and hence, should always be inquired. In absence of any such affection, diagnosis of functional disorder is obvious. It is only with such a rational approach to history taking that undue delay in the diagnosis and unnecessary investigation and drug therapy can be avoided.

Take Home Message

Treating cough should not be a challenge as proper diagnosis is possible with analysis of detailed history and thorough physical examination. It leads to a probable anatomical and pathological diagnosis while etiological diagnosis is a rational guess. Tests are not commonly required unless specific diagnosis is being considered. CBC and eosinophilia in particular are not very useful for specific etiology. Chest X-ray is ideal for lung parenchymal disease but it is not so useful in airway or interstitial diseases. Chest USG is good for pleural effusion. CT scan should be avoided unless for specific reasons as it exposes the child to significant radiation with possible side effects in future. Symptomatic therapy has major limitations and parents must be properly counselled to accept time-bound natural relief, partially aided by drugs. It is doctor's duty to convince a patient and avoid prescribing unnecessary tests and drugs.

MCQs

1. **In which of the following condition, cough continues for about two weeks in spite of fever getting better within 3-4 days.**

A) Acute viral infection
B) Hyper-reactive airways triggered by acute viral infection
C) Chronic viral respiratory infection
D) Secondary bacterial infection

2. **Which of the following statements is wrong? Cough persisting for several weeks may be due to**

A) Pertussis – whooping cough
B) Pneumonia
C) Tuberculosis
D) Inhaled foreign body

3. **Which of the following statements is wrong? Primary complex due to tuberculosis may present with**

A) Severe cough
B) Mild cough
C) No cough
D) Breathlessness

4. Which of the following statements is wrong? Recurrent respiratory infections occur in

A) Allergic rhinosinusitis
B) Viral respiratory infections
C) Tuberculosis
D) Inhaled foreign body

5. Which of the following statements are right? Child may not look sick in spite of severe cough in

A) Asthma
B) Inhaled foreign body
C) Habit cough
D) All of the above

Answers to MCQs

Correct answers as follows:

Q1 B	Q2 B	Q3 D	Q4 C	Q5 D

34 Diarrhea – When Solid Waste Becomes Liquid

Back to Basics – Understanding Diarrhea

What is Diarrhea?

It is defined as change in bowel pattern that results in loose stools with increased frequency and child appears sick. Stool of normal consistency but passed more than 1-2 times a day may not justify definition of diarrhea and so also an occasional loose stool with normal frequency does not mean diarrhea. First part of the definition – change in bowel pattern - is also important. This is because young infant on exclusive breast feeds may pass as many as 10-15 loose, often watery stools per day and is not considered to be abnormal as there is no change in bowel pattern. Such infant has always been passing loose frequent stools and it is physiological, not pathological. It is substantiated by infant being happy in spite of many loose stools, feeds well and also gain weight well. Generally pathological stools – diarrhea – makes a child sick and not happy, often with loss of appetite and dehydration depending on amount of water loss.

What is Dysentery?

Diarrhea associated with stools containing mucous and/or blood is referred to as dysentery. It is usually a disease of large intestine – colon and is accompanied with abdominal pain. It represents severe inflammation and so child is quite sick. However small amount of mucous in stools without blood or abdominal pain may not be called as dysentery and such a patient may not be sick. Mucous in stools indicates any source of irritation and not necessarily an infection.

What is Indigestion?

This term is used loosely by lay person and may represent different problems related to gastrointestinal dysfunction. It may not even relate to digestion problem and really does not connote any specific disease or defect. If digestion is affected, it should be ideally be called as maldigestion – meaning abnormal digestion. Digestion refers to breaking down of nutrients to smaller molecules that can be further absorbed. Proteins have to be hydrolyzed to aminoacids, complex carbohydrates to simple sugars referred to as monosaccharide and fats to small molecules of fatty acids. Digestion starts with chewing of food and salivary amylase helping in first phase of carbohydrate digestion. Stomach helps in digestion of proteins and pancreatic enzymes and bile along with small intestinal enzymes are responsible for final process of digestion. If food is not digested, it cannot be properly absorbed and so results in diarrhea.,

How Does Diarrhea Occur?

Diarrhea results when normal process of digestion or absorption is disturbed. Small intestine receives consumed food partly after digestion. If food is not digested properly, it is not absorbed and even if food is digested but If small intestines are unable to absorb properly, diarrhea results. Jejunum is the site of absorption of most nutrients except Vitamin B12 and bile acids that are absorbed in ileum. Besides amount of consumed food or fluid, much larger amounts of fluid is secreted by small intestine. Adult may consume about 1.5 litres of fluid in a day but small intestine of an adult secrets another 8.5 litres of fluid and hence small intestine has a load of about 10 litres of fluid to be absorbed every day. Normally, 80-85% of fluids are absorbed by small intestine and only small amount is delivered to large intestine. If small intestine fails to absorb fluids, it results in large amount of watery diarrhea. If small intestine secretes larger amount of fluids than normal due to any disease as happens in cholera, even normal small intestinal absorptive capacity cannot cope up with such a huge amount of secreted fluid, resulting in profuse diarrhea with serious consequences such as hypovolemic shock. Large intestine receives only 10-15% of fluids that are further absorbed. Thus, small intestinal diarrhea presents with large amount of watery stools while large intestinal diarrhea presents with frequent small amount of stools often with mucous and/or blood.

How to Know Which Nutrients are not Absorbed?

If weight loss is significant, it is calories that are not absorbed. Carbohydrates are main source of calories and its malabsorption results in diarrhea with gaseous abdominal distension and anal excoriation due to acidic stools. This is due to fermentation of unabsorbed carbohydrates in colon by bacteria that produces gas and acidic stools. Protein malabsorption leads to edema. Stools due to fat malabsorption are greyish white and foul smelling, often large in volume. Anemia may be a feature of iron, vitamin B12 or folic acid malabsorption. Calcium deficiency causes tetany, vitamin D deficiency results in rickets and vitamin K deficiency leads to bleeding. Of course, all such deficiencies occur commonly due to deficient food intake of these substances rather than malabsorption. Type of stools and resulting deficiency signs may suggest which nutrients are not absorbed from intestine. This helps especially when nutrient intake is normal and still deficiency signs appear suggesting abnormal intestinal function. At times, intestinal disease may result in deficiency of a specific nutrient while all other nutrients are well absorbed.

What are Causes of Diarrhea?

Infective Causes

Acute diarrhea is commonly caused by enteroviral infections in healthy infants and toddlers. Such infections are rare beyond toddler age and are not preventable even with good hygienic care. They are referred to as democratic infections as they occur in all socioeconomic groups. Rota viral diarrhea is a classic example. Bacterial infections such as E.coli, salmonella or campylobacter are seen in malnourished children as well those who are exposed to contaminated food. Toxins produced by vibrio cholera results in most severe form of diarrhea. Diarrhea is caused by toxins produced by bacterial infections such as shigella but also may result from infection at sites other than intestines such as urinary tract infection (UTI) and is referred to as parenteral diarrhea – meaning other than enteral infection. It occurs typically in infants and young children. Other infections causing diarrhea include parasites such as giardiasis and cryptosporidium and fungal infection mostly in immunocompromised patients. Tuberculosis does not present with diarrhea as major symptom.

Non-Infective Inflammatory Causes

Autoimmune disorders such as inflammatory bowel disease – commonly Crohn's disease in children and ulcerative colitis in adults are not uncommon in children. They mimic infections as they also present with fever, stool microscopy showing pus cells and neutrophilic leukocytosis. Kawasaki disease – generalized autoimmune multisystem disease – may also present with diarrhea.

Non-Inflammatory Causes

Acute malabsorption of carbohydrates as in case of transient lactose intolerance commonly occurs after viral infection. As lactase enzyme resides in most superficial part of mucosa, it is first to be disturbed resulting in lactose malabsorption as happens in viral infection. However, it is self-limiting and does not need lactose free diet. Congenital lactase deficiency is extremely rare. Children and adults who are not used to consume milk or milk products are likely to cause diarrhea when exposed to excess of such products. It is due to disuse atrophy of enzyme – lactase. Drugs such as magnesium containing antacids, H2 receptor antagonist such as cimetidine and ranitidine, proton pump inhibitor such as lansoprazole and omeprazole, digoxin and methyldopa are known to cause diarrhea. Irritable bowel syndrome refers to diarrhea due to psychological factors such as stress, anxiety etc. Hunger diarrhea occurs in infants who are poorly fed and greenish stools, besides intestinal hurry also produces greenish stools. Rarely hormonal disorders such as thyrotoxicosis and VIPoma also cause diarrhea.

Limitations of Laboratory Tests in Acute Diarrhea

Routine stool microscopy is not helpful in diarrhea as presence of mucous, few pus cells or even RBCs are non-specific abnormalities that are present in infections, non-infective inflammation as well as any other cause of intestinal irritation. It may pick up parasitic infection though it is not related to acute diarrhea. Stool should not be tested for lactose in acute diarrhea as its presence does not equate to lactose intolerance. Stool culture has no place in routine clinical practice. Specific tests may be required for conditions such as celiac disease or inflammatory bowel disease. Stool examination may be necessary in chronic diarrhea.

Should Diarrhea be Controlled?

Infections being commonest causes of diarrhea, it is nature's attempt to expel irritants – germs and inflammatory exudates – for effective cure. Hence it is not logical to attempt control of diarrhea and in fact it may be harmful. But useful constituents for the body that are lost in diarrhea must be replaced and they include water and electrolytes. It is best done by oral rehydrating solution (ORS) or any equivalent home-made solution that contains ideal composition of sugar with sodium, potassium and bicarbonates as in "limbu-pani" – a glass of water with one teaspoonful sugar, pinch of salt and dash of lemon. Coconut water is another natural alternative. Soft drinks are harmful as they contain large amount of sugar that would worsen diarrhea. Zinc is known to hasten recovery from diarrhea and is the only drug to be prescribed in addition to ORS and can be given for 14 days in each episode of diarrhea. It is most important in malnourished children. Probiotics may help to small extent but are not necessary in acute diarrhea. There is no need for diet restriction. Soya milk formula is not necessary in acute diarrhea. Of course, specific therapy for bacterial or parasitic infections is obviously necessary.

Chronic Diarrhea

It is a multifactorial problem contributed by malnutrition, persistent infection, allergy to animal proteins, malabsorption, bile acid irritation and often worsened by drugs and hence must be properly evaluated. It is beyond the scope of this article. Recurrent episodes of infective diarrhea (due to poor food hygiene) may be mistaken for chronic diarrhea but a child with recurrent diarrhea does recover completely in between episodes as against chronic diarrhea that is persistent and so presents with progressive loss of weight.

Take Home Message

Diarrhea may result from maldigestion (affection of stomach, liver or pancreas), malabsorption (affection of intestines) or intestinal hurry (affection of intestines through local, hormonal or neurogenic disorders) and hence it is rational to make an anatomical diagnosis before proceeding with pathological or etiological diagnosis. At times, chronic constipation can masquerade as loose stools as happens in habitual constipation or congenital megacolon. Detailed history and distended abdomen loaded with feces can point to constipation as an underlying symptom. Evaluation of what is being lost in diarrheal stool is important such as water, electrolytes and nutritional elements. One should not attempt to stop diarrhea with drugs that may also be dangerous.

MCQs

1. Which of the following statements is right? Stool pattern is considered abnormal if

A) 2-3 stools a day of normal consistency
B) Passing stools immediately after food
C) Change in bowel pattern
D) All of the above

2. Which of the following statements are right? Small intestinal disease may present with

A) Profuse watery stools
B) Stools with mucous
C) Stools with mucous and blood
D) All of the above

3. Diarrhea is the result of

A) Increased intestinal secretions
B) Decreased intestinal absorption
C) Indigestion
D) All of the above

4. Which of the following statements is wrong? Diarrhea may be secondary to

A) Urinary tract infection
B) Endocrine disorder
C) Tuberculosis
D) Bacterial otitis media

5. Which of the following statements is wrong? Lactose malabsorption presents as

A) Watery diarrhea
B) Gaseous abdominal distension
C) Stools with mucous
D) Anal excoriation

Answers to MCQs

Correct answers as follows:

Q1 C	Q2 D	Q3 D	Q4 C	Q5 C

35 Diarrhea Beyond Infections

Clinical Application of Basic Concepts of Diarrhea

Exclusively breast-fed infant never suffers from diarrhea with rare exception of immune deficiency disorders. However acute bacterial infection such as urinary tract infection may present with parenteral diarrhea in young infants. Diarrhea is more common in malnourished infants and children and in turn worsens nutritional status. Well -nourished infant and toddler often suffers from self-limiting viral diarrhea as a result of small intestinal infection while older children often suffer from bacillary dysentery or parasitic infections such as amebiasis or giardiasis as a result of large intestinal infection due to ingestion of contaminated food. Non-infective diarrhea such as inflammatory bowel disease is more common in older children. Thus, age, nutritional status and type of stools suggest probable etiology and in routine practice, even stool examination is rarely necessary in acute diarrhea. Physical examination is aimed at suspecting probable complications such as dehydration or local complications such as paralytic ileus as evident by abdominal distension.

Case-Based Study

Case 1

Two month old infant presented with loose stools for last two weeks. He was on exclusive breast feeds since birth. Prior to onset of diarrhea, he used to pass stools 3-4 times a day which were golden yellow in color. But since last two weeks, he passed 8-10 stools per day. However, he had been feeding well and also gained weight in spite of diarrhea. Physical examination did not reveal any abnormality. There has been change in stool pattern and so needs proper evaluation. However, infant is not sick and feeds well with normal weight gain. This may suggest it may not be pathological. What is then a probable cause of change in stool pattern? Breast milk consists of foremilk – first part of milk-feed which is watery and contains large amount of sugar while hindmilk – later part of milk-feed – contains fat. When infant takes a full feed – both foremilk and hindmilk – stools are formed and infrequent but when infant stops sucking after taking only foremilk and does so at every feed, stools are watery and frequent. So, this infant must be getting distracted while feeding and so takes only foremilk. As it is not sufficient for him, he feeds more frequently and takes again foremilk each time. This is the cause of this infant's loose stools – **foremilk without hindmilk.** There is no need of any tests or drug treatment but mother must be counselled to feed for a longer period at each feeding time without distraction so that infant consumes both foremilk and hindmilk. Many young infants stop sucking even with half stomach full and then doze off to sleep. Such an infant should be gently tickled to wake up again from slumbar and this is the way, infant can be trained to complete a full feed at one time. Detailed inquiry about feeding pattern is necessary to pick-up such problems.

Case 2

Eight month old infant presented with greenish loose stools since last one month. Prior to onset of this problem, he used to pass stools 1-2 times a day with normal color. There were no other complaints. On direct questioning, mother informed that infant would refuse semisolid food even when she had been trying to introduce it since last two months and he was only on breast feeds. He had not gained weight over last two months. However, he was happy and playful but ever hungry. Physical examination did not reveal any abnormality. Similar to previous case, there is change in stool pattern but infant is happy and so, it must not have been pathological. What then must be cause of diarrhea in this child? Green stools suggest unused bile getting excreted in stools. It could result from intestinal hurry due to infection that does not allow enough time for bile to mix with food but this infant is not sick and so it is unlikely to be an infection. Other cause is **inadequate food intake** because of which unused bile is excreted in stools. This infant is happy feeding on breast all the time, in fact, happy sucking even without adequate intake and is not used to intake any semisolid food. Few infants when exposed to semisolid food reject to begin with but persistence makes the infant accept it. However, if mother gives in to frequent demand on breast feeding, infant does not learn to eat semisolid food. He gets breast addicted and looks satisfied just by sucking even an empty breast resulting in inadequate intake. So this child does not need any tests or drug treatment for diarrhea but just counselling parents to offer semisolid food while mother eats. It is a stimulus for the infant to imitate and learn to eat well. Children learn best by imitation. Breast addiction is not uncommon and is the cause of underweight, constipation as well "hunger diarrhea". Such a child is for ever hungry but refuses to accept other than breast milk. It is only on direct questioning that such a problem comes to attention.

Case 3

Ten year old child was seen for frequent stools for last two weeks. Stools were of normal consistency and color but frequent. He used to pass stools once or twice a day but last two weeks, he has been passing stools 5-6 times a day. He continued to be happy and playful. Physical examination did not reveal any abnormality. So, there is change in stool pattern in terms of frequency but color is normal and so also child is happy and not sick. It indicates that food is well digested and his food intake is normal but there is intestinal hurry. As there is no evidence of infection, intestinal hurry is likely to be due to **stress.** Parents need counselling and no tests or drugs are required. Many may have experienced desire to pass stools when stressed as happens in a child going for examination. Similarly, strong gastro-colic reflex makes a child pass stools after eating but in both these situations, stools are normal though frequent.

Case 4

One year old child presented with recurrent episodes of loose stools for last 6 months. Each episode starts with fever and loose stools with mucous and foul smell. Every time he is prescribed different antibiotics and gets well but only to recur after few days. In between episodes, he feeds well, remains active and also gains weight. Though over last 6 months, he has gained only one kg of weight. Physical examination did not reveal any significant abnormality. It is likely to be repeated bacterial infections as suggested by fever and stools with mucous and foul smell. Parasitic infection such as amebiasis is rare in young children besides it rarely presents as an acute diarrhea. At any age, repeated bacterial infections strongly suggest either abnormality in the host such as immune deficiency or cystic fibrosis or due to unhygienic conditions. As this child remains well in between episodes and also gains weight, it rules out any significant host abnormality and so it must be due to **poor hygiene**. Thus, treatment of each episode by antibiotics is not going to solve the problem unless parents are counselled about taking adequate care of hygiene. Bottle feeding is the main culprit for poor hygiene and so also ingestion of contaminated food. Hand hygiene is equally important to prevent food borne infections. Gastro-intestinal infections are largely preventable and hence, besides treating infection, one must find the root cause behind such an infection. This is the only way recurrence can be prevented.

Case 5

Two year old child presented with abdominal distension, loose stools off and on and loss of weight and appetite over last one year. Frequency of stools varied from 2-4 per day with changing consistency. There was no fever or vomiting. He was treated with antibiotics, anti-parasitic drugs and also enzymes, digestives. Physical examination revealed chronically sick child with gaseous abdominal distension but without any other signs. It is obviously a chronic progressive disease starting around one year of age. Absence of fever suggests non-infective etiology. However parasitic infections may present without fever but he has failed to get better in spite of anti-parasitic therapy. Parasitic infections are not difficult to treat though they may recur off and on due to poor food hygiene. So, they are recurrent but this child has a persistent disease, as evident by progressive loss of weight. This may be due to chronic malabsorption due to deficient intestinal enzymes. However, such a child would have normal or voracious appetite. As this child has loss of appetite, this malabsorption must have resulted from chronic inflammation. This inflammation is unlikely due to infection as it would have at least partially responded to antibiotics and so it is likely to be due to non-infective inflammation. As it has started around one year of age, on direct questioning to parents, it was revealed that it coincided with introduction of wheat. This gives a clue that it may be **celiac disease** due to gluten sensitivity or allergy. Serum antibody test and intestinal biopsy can confirm the diagnosis and is managed by avoidance of wheat products as well as rye and barley. Celiac disease is not uncommon. It may present at any age even after months or years of consumption of gluten-containing foods, wheat, rye, barley besides canned fruits, flavoured milk or yoghurt and many processed food items.

Case 6

Eight year old child presented with loose stools with mucous, abdominal pain and poor appetite for last one month and fever off and on for last three weeks. Stools vary in number from 2-5 times a day. Abdominal pain was dull and generalized all over. Fever was mild to moderate. He had lost two kg of weight. Physical examination revealed sick looking child with abdominal distension and mild pallor. There was vague tenderness all over the abdomen. Other systems were normal. This child has subacute progressive intestinal inflammatory disease as evident by mucous in stools but not so frequent suggesting probably both small and large intestine involved. It is unlikely to be infection as uncontrolled infection would have developed local or systemic complications. Thus, it is mostly non-infective inflammation such as **Crohn's disease.** Neutrophilic leukocytosis with thrombocytosis and hypo-albuminea are investigatory correlates of such a disease. Intestinal biopsy would prove the diagnosis and is treated with steroids and anti-inflammatory drugs. Inflammatory bowel disease resembles intestinal infection though subtle points and progress can differentiate one from the other. Etiology remains obscure and role of heredity, stress and diet is considered in causation of this disease. Ulcerative colitis is more common in adults.

Case 7

Eight year old child presented with loose stools and abdominal pain off and on for last 4 months. Stool frequency varies from 2-4 times a day and at times contains mucous. However, appetite activity, play and sleep are unaffected, he has gained one kg of weight over last 4 months in spite of loose stools. Physical examination did not reveal any abnormality. Several tests were carried out without clue to diagnosis and so also drugs were tried but failed. There is change in bowel pattern since last 4 months but it has not affected general well-being of the child. This fact is important to note and it excludes all pathological conditions. Diagnosis of **irritable bowel syndrome** was made based on circumstantial evidence. Irritable bowel syndrome is related to stress in a susceptible child and one must find out by discussion what stress the child at this age must be undergoing. Stress may arise from school, home or friends. Parents need to be counselled to observe common areas of stress with friends or at school and they should avoid undue stress at home.

Case 8

Four year old child presented with soiling underwear with small volume of loose stools few times a day for last one month. He was treated for loose stools without any benefit. Physical examination did not reveal any abnormality. On direct questioning, parents informed that besides frequent passing stools with soiling, he would pass good volume of hard stools once in 2-3 days. So, he was constipated as evident by-passing hard stools infrequently. But also. he was passing small volume of loose stools few times a day. As parents were more concerned about loose stools and soiling underwear, history of constipation did not come out as main problem. This is typical of **habitual constipation masquerading as diarrhea.** Habitual constipation results from diet poor in roughage in a child who has irregular bowel habits. It is often compounded by hurry to go to school in the morning and unhygienic toilet facilities at school that makes a child hold back stools. Retained hard stool leads to stretching and weakness of rectal muscles that makes it more difficult to pass stools. It becomes a vicious cycle. Loose stool proximal to retained hard stool leaks from side of hard stool and keeps on soiling underwear. Diarrhea is not the problem of this child and he needs management of constipation that is beyond the scope of present article on diarrhea.

> **Take Home Message**
>
> First three cases are examples of diarrhea due to non-pathological causes. What is common to all these cases is that child is not sick and happy. It is a clue to search for non-pathological causes. Last case masquerades as diarrhea but actually it is constipation due to poor habits. Other four cases can be diagnosed by analyzing history though physical findings are mostly scarce. These cases emphasise importance of detailed history taking. Laboratory tests have limitation and should be reserved for specific diseases.

MCQs

1. Which of the following statement is wrong? Breast-fed infant may pass

A) Watery stools
B) Frequent stools
C) Hard stools
D) Infrequent but soft stools

2. Green stools may suggest

A) Infection
B) Underfeeding
C) Intestinal hurry
D) All of the above

3. Most common cause of recurrent GI infection in infant is

A) Immune deficiency
B) Cystic fibrosis
C) Bottle feeding
D) All of the above

4. Which of the following statement is wrong? Blood and mucous in stools is seen in

A) Bacillary dysentery
B) Inflammatory bowel disease
C) Intestinal viral infection
D) Intussusception

5. Which of the following modality is most useful in evaluation of diarrhea?

A) Detailed history
B) Physical examination
C) Laboratory tests
D) All of the above

Answers to MCQs

Correct answers as follows:

Q1 C	Q2 D	Q3 C	Q4 C	Q5 A

36 Constipation
Gut in Slow Motion, Constant Anticipation without Culmination is Constipation

Back to Basics – Understanding Constipation

What is Constipation?

Change in bowel pattern resulting in infrequent passage of stools, often hard and at times accompanied with painful defecation and may be stool smeared with blood. Incomplete evacuation of stool with frequent desire to pass stools must also be seen as constipation. Frequency of passing stools varies in normal individuals from 2-3 times a day to once in two days. It is the change in frequency and/or consistency that is to be considered. Individual passing stools three times a day, suddenly passes one stool a day is a change that needs to be noted. Infant on exclusive breast feeding may pass a stool once in few days but it is soft, painless and infant is happy growing well, it is not considered as constipation because it is not hard and frequency has remained the same.

Physiology of Bowel Movements

After food is digested and absorbed by small intestines, it is passed on to large intestine. Colon and rectum function together to provide absorption of water, electrolytes and short chain fatty acids, to dehydrate the fecal matter, to store unwanted part and help in evacuation in a socially appropriate manner when reflex urge sets in. If stool matter remains in colon and rectum for longer time, it becomes harder and more difficult to expel. Continence is maintained by coordinated function of pelvic floor, rectum and anal sphincters. Evacuation occurs through relaxation of pelvic floor. Rectum acts to store as well as expel stool matter, both actions require cortical sensory awareness acting in conjunction with intramural and spinal reflexes that ensure timely defecation. Anal sphincters act individually and in unison in response to rectal distension and sensation of rectal filling. There has to be adequate amount of stool matter for rectal distension enough to feel sensation of filling. Reflex relaxation of internal sphincter has an additional sensory function that allows rectal stool matter to move into upper anal canal. Voluntary control of external sphincter allows deferring evacuation till opportunity exists.

Prerequisites for Normal Bowel Movements

Consumption of adequate amount of food is necessary to form volume of stool enough to distend rectum so that sensation of rectal filling is perceived by cortex. There has to be enough insoluble fiber in diet to form bulk of soft stool matter so that it moves smoothly through colon and rectum and is expelled without difficulty. Bowel movements depend upon normal intestinal muscle function leading to peristalsis. Once rectal filling results in urge to pass stools, intact nervous system acts through reflex action to relax internal sphincter and pelvic floor muscles and move the stool matter into upper anal canal, possible with good anorectal tone. Finally intact voluntary control of external anal sphincter is necessary to defer evacuation to right moment. Thus, multiple factors contribute to normal bowel movements and disturbance of any of these factors may result in constipation.

Types of Constipation

Primary constipation that is due to intrinsic problem in colon and anorectum related to abnormal function of normally innervated and structurally intact muscle. This may result from dyssynergia between external sphincter and puborectalis muscle. In such a case, there is incomplete emptying of rectum in spite of soft stools. *Functional constipation* is a result of gut-brain interaction. It is contributed by altered motility, visceral hypersensitivity, altered mucosal and immune functions and change in intestinal microbiota; It could be worsened by stress. *Habitual constipation* is a type of primary constipation and is known as constipation of modern civilization. It is due to improper eating habits (inadequate intake of fiber and water), poor physical exercise and defecation without squatting (use of toilet seat) resulting in anorectal angle that is not conducive for smooth expulsion. Irregular bowel habits due to rush in the morning to go to school and holding back stools through school period adds to habitual constipation. As passage of stools become painful, child learns to hold back the stool in spite of an urge and it worsens the problem. *Secondary constipation* is due to structural defects (Hirschsprung disease), chronic systemic illness (inflammatory bowel disease, intestinal TB, chronic diverticulitis), neurological (spinal or cortical disorders), hormonal (hypothyroidism, hyperparathyroidism), metabolic disorders (hypercalcemia, cystic fibrosis), lead poisoning and also side effect of few commonly used medications (calcium and iron supplements, anti-spasmodic like dicyclomine, pain relievers such as NSAIDs, propranolol etc.)

Red Flags in Constipation

Following symptoms and signs are indicators of need for prompt action and further investigations. They include sudden development of constipation for no apparent reason, weight loss, severe abdominal pain, significant rectal bleeding and recent onset of severe constipation lasting for more than two weeks in spite of proper management. Delayed passage of meconium on first day of life may be initial symptom of secondary constipation such as in hypothyroidism or Hirschsprung disease. Breast fed infant always passes soft stools irrespective of frequency and hence if constipated, always needs further investigations.

Harmful Effects of Persistent Constipation

Constipation in children must be successfully treated without delay because persistent constipation results in loss of rectal tone and perpetuates worsening constipation. Urinary tract infection often results from constipation due to pressure over lower urinary tract by distended rectum. Besides, such harmful effects, constipation also causes significant discomfort due to bloating of abdomen and pain and appetite may be disturbed leading to undernutrition. Thus, constipation in children must be viewed as potential permanent harm and must be addressed promptly.

Management of Constipation

Causes of secondary constipation should be ruled out clinically and in case of suspicion should be investigated as these problems can be treated effectively with appropriate intervention. Immediate short-term aim in management of primary constipation is to ensure bowel movement every day to avoid permanent damage, for which drugs may be necessary. However, drugs must be used sparingly. Balanced diet with adequate fiber and intake of water, life style change with proper toilet habits and physical exercise and behavioral modification with coping with stress form the mainstay of long-term management. Fiber is a natural bulk laxative that works by increasing bulk of stools. Prunes have lots of insoluble fiber and also has sorbitol that is laxative. Besides, it also has soluble fiber that is fermented in colon to produce short chain fatty acids that add bulk to stools. Prunes also stimulate beneficial gut bacteria. Apple, pear, kiwi, figs, citrus fruits, spinach and greens, sweet potato, beans, peas, lentils, flaxseeds, whole grain and oats are some of the food items that are very useful. One must avoid fried food, chips, cookies, lots of dairy products and red meat. There are different types of laxatives used in management of primary constipation. They include lubricating laxatives such as mineral oil, emollient laxatives or stool softeners such as lactulose, osmotic laxatives such as milk of magnesia, sorbitol and polyethylene glycol and stimulant laxatives such as senna. Increasing fiber in the diet as bulk laxative along with stool softeners are first line drugs. Osmotic laxatives may have to be added in case of stubborn constipation. Rectal suppository or enema should be reserved only for emergency situation for temporary use. They are not ideal for long-term use as they induce fear in children.

Prevention of Constipation

Exclusive breast feeding for first 6 months followed by complementary feeds consisting of suitably modified family food, continuing breast feeds for at least first year of life promotes ideal bowel movements. Good eating habits with consumption of vegetables and fruits, adequate water intake, physical exercise with outdoor activities and ideal toilet habits help in prevention of constipation. Once such habits are established in early childhood, they are sustained over subsequent years.

Take Home Message

Constipation is a common problem in children and is often ignored in initial stages till it becomes troublesome. Ideal habits promote good bowel movements. Secondary constipation must be suspected clinically and treated accordingly while primary constipation is managed by diet and life style modification with stool softeners or osmotic laxatives as per the need. Long term use of drugs must be avoided.

MCQs

1. What is constipation?

A) Change in usual bowel pattern
B) Soft stool with poor emptying in spite of straining
C) Hard stools with difficulty in evacuation
D) All of above

2. Which of the following mechanisms are not under voluntary control?

A) Rectal distension
B) Relaxation of internal sphincter
C) Relaxation of pelvic floor muscles
D) None of the above

3. Which of the following type of constipation presents with soiling of underwear?

A) Secondary constipation
B) Habitual constipation
C) Functional constipation
D) None of the above

4. Which of the following conditions need urgent action?

A) Acute onset of constipation
B) Severe abdominal pain
C) Weight loss
D) All of the above

5. Which of the following statement is wrong? To prevent constipation,

A) Diet must contain enough fiber
B) Plenty of dairy products are useful
C) Ideal physical exercise
D) Good toilet habits

Answers to MCQs

Correct answers as follows:

Q1 D	Q2 D	Q3 B	Q4 D	Q5 B

37 Constipation – A Challenge in Diagnosis and Management

Clinical Application of Basic Concepts of Constipation

Acute onset of constipation is brought to the notice of a doctor but patient complains of chronic constipation only when it becomes troublesome and painful. History in every case should include inquiry about stooling as a routine part of personal history. Incomplete emptying of rectum resulting in frequent urge to pass stools is also a part of constipation and at times, habitual constipation presents as frequent soiling of underwear with loose stools and mistaken for diarrhea. Constipation is an emergency because of potential dangers of chronic persistent constipation. Early diagnosis of constipation and timely successful management are important.

Case-Based Study

Case 1

Two year old child presented with history of progressive abdominal distension and constipation since early infancy. It was gradually getting worse. He had poor appetite and had lost weight over last one year. There was no vomiting though had occasional episodes of diarrhea and had no other symptoms. His development (milestones) was normal. He was breast-fed during first 6 months followed by introduction of complementary feeds. It is chronic progressive constipation starting early in life. Infant on exclusive breast feeding never suffers from constipation and hence it is certainly a pathological disorder. Abdominal distension with constipation without vomiting suggests chronic colonic obstruction. Prolonged constipation may lead to occasional diarrhea as stagnated excreta promotes infection. Physical examination revealed marked abdominal distension loaded with feces. Per-rectal examination led to ribbon like stool coming out indicating narrow colonic passage leading to obstruction.

This is typical of congenital megacolon – **Hirschsprung disease**. It is due to absence of nerve cells in the muscles of colon because of which colon can't evacuate stool. Diagnosis can be confirmed by barium enema and rectal biopsy and is managed surgically. Exclusively breast-fed infant never is constipated though stooling may be infrequent but soft. Chronic intestinal obstruction at that age is due to congenital megacolon. One may be able to suspect it even close to birth because of delayed passage of meconium. Normally meconium is passed within first 24-48 hours. Hirschsprung disease may be easily missed in initial years depending upon length of colon affected by absence of ganglion cells.

Smaller the segment involved, later is the diagnosis made. This is because constipation is initially manageable but over time, abdominal distension and failure to gain adequate weight attract attention to facilitate correct diagnosis.

Case 2

Two year old child presented with gradually progressive abdominal distension and constipation since early infancy. He was gaining weight well though was short in length/ height. He was lethargic, not active and had delayed milestones. At two years of age, he was not able to speak even few words. Physical examination showed dull looking child with puffiness of face, dry skin, hoarseness of voice, bradycardia, abdominal distension and umbilical hernia. Per rectal examination was normal. This child besides being chronically constipated, has delayed development and lethargy. It suggests **congenital hypothyroidism** or cretinism. This case is similar to previous one but there are many subtle differences. Child with congenital megacolon fails to gain weight but mentally normal while hypothyroid child fails to gain height and mentally subnormal. Both conditions can be suspected within first 2 days of birth by delayed passage of meconium. In case of congenital megacolon, meconium passage is delayed because of colonic obstruction while in hypothyroidism, it is due to sluggishness of intestinal muscle and so poor peristalsis. Both conditions should be suspected early in life to avoid permanent damage. It is most important in case of hypothyroidism as even small amount of delay in diagnosis and treatment may lead to permanent brain damage. In fact, in most centers in the country, cord blood is tested for TSH to screen for congenital hypothyroidism so as to prevent permanent brain damage. If TSH is high, further tests should be carried out to confirm the diagnosis. Incidence of congenital hypothyroidism is 1 in 2500 births and it is very high but preventable.

Case 3

Two year old child presented with gradually progressive constipation since the age of 9 month. He was consuming one litre of milk every day but was reluctant to eat solid food. His weight gain had slowed down in second year though he was very active and alert. Prior to development of constipation, he used to pass normal soft stools. Physical examination showed mild abdominal distension but no other abnormalities. Constipation in this child has started later in first year of life and has been slowly progressive without much disturbance to child's health and activity. Thus, it is not likely to be due to any defect or disease but result of **excessive milk intake and poor eating habits.** He has good appetite but his intake is restricted only to milk. This is because of feeding bottle addiction as he would consume 6-8 ounces of milk twice through the night while half asleep. Further attempt to force feed the child by mother had made this child stubborn and would just starve and cry for milk. Thus, sole cause of constipation in this child is faulty eating habits due to bottle addiction. This child would not improve unless his habits are changed.

Temporary stool softeners may be necessary. It is important to cultivate ideal eating habits right from 6 months of age. At that age, infant is eager and ready to put anything in mouth – it is a normal reflex. By about one year of age, most infants develop addiction either to breast or bottle feeding and this is the time to wean off gradually. If not done at that right time, child refuses to eat solid food and gets hooked on to milk feeds only. Further forced feeding should be always avoided. It is best to allow the child to starve but not to offer milk more than 2-3 times a day.

Case 4

Five year old child presented with gradually progressive constipation over last 2 years. Initially he would pass hard stools though each day, gradually frequency reduced to once in 2-3 days and stool was getting more difficult to pass with pain and occasional stool smeared with blood. He had no other significant symptoms. His appetite was average and so also his weight. He was active and playful. Physical examination did not reveal any significant abnormality. Constipation in this child has started around 3 years of age and has been very slowly worsening but without significant disturbance in his health or activity. Thus, it is unlikely to be due to defect or disease. On direct questioning, it was found that he was consuming imbalanced diet as it contained very little fiber. He also drank little water. He was often consuming "junk" food and had poor intake of vegetables and fruits. This is known as **habitual constipation**. In addition, he would have to rush to school in the morning without passing stools and would withhold stool in school due to unclean toilet. This worsened his constipation. His diet needs drastic change and he should make a habit of passing stool every morning. Western toilet is not ideal to pass stools easily as against Indian type of squatting that maintains anorectal position straight facilitating easy expulsion of stool. Such constipation is a symbol of modern civilization. This case is similar to previous one as eating habits came in the way of constipation in both these children. Parents are totally responsible for inculcating right eating habits in early childhood to ensure good health. Management of constipation in such children revolve around parental cooperation to change habits. However, it is ideal to ensure right eating habits right from one year of age, Otherwise, habits die hard.

Case 5

10 year old child presented with constipation and abdominal pain off and on for last one year. His stooling pattern would vary in frequency and consistency and also in timing of passing stools. Most of the time he would tend to be constipated with occasional normal stool. He also had abdominal pain that also varied in frequency and severity with irregular pattern. His appetite was average and had not lost weight. His diet was essentially normal and so also his water intake. Physical examination did not reveal any significant abnormality. Constipation in this child obviously is not due to any defect or disease but

also not a result of poor diet or toilet habits. On direct questioning, it was realized that this child was always stressed and worried about his performance in every field. This is typically referred to as **functional constipation**. It is a result of gut-brain interaction. It is now well known that intestines govern brain emotions. If one sees something frightful, intestines cramp first before brain realizes danger. When one goes to attend an examination or similar stressful event, one gets an urge to use toilet once more. And finally in colloquial language, we use the term – gut feeling that is superior to brain feeling. Intestinal complaints are most common due to such functional disorder and they may present with change in bowel pattern and abdominal pain. Such a child as well as parents need counselling and if necessary, psychological help.

Case 6

10 year old child presented with episodes of constipation, vomiting and abdominal distension three times over last 6 months. Each time he received conservative treatment with IV fluids and rest to intestines that recovered him within 3-4 days. In between these episodes, he did not have any symptoms referable to abdomen but had poor appetite, felt generally weak and had lost 2 kg weight over last 6 months. Physical examination during last episode showed abdominal distension with poor peristalsis and mild tenderness without any lump in abdomen. It suggested intestinal obstruction. Recurrent episodes of intestinal obstruction with intervening period of feeling unwell and loss of weight indicated persistent slowly progressive disease with intermittent symptoms of intestinal obstruction. It favors diagnosis of **intestinal Tuberculosis**. Barium meal would demonstrate narrowing of intestinal segments and biopsy may confirm diagnosis of tuberculosis. Intestinal tuberculosis affects submucosa and not mucosa and hence does not present with diarrhea. As disease progresses, attempt at natural healing leads to fibrosis of affected submucosal lesion resulting in partial intestinal obstruction. It may be relieved temporarily with conservative treatment only to recur again. Occasionally, constipation may alternate with loose stools due to transient mucosal inflammation though constipation is the major symptom in such cases.

Case 7

10 year old child presented with recurrent episodes of constipation, abdominal distension and vomiting three times over last one year. Each time he would recover with conservative treatment and in between episodes, he would be fully normal, had gained weight and remained active. Two year prior to these episodes, he had undergone abdominal surgery for Meckel's diverticulum. Physical examination during last episode showed signs of intestinal obstruction. As this child has remained well during intervening period, it looks like a mechanical problem rather than inflammatory cause. Thus, it may be due to development of adhesions following previous surgery. Such a child may need re-exploration though with

a possibility of **recurring adhesions**. This case is similar to previous one except that this child has been normal in between episodes as against previous child who was unwell during intervening period. It clearly indicates that this child has recurrent problem with recurrent symptoms whereas previous child had persistent problem with recurrent symptoms. Thus, it is important to differentiate persistent disease with recurrent symptoms from recurrent disease with recurrent symptoms. Sickness or wellness during Intervening period helps to differentiate the two conditions.

Case 8

10 years old child presented with constipation and abdominal pain over last two months. A year ago, he was diagnosed to be suffering from inflammatory bowel disease and was on treatment for the same. His main symptoms then were loose stools with mucous and abdominal pain. His disease was partially controlled with anti-inflammatory drugs and diet modification. Physical examination showed abdominal distension with colon loaded with feces. It is clear that constipation in this child should be related to his pre-existent inflammatory bowel disease. It may be aggravated by drugs prescribed for IBD or low fiber diet and/or poor intake of water. However, one must rule out any evidence of stricture formation due to intestinal inflammation that may need surgical intervention. It can be confirmed by intestinal imaging study. This case illustrates possibility of constipation in diseases that generally present as loose stools such as inflammatory bowel disease or irritable bowel syndrome. On the other hand, diseases that present with constipation as major symptom may also present with occasional loose stools as happens in intestinal tuberculosis or Hirschsprung's disease.

Take Home Message

Constipation may present with varied causes. Some of them may just need modification of diet or life style while others require specific intervention to cure it. Early diagnosis and treatment would avoid long-term damage. Thus, constipation should not be taken lightly and every attempt must be made to find right cause. Laxatives or stool softeners are only temporary measures till the problem is permanently solved.

MCQs

1. **Which of the following statement is wrong? Constipation in early infancy may be caused by**

A) Formula feeding
B) Poor intake of water
C) Congenital hypothyroidism
D) Congenital megacolon

2. Besides abdominal symptoms, evaluation of constipation must include

A) Diet and life style
B) General well-being
C) Mental milestones
D) All of the above

3. Which of the following statement is wrong? Modern civilization has contributed to constipation because of

A) Junk food
B) Electronic media
C) Western toilet
D) None of the above

4. Which of the following statement is wrong? Constipation and loose stools may coexist in

A) Inflammatory bowel disease
B) Congenital megacolon
C) Congenital hypothyroidism
D) Intestinal tuberculosis

5. Which of the following statement is right? Drug of first choice in constipation is

A) Lubricating laxative such as mineral oil
B) Stimulant laxative such as senna
C) Stool softeners such as lactulose
D) Osmotic laxatives such as milk of magnesia

Answers to MCQs

Correct answers as follows:

Q1 B	Q2 D	Q3 D	Q4 C	Q5 C

38 Vomiting - Look Beyond GI System

Back to Basics – Vomiting

What is Vomiting

Vomiting is involuntary forceful expulsion of contents of stomach and intestine while regurgitation is return of ingested food from stomach into esophagus and mouth without force. It is important to differentiate one from the other because regurgitation is a common natural event in young infants and should not be confused with vomiting. Nausea is merely a sensation of vomiting and may precede act of vomiting but may not end up with vomiting.

Pathogenesis of Vomiting

Vomiting may be a symptom arising from many organs. Typically, vomiting due to gastro-intestinal system disorder is caused by obstruction or inflammation in upper GI tract. Besides GI disorders, receptors in the floor of fourth ventricle in the brain represents chemoreceptor trigger zone (CTZ) known as area of postrena which if stimulated causes vomiting. CTZ may be stimulated by either raised intracranial pressure or by abnormal metabolites arising from disturbed metabolic functions in the body as happens in liver disease (acute hepatitis), chronic renal disease and inborn errors of metabolism. Autonomic nervous system through its network may also lead to vomiting as may happen in case of acute stress of any kind such as acute cardiac disorder or extreme physical stress as in a long distance marathon and also due to adrenal disorders. Stimulation of vestibular part of 8th cranial nerve is responsible for vomiting in motion sickness and stimulation of vagus – 10th cranial nerve due to pharyngeal or gastric mucosal irritation leads to vomiting. Some drugs also lead to vomiting, in particular, anti-cancer drugs. Severe bout of cough often ends up in vomiting. It is clear that cause of vomiting may lie in various different organs and not just in GI system, though vomit finally comes out of GI tract.

Natural Response to Vomiting

There is an increased salivation as nature's attempt to protect enamel of teeth from coming in contact with acid from stomach. Retroperistalsis starts from intestines sweeping all the contents upwards with relaxation of pyloric sphincter. Intrathoracic pressure lowers with deep inspiration and glottis is closed that prevents aspiration. Intra-abdominal pressure is increased with relaxation of lower esophageal sphincter facilitating expulsion of stomach contents. It is often accompanied with sympathetic response leading to sweating and tachycardia.

Contents of Vomitus

Commonly vomitus contains ingested food particles. Once stomach empties after repeated vomiting, all that vomitus contains is just small amount of mucous. Problem arising from obstruction beyond second part of duodenum results in bile-stained vomit. Repeated attempts to vomit with an empty stomach may cause retching that may also end up with greenish vomit due to forceful expulsion of duodenal contents. Occasionally, such a retching episode injures small blood capillaries in esophagus resulting in streaks of blood. It is referred to as Mallory-Weiss tear. It is caused by mechanical force of vomiting and is self-limiting. At times vomitus may contain large amount of blood as commonly happens in case of esophageal varices due to portal hypertension. Coffee ground vomit indicates that blood has stayed in the stomach for some time before vomiting and is due to iron in blood getting oxidized. Blood in vomitus may also be a result of severe gastritis or in adults due to stomach cancer. Fecal vomit may suggest gastrocolic fistula.

Complications in Vomiting

Frequent episodes of vomiting may lead to destruction of enamel of teeth due to acid contact. In young children, senior citizens and patients with neurological diseases, aspiration of vomitus is a risk. Severe vomiting may result in dehydration and electrolyte disturbances leading to hyponatremia, hypochloremia and metabolic alkalosis. Resultant metabolic alkalosis may cause hypocalcemia. Persistent vomiting for several days cause malnutrition and constipation.

Red Flags in Vomiting

Vomiting occurring few days after onset of other symptoms suggests a serious underlying cause that must be promptly diagnosed and treated appropriately. On the other hand, vomiting at the onset of the disease generally indicates local upper gastrointestinal problem and often self-limiting as in case of gastroenteritis. However persistent vomiting beyond two days in such a scenario indicates serious nature of disease. Reduced urine output suggests dehydration that needs correction and so also electrolyte disturbances. Significant abdominal distension may be due to intestinal obstruction or paralytic ileus. Severe abdominal pain indicates either inflammatory or vascular disease (due to intestinal ischemia). Accompanying neurological symptoms such as headache, drowsiness or seizures signify serious neurological disease.

Management

It is most important to find out cause of vomiting that would lead to rational therapy of the disease. However, symptomatic control of vomiting may be tried for first one or two days. Generally symptomatic treatment does not work well though vomiting is controlled in benign conditions often on its own. Hence it is not rational to continue anti-emetic drugs for more than few days at most, exception being vomiting due to chemotherapeutic drugs. Ondansetron, metaclopramide or domperidone are the drugs used for symptomatic control and rarely injectable form may be used in case of drug not being retained orally. Common side effect of most antiemetic is extra-pyramidal syndrome leading to dystonia and abnormal movements.

Take Home Message

Vomiting occurring few days after onset of other symptoms usually has underlying serious disease while vomiting that starts at the onset of disease is usually of gastrointestinal origin and often benign though may continue as well. Persistent vomiting demands proper evaluation. Symptomatic treatment is not much effective and should not be continued beyond first two days, instead demands proper diagnosis and management of primary disease.

MCQs

1. Vomiting is not a symptom of affection of this system in the body

A) Endocrine
B) Hematology
C) Respiratory
D) Renal

2. Which of the following diseases trigger vomiting centre in the brain

A) Epilepsy
B) Whooping cough
C) Uremia
D) Arterial stroke

3. This type of vomiting is not likely to be serious

A) Vomiting as first symptom with abdominal distension
B) Vomiting as first symptom without abdominal distension
C) Vomiting occurring after few days of onset of disease
D) Persistent vomiting beyond 2 days

4. Which of the following statement is right? Persistent/severe vomiting may lead to

A) Hypochloremia
B) Hypocalcemia
C) Hyponatremia
D) All of the above

5. Which of the following antiemetic drugs can stop vomiting completely?

A) Ondansetron

B) Metoclopramide

C) Domperidone

D) None of the above

Answers to MCQs

Correct answers as follows:

Q1 B	Q2 C	Q3 B	Q4 D	Q5 D

39 Vomiting – Need for Urgent Diagnosis

Clinical Application of Basic Concepts in Vomiting

Vomiting may not be considered only as primary gastrointestinal disorder as it is caused by diseases of almost every system in the body, though finally it is mediated through GI system. Thus, attention should be given to every organ in the body that may be responsible for vomiting. Self-limiting vomiting due to transient gastritis generally stops within first two days. Vomiting persisting beyond 48 hours is unlikely to settle by itself and merely continuing anti-emetic drugs is irrational. Acute onset of vomiting due to metabolic disorders may not reveal any abnormal physical findings and need clinical suspicion based on exclusion of other causes.

Case-Based Study

Case 1

Two month old infant presented with history of vomiting for last two weeks. Infant was well till the onset of this symptom and was on exclusive breast feeds and growing well. Vomit is forceful and contains large amount of curdled milk. Prior to vomiting, infant is restless but feels relieved after a vomit and takes feeds well. However, vomiting recurs after few hours again. Last two weeks, he passes stools infrequently and has not gained weight since then. Physical examination showed mild dehydration and distension of upper abdomen more in left hypochondrium and epigastrium. There were no other abnormalities. In view of forceful vomiting containing curdled milk without bile and distension of upper abdomen, it suggests pyloric obstruction. As infant is otherwise asymptomatic, it is due to mechanical cause that must have been present since birth. Hence it is **congenital pyloric stenosis**. Question arises why it did not present at birth. It is not a complete obstruction as in atresia but partial obstruction and hence referred to as stenosis. Over first few weeks, due to partial obstruction, curdled milk is retained in stomach for longer time that causes chemical inflammation of pylorus due to acidic nature of curdled milk. Thus, over time, congenital partial obstruction becomes complete and hence there is delayed presentation. Rarely if pyloric obstruction is near complete at birth, neonate may present with pyloric stenosis within few days. Diagnosis can be easily confirmed by imaging study and needs surgical correction of the defect. Absence of general symptoms such as fever in an otherwise well infant indicates mechanical cause. Forceful vomit suggests obstruction. Vomitus not containing bile localizes obstruction proximal to second part of duodenum. Presenting so early in life favors a congenital lesion. Hence diagnosis is easy to arrive at and is totally curable with surgery. It is important to diagnose early enough to avoid dehydration and malnutrition. It is ideal to confirm the diagnosis as other causes of obstruction proximal to second part of duodenum may simulate pyloric stenosis.

Case 2

Two month old infant presented with history of acute onset of vomiting followed by drowsiness. He was apparently well prior to onset of this illness. He was on exclusive breast feeding and was gaining weight well. Physical examination showed drowsy infant barely responding to painful stimuli. There were no other abnormal findings. What starts acutely may be due to mechanical, neurological, vasogenic, metabolic or immune mediated disorder. There has been no history of trauma. Vascular etiology affects localized part of the brain related to the vascular supply and hence not likely in this child. Immune mediated disorders are rare at this age and are often accompanied with general symptoms such as fever or skin rash. Primary neurological condition that may result in acute onset of drowsiness is viral encephalitis but would have presented with fever, seizures and other prodrome of viral infection such as cold, cough etc. Thus, it is mostly a **metabolic disorder due to inborn metabolic defect.** It is not possible to guess which metabolic disorder it could be. This infant was hospitalized and put on IV fluids and some laboratory tests were ordered. Within 24 hours, infant improved dramatically and seemed to be normal. This is typical of metabolic disorder as oral feeds were stopped, offending agent coming through feed was withdrawn and resulting in fast improvement. Further laboratory tests confirmed it to galactosemia. Infant is born with this type of metabolic error. It is treated with lactose and galactose free diet. Early diagnosis and treatment prevent permanent neurological handicap. Acute onset of vomiting and drowsiness clearly denotes central cause of vomiting. Sudden onset and equally sudden recovery on withdrawal of oral feeds indicates metabolic disorder. Further laboratory tests help in pinpointing a cause.

Case 3

8 month old infant presented with vomiting since last one month and cough off and on. He was apparently well till onset of present problem. He would start feeding but would vomit while feeding and vomitus contained milk as such. Occasionally, he would suddenly chock while feeding with severe cough. It kept on happening over last one month. At times, milk would go down the stomach without vomiting. Physical examination did not show any abnormality. As vomitus contains milk as such and not curdled milk, it is clear that milk does not reach stomach at all and so problem lies in esophagus. When liquids cannot go down esophagus, it is unlikely to be due to mechanical obstruction and hence it must be because of functional obstruction. It suggests malfunction of esophageal muscle that does not allow liquids to travel down. Retained milk is mostly vomited out but occasionally would be inhaled into airways and result in severe chocking and cough.

Further investigations demonstrated **achalasia cardia** – failure of esophagus to relax and so remains mostly contracted. It is managed by repeated dilatation. When solid food can't go down the stomach, it is likely to be mechanical obstruction but when solid food can go down due to gravity but liquids can't do down, it is often a symptom of muscle dysfunction, often of neurological abnormality. Achalasia is a condition in which esophagus does not relax and so obstructs the passage of ingested material. It may lead to aspiration of ingested material into the airways. Chalasia is just the opposite of achalasia in which esophagus remains dilated facilitating acid reflux from stomach and also aspiration into the airways. Older child and adult would also present with retrosternal burning sensation.

Case 4

8 month old infant presented with history of vomiting for last 2 months. He was well prior to onset of this illness. He was growing well. He vomits each time he feeds and in general reluctant to feed. He had lost 2 kg weight. Apparently, there was no other symptoms. Several tests and trials with medicines had failed. Physical examination revealed malnourished sick looking infant, weighing 5.2 kg but with no other abnormal findings. On direct questioning, it was found out that he was very irritable, constipated but passing lots of urine in spite of vomiting and severe anorexia. So, he had polyuria. Thus, it was due to **renal tubular disorder**. Further tests confirmed the diagnosis of hypercalcemia. It was a result of vitamin D toxicity. This case demonstrates importance of detailed personal history that pointed to polyuria. Generally, one tends to ask for oliguria as a marker of renal disease but renal tubular disorder presents as polyuria besides other metabolic defects. There are no abnormal physical findings in such a metabolic disorder and it is only a detailed history that gives a clue to probable diagnosis. It is an abnormal metabolite that stimulates central trigger zone to cause vomiting.

Case 5

4 year old child presented with vomiting for last two months. He was well prior to onset of this illness. He would vomit off and on and vomitus would contain ingested food. There was no history of headache or any other symptoms. Physical examination did not reveal any abnormality. It suggests central cause of vomiting. In absence of any other clue, one may have to investigate for metabolic disorder. Initial screening tests showed low serum sodium and high potassium. It suggests an adrenal disorder. Few days later this child developed neurological abnormality in the form of spasticity and deterioration of milestones. MRI of brain confirmed the diagnosis of **adrenoleukodystrophy.** It is a rare disease but this case emphasises a point that few diseases evolve over time to reveal a final diagnosis. However, it was easy to consider that vomiting in this child was due to chronic adrenal disorder. Acute adrenal disorder presents as shock. Rarely, adrenal tuberculosis may also present similarly but would have other symptoms such as low grade fever and

loss of appetite and weight with evidence of primary lung disease. Diseases with multiple symptoms may start with only one symptom and then come out with other symptoms. In such a case, one may have to keep in mind an evolving disease and even search for it with a single symptom at presentation.

Case 6

8 year old child presented with history of vomiting, severe abdominal pain and mild fever for last 24 hours. It started with vomiting followed by abdominal pain. Pain was periumbilical, dull and poorly localized. He had not passed stools for a day. Vomitus contained ingested material. He developed mild fever on D2. At this juncture, it was clear that as pain was the major symptom, there was intra-abdominal inflammatory pathology evolving without obvious localization. It is unlikely to be intestinal obstruction as there was no bile-stained vomit. By next day, pain had increased in severity and was localized to right iliac fossa. It clearly meant localization now to appendix and hence diagnosis of **acute appendicitis** was made. It can be confirmed with USG. He was operated and recovered fully. This case illustrates importance of inquiring about chief complaint. This child's chief complaint was abdominal pain but parents were worried about vomiting more than abdominal pain. Vomiting in such a case is related to autonomic response to pain. Visceral abdominal pain – related to viscera – is often periumbilical and dull with poor localization till it localizes to the site of inflammation with involvement of peritoneum and leads to increased severity of pain.

Case 7

10 year old healthy child presented with episodes of vomiting and headache on getting up in the morning that would ease over time only to recur next morning again. Severity and duration of these episodes went on increasing over next two weeks. There was no fever. These symptoms suggest increased intracranial pressure that is gradually worsening. And hence it is likely to be space-occupying intracranial lesion. Physical examination revealed papilledema on fundus examination and increased tone and brisk deep tendon reflexes in both lower limbs. It suggests slowly increasing hydrocephalus that was proved to be due to **cerebral aqueduct obstruction**. This child was operated for the same and had ventriculo-peritoneal shunt placed. Vomiting accompanied with headache is classic of raised intracranial pressure. Slow onset of raised ICP manifests first on waking up in the morning as during lying down position, there is venous stasis in intracranial compartment that adds to the borderline increased pressure and hence manifests on waking up. With routine movements, intracranial stasis gets reduced and so symptoms of vomiting and headache subside temporarily till pressure further increases and then symptoms get worst through the day.

Case 8

5 month old infant presented with vomiting since last 2 months. Prior to onset of vomiting, he was happy and growing well on exclusive breast feeds. For first three months, mother was at her mother's place with her infant. Since she came back to her home, vomiting started and it continued. Physical examination did not reveal any abnormality though infant had not gained any weight over last two months and was irritable. Several tests done were all negative and so also empirical therapeutic trials had failed. History of change in place coincided with onset of symptoms and hence it was decided to go into further details.

On further discussion with the family, psychologist found out the cause of **disturbed mother-infant relation** as the cause of vomiting. Elder aunt of the infant had taken charge of the baby and mother was allowed to handle the baby only during breast feeding. This infant was craving for mother's bonding. Father of the infant was taken into confidence and he managed to send his elder sister out of town on some pretext and from the very day, infant stopped vomiting. So, it was a functional disorder and not any organic disease. This case illustrates possibility of functional disorders even in a young infant. Mother-infant relationship is vital for infant's secured feeling and it promotes not only sound health but also ideal psychological development. Health is not just physical well-being but also mental, psychological and emotional well-being. Factors disturbing any of these components would affect health and manifest with physical symptoms simulating organic disorder.

Take Home Message

Vomiting is a symptom that may arise from almost every system in the body. Thus, anatomical diagnosis is a must. Disease may evolve over first few days to suggest a diagnosis. As a rule, persistent vomiting beyond first two days definitely needs further evaluation and mere continuation of anti-emetic drug is not justified. Vomiting due to metabolic disorders present often without any abnormal physical findings and diagnosis depends on strong clinical suspicion based on analysis of history.

MCQs

1. Which of the following statement about congenital pyloric stenosis is wrong?

A) May present at birth
B) May present at 4 weeks of age
C) May present at 8 weeks of age
D) May present after one year of age

2. Which of the following statement is wrong? Vomiting due to upper GI obstruction may be caused by

A) Congenital malformation
B) Muscle dysfunction
C) Infection
D) Neurological disorder

3. In this condition, child recovers completely within a day if not fed orally but recurs shortly

A) Pyloric stenosis
B) Inborn error of metabolism
C) Acute appendicitis
D) None of the above

4. In this condition, vomiting is the most predominant symptom

A) Raised intracranial pressure
B) Acute appendicitis
C) Metabolic disorders
D) All of the above

5. Which of the following symptoms must be inquired when child presents with vomiting?

A) Oliguria
B) Polyuria
C) Both of the above
D) None of the above

Answers to MCQs

Correct answers as follows:

Q1 D	Q2 C	Q3 B	Q4 C	Q5 C

40 Abdominal Pain – A Varied Pathogenesis

Back to Basics – Abdominal Pain

What is Pain?

Pain is an unpleasant sensory and emotional experience arising out of an underlying cause. It helps an individual to guard against it. Pain stimulates pain receptors that are present in all organs (except brain, lung parenchyma). It is transmitted via nerves to spinal cord and then to brain where it is processed. Brain thereafter sends message down the spinal cord via specific nerves to initiate desired action. It is also important to note that pain can arise from diseases of nerves as well and such a pain is burning or like an electric shock.

Anatomy and Physiology Related to Abdominal Pain

Abdominal contents are divided into foregut, midgut and hindgut. Foregut represents pharynx, esophagus, stomach, liver, gall bladder, pancreas while midgut represents duodenum, cecum, and appendix while hindgut represents colon, rectum and part of anal canal. Each section has visceral afferent nerve that transmits pain to spinal cord via autonomic sympathetic nerve. Visceral afferent nerve thus represents non-specific area. There is an overlap between visceral nerve and somatic nerve that is specific to a particular area. That is how pain from visceral organ is first felt at the distribution of somatic afferent and hence pain from inflamed appendix is first felt at periumbilical region – T10 level and then shifts to right iliac fossa at T12 level where appendix is situated. Specific quadrant pain is related to the organ situated in that quadrant. However, some quadrants contain more than one organ. At times, pain in right hypochondrium may represent lower lobe pneumonia and may be mistaken for pain arising from liver. Similarly, as kidney lies in posterior compartment, pain manifests at renal angle on the back.

Type of Abdominal Pain

Visceral pain arises from abdominal organs as a result of stretch, inflammation or ischemia. It is dull, poorly localized superficial, often referred to distant area from the site of involved organ. It is accompanied with autonomic symptoms such as nausea, vomiting, sweating and feeling sick. As against **parietal pain** represents involvement of peritoneum, it is sharp, severe and well localized to the site of involved organ. This is how as mentioned above, appendicular pain starts in midline and gets localized to right iliac fossa with increasing severity once the peritoneum is affected. If hollow organ is involved, pain is colicky with intermittent pain-free period and if solid organ is involved, pain is dull and continuous.

Pathogenesis of Pain

Most common cause of pain is **inflammation**. Inflammation is mostly a result of infection but also due to non-infectious causes such as systemic inflammatory diseases and malignancy. **Vascular pain** results from ischemia and is localized to the part supplied by affected artery. **Stretch** leads to pain as happens if liver or lymph node capsule is stretched. **Psychogenic abdominal pain** is common in older children and is caused by stress. **Referred pain** may present at the distant site from affected organ as happens in back pain arising from renal disease or shoulder pain in adults due to myocardial ischemia. **Neurogenic pain** is localized to area supplied by affected nerve and usually seen in affection of peripheral nerves, thus not applied to abdominal pain (rarely herpes zoster may present with severe superficial burning pain in a localized part innervated by a single nerve and diagnosis becomes apparent only after vesicular skin rash appears a day or two later)

Onset, Duration and Progress: a Good Guide

Sudden onset of severe pain is often mechanical (renal or biliary calculus, intestinal obstruction, ovarian torsion – mostly surgical) or vascular (include five types of lesions - vasculitis, vasculospasm, thrombosis, embolism and hemorrhage – mostly medical). Onset of pain over few days preceded by fever is typically an inflammatory pain and may also have additional symptoms depending on which organ is involved. (Loose stools with blood and mucous in bacillary dysentery, nausea, vomiting followed by jaundice in viral hepatitis, severe periumbilical pain with vomiting in appendicitis). Severity of pain suggests severe inflammation as in case of liver abscess or appendicitis while viral hepatitis often has mild pain. Recurrent pain with intervening normal period suggests colicky pain coming from hollow tubular structures such as intestines, ureter or bile ducts. Persistent pain worsening over few hours may indicate surgical cause while persistent pain over days or weeks may be due to gastritis or peptic ulcer (rare in children) and may be psychological, especially if it does not hinder routine activities. It is generally "pain of convenience" – it comes whenever need arises and disappears completely when child is engrossed in what he likes to do. Worsening pain or one that disturbs health needs cautious evaluation.

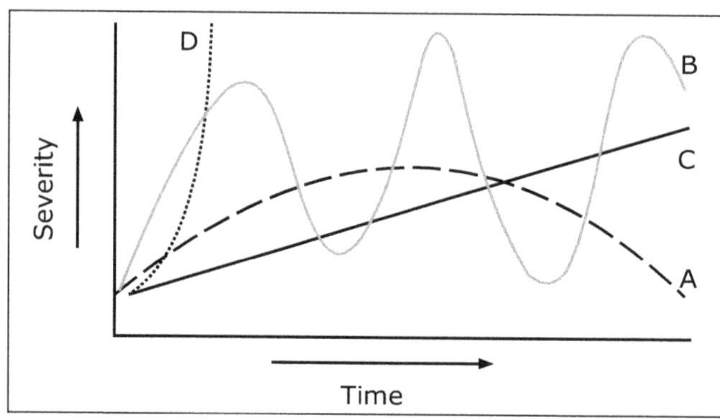

A – Self-limiting mild-moderate pain
B – Colicky pain
C – Slowly worsening pain
D – Acute severe worsening pain

Physical Examination

Inflammatory pain is accompanied with tenderness besides other localizing signs such as guarding or rigidity and such a child is very sick looking. Mechanical causes may or may not present with abnormal physical findings. There are no physical findings in renal or biliary colic so also lead colic. Vascular pathology causing pain is devoid of any local tenderness and they include vasculitis, intestinal ischemia as happens in dengue capillary leak syndrome and shock, sickle cell hemolytic anemia or Henoch-Schoenlein purpura (IgA vasculitis). In adults, diabetes may present with abdominal pain without any local physical abnormality though in children it is a rare manifestation of diabetes. Abdominal migraine and abdominal epilepsy also present without any physical findings. Generally these two conditions are considered when other causes are excluded. Besides local abdominal examination, findings away from abdomen should not be ignored. Degree of sickness, dehydration or electrolyte – acid-base imbalance must be noted in every child. Affection of other systems offers clue to a disease with multiorgan involvement as seen in inflammatory bowel disease with arthritis or sickle cell anemia with pallor and splenomegaly.

When Physical Examination is Normal!

In presence of abnormal physical findings such as localized tenderness, guarding and rigidity or a palpable lump make diagnosis rather easy. But real challenge is when there are no abnormal physical findings. In such situations, one must look at personal history in details. Appetite, sleep, playfulness, energy and activity, behavior besides bowel movements and urination. If all these points in the history are negative, one is nearly certain it to be a functional pain. However. any of the above mentioned symptoms are subtly upset, one needs to be cautious. Severity of pain and especially if pain awakens the child, one must find organic cause. Rare conditions such as Meckel's diverticulum, lead poisoning, porphyria, abdominal migraine and abdominal epilepsy are some of the conditions where there may be paucity of abdominal findings.

Red Flags

Sudden acute severe abdominal pain with abdominal distension and vomiting is usually an emergency and there is a need to find the cause to initiate appropriate action. For example, there may be an urgent need for surgical intervention as in case of intestinal obstruction. Bile-stained vomit signifies intestinal obstruction till proved otherwise. Blood in vomit, blood passed per rectum or purpuric skin rash needs proper assessment as it often signifies underlying serious illness. Unanticipated severe abdominal pain presenting few days after the onset of fever indicates complication as happens typically in dengue fever. When fever in such a case is on the wane, sudden appearance of severe abdominal pain suggests capillary leak syndrome with shock during which intestines are not perfused with adequate blood and so suffer ischemic pain. If neglected for a day, it may endanger life. Loss of weight in persistent abdominal pain needs evaluation. Finally, if child wakes up from deep sleep with severe pain, it definitely deserves further investigations even in absence of abnormal physical findings. Though one may come across a child who wakes up happily only to fake severe abdominal pain. Guarding, rigidity, toxic or sick look and signs of shock or sepsis are obvious serious signs.

Investigations

Tests must be ordered only after considering a provisional diagnosis. Though unfortunately tests are carried out because one has no clue to any diagnosis. But in such a case, which tests would you order? “So called routine” tests are irrational. CBC and routine stool examination mostly do not add any value to a diagnosis. In an inflammatory pain. CBC is bound to be abnormal but one has made out inflammation even without CBC. And CBC in such a case fails to define cause of inflammation. Serum amylase or lipase are markedly increased in acute pancreatitis but moderate increase may also be seen in intestinal ischemia or strangulated hernia. Similarly, stool examination has little value though presence of occult blood may need cautious interpretation. Stool microscopy showing worm infestation may not be related to the cause of abdominal pain. Abdominal USG is not necessary if liver or spleen in enlarged on physical examination as it adds not much greater value to diagnosis unless one suspects liver abscess or any other space occupying lesion. Same is true with CT or MRI scan. USG showing “probe tenderness on right iliac fossa” or distended loops of intestine or thickened bladder wall need correlation with clinical profile and recently it is an established trend that all tests come with a rider “correlate clinically”. Imaging report often have “?” as prefix to a probable interpretation! But clinicians are supposed to offer definite opinion and not a probable diagnosis. Thus. prerequisite for ordering tests is provisional bedside diagnosis and test results must be correlated with clinical profile.

Take Home Message

Abdominal pain is often a challenging symptom. Acute onset of severe abdominal pain needs cautious attempt at early diagnosis for better outcome. Similarly, one must rule out potential serious diseases. Tests must be ordered with specific aim of getting more relevant information. There are no “routine” tests. Management has to be more specific for rational outcome. Empirical treatment must have a justification and should not be polytherapy hoping one of the drugs may work.

MCQs

1. Which of the following statement is wrong? Pathogenesis of pain includes

A) Vasogenic
B) Neurogenic
C) Degenerative
D) Inflammatory

2. Disease involving this system may cause abdominal pain

A) Respiratory system
B) Hematological system
C) None of the above
D) Both of the above systems

3. Which of the following statement is wrong? There are no abdominal findings in this condition

A) Lead colic
B) Abdominal migraine
C) Vasculitis
D) All of the above

4. This may not suggest "Red flag" in case of abdominal pain

A) Blood per rectum
B) Bile-stained vomit
C) Severe pain
D) Pain disturbing sleep

5. Which of the following test would you order first when there is no clue to the cause of abdominal pain?

A) Stool microscopy
B) Urinalysis
C) None of the above
D) Both the tests

Ans to MCQs

Correct answers as follows:

Q1 C	Q2 D	Q3 D	Q4 C	Q5 C

41 Beware of Abdominal Pain – it is in a Pandora's Box

Clinical Application of Basic Concepts of Abdominal Pain

Detailed history offers a probable clue to the diagnosis. Comfortable or sick looking child, distended or flat abdomen, tender or not can differentiate few conditions from others. Other signs of specific organ involvement would help to narrow down anatomy of the disease. It is not difficult to decide probable pathology as mechanical and vascular causes have sudden onset while inflammatory disorders would have onset over few days. Progress and duration add to analyze probable cause.

Case Based Study

Case 1

Eight month old infant presented with acute onset of vomiting that was followed within hours with recurrent severe crying episodes. It was followed with passing blood and mucous per rectum. There was no fever. Physical examination showed mild abdominal distension and no other abnormal findings. Considering acute bacillary dysentery, he was treated with antibiotics. Acute onset of severe abdominal pain with vomiting without fever or diarrhea suggests surgical cause and blood and mucous passed through rectum indicates vascular compromise as in **intussusception.** Over next few hours, he looked sicker with increasing abdominal distension. USG confirmed intussusception and he was operated. Fortunately, intestines did not show gangrene and so could be salvaged. Acute onset of abdominal pain with vomiting and abdominal distension is clear indication of surgical problem. Absence of fever and sudden onset rules out medical cause of inflammation such as acute bacillary dysentery. Blood and mucous passed through rectum was not accompanied with passage of stools and so it was not intestinal infection. Delay in diagnosis may result in gangrene that may endanger life and need resection of some part of the bowel.

Case 2

Eight year old child presented with fever and loose stools for 2 days, better with symptomatic treatment for few hours but fever recurred with stools with blood and mucous and abdominal pain. Physical examination showed mild abdominal distension and vague tenderness all over abdomen. CBC showed neutrophilic leukocytosis and RBCs and pus cells in stool microscopy. Considering it to be acute bacillary dysentery, he was treated with antibiotics without benefit. Afebrile period after initial fever rules out acute infection and so it is non-infective inflammation. Diagnosis of **inflammatory bowel disease** was confirmed. Fever in acute infection does not subside unless infection gets cured. As this child's fever abated for few days before coming on again, it is not an infection. However, fever, blood and mucous in stools and abdominal pain are all symptoms of inflammation and hence diagnosis of non-infective inflammation would be considered. Rational analysis of history is necessary for proper assessment.

Case 3

Three month old infant was diagnosed as inguinal hernia and was scheduled for surgery in next few days. Meanwhile he suddenly started crying and inguinal swelling increased. He also had mild fever. Surgeon tried to reduce hernia and he succeeded but crying would not stop. Thinking about rare situation where hernia is reduced but without relieving obstruction, urgent surgery was considered. At that time pediatrician's opinion was asked for to rule out any other condition responsible for continued crying. As this child had fever at onset of crying, acute intestinal infection was possible. Per rectal examination led to passing of stools with blood and mucous confirming diagnosis of **acute bacillary dysentery.** Any disease with fever at onset indicates most likely an infection. Obstructed hernia should not have presented with fever. Abdominal pain in this child led to crying that in turn increased scrotal swelling that was easily reduced and so it was not an obstructed hernia. Acute bacillary dysentery may start with fever and at times followed by generalized convulsion due to toxic encephalopathy even before onset of abnormal stools with blood and mucous.

Case 4

Eight year old child presented with episodes of recurrent severe abdominal pain over last one year. Each episode started with poorly localized abdominal pain, not controlled by any drugs but getting relieved by itself. Mild abdominal discomfort remained for few more hours. Physical examination was totally normal even during the attack. Routine tests were also normal. Poorly localized abdominal pain suggested visceral affection likely to be intestinal, without peritoneal involvement and it has been recurrent but non-progressive. It has not been a colicky pain but dull ache. It suggests persistent intestinal lesion with recurrent pain. It was finally diagnosed as **Meckel's diverticulum**. It represents a localized acidic patch in some part of intestine, presenting same way as gastric ulcer does. It is suspected by microscopic blood in stools and further confirmed by radionuclide scan. It is not a common disorder but sound analysis of history paves the way to a probable diagnosis even in absence of any physical signs. Recurrent abdominal dull pain is rare and is likely to be non-infective inflammatory disorder. It may be due to immune-mediated vasculitis or chemically mediated disorder. Vasculitis is a general disease and so absence of involvement of other sites makes it less likely. Microscopic blood in stools was a clue in this child suggesting an inflammatory disorder.

Case 5

Three year old child presented with acute onset of severe abdominal pain for last two weeks. There was moderate fever at the onset that settled within two days but pain continued though varying in severity but present most of the times and gradually getting more severe. There were no other symptoms. Physical examination showed healthy child but miserable with pain and mild abdominal distension without tenderness. Sudden onset of severe generalized abdominal pain worsening over time suggests progressive disorder of non-infective etiology. Infection does not present with sudden onset abdominal pain and hence fever in this child would favor immune mediated disease. Such a disease could be vasculitis. It was proved to be **Hennoch-Schonlein purpura**. Within next few days, this child developed purpuric skin rash and also developed arthritis and hematuria. Sudden onset of a symptom could be either mechanical (traumatic), vascular, neurogenic, metabolic or immunological but not infective. Abdominal pain in this child is obviously not traumatic, neurological or metabolic. Fever leads to a probable immunological cause and hence diagnosis of general vasculitis. Primary vascular lesion is restricted to small area supplied by affected blood vessel as happens in myocardial infarct but this child had generalized vasculitis affecting multiple organs – intestine, kidney and skin. It could also involve any other organs as well.

Case 6

Ten years old child developed severe abdominal pain localized to lumbar region of abdomen on one side that was described by him as burning. There were no other symptoms. Physical examination did not reveal any abnormality. Abdominal pain if visceral is dull ache and poorly localized while if it is parietal, it is sharp and well localized. This did not fit in either of these two types. This was well localized but burning. It suggests neurogenic pain. Next day this child came up with vesicular skin rash over the area of abdominal wall where child was describing burning pain. Diagnosis of **herpes zoster** was evident. Character of pain gives a clue to probable diagnosis. Colicky pain arises from tubular structures such as intestine, Ureter or bile duct. Dull ache usually refers to solid organs and burning pain characteristic of neurogenic pain.

Case 7

Eight year old child presented with history of abdominal pain, loose stools with mucous and fever off and on for last three months. He was treated with antibiotics without improvement. Physical examination showed chronically sick looking child with abdominal distension and vague generalized abdominal tenderness. Finally, endoscopy was performed and biopsy showed changes suggestive of intestinal tuberculosis. He was put on anti-TB treatment with steroids and he improved. As steroids were tapered over next few weeks, his symptoms recurred in spite of continuing anti-TB treatment. He was reviewed again with another endoscopy and biopsy that this time revealed diagnosis of **inflammatory bowel disease.** Anatomical lesion in intestinal tuberculosis is submucosal and not mucosal and hence loose stools is not the primary manifestation of such a disease. In fact, classically, intestinal tuberculosis presents as subacute intestinal obstruction resulting in vomiting and at times overflow loose stools. But primary symptom is constipation and vomiting and not loose stools – described as alternating constipation and diarrhea. This case also highlights limitation of laboratory results if considered without clinical correlation. Histopathology of intestinal tuberculosis is often confused with that of inflammatory bowel disease but clinical profile of two diseases is different.

Case 8

Six year old child presented with acute onset of high fever and severe abdominal pain that was followed within next eight hours with generalized convulsion. Physical examination showed highly febrile, drowsy child with abdominal distension. Next day he passed stools with mucous and blood. Diagnosis of **acute bacillary dysentery** with toxic encephalopathy was made and child recovered after treatment with antibiotics. Generalized convulsion within few hours of onset of fever rules out meningitis that would have presented as headache, irritability and vomiting without convulsion. So, convulsion is likely to be due to either metabolic or immunological disorder. Metabolic disorders do not start with high fever with abdominal pain and so unlikely. Combination of high fever, abdominal pain and convulsion all within few hours is rare in immunological disorder. Hence one must consider toxin mediated disorder as was in this child. Shigella infection produces toxin that may result from several complications and at times complication presents before local intestinal symptoms. Such a presentation of shigella dysentery is not uncommon.

Take Home Message

It is important to follow simple basic rules of history taking. Site of abdominal pain, type and severity, besides origin, duration and progress and accompanying symptoms offer a clue to diagnosis. Detailed history alone can be helpful even in the absence of abnormal physical findings. Investigations need clinical correlation, especially in case of abdominal USG that often reports non-specific findings such as mesenteric lymph nodes, dilated local intestinal loop or thickened bladder wall.

MCQs

1. Which of the following statement related to abdominal pain is wrong?

A) It may be due to primary renal disease
B) It may be due to primary lung disease
C) It may be due to primary hematological disease
D) None of the above

2. Which of the following symptoms may not be due to primary intestinal problem?

A) Abdominal distension
B) Constipation
C) Loose stools
D) All of the above

3. Child passing blood in stools often suffers from pain except in this condition

A) Bacillary dysentery
B) Intussusception
C) Intestinal polyps
D) Inflammatory bowel disease

4. Physical examination of abdomen is normal except in this condition

A) Inflammatory bowel disease
B) Meckel's diverticulum
C) Intestinal vasculitis
D) Renal calculus

5. These abnormal test results may not correlate with cause of abdominal pain

A) Stool microscopy showing ova of roundworms
B) USG showing mesenteric lymph nodes of 1.5 cm in size
C) Plain X-ray of abdomen showing calcified spot in the liver
D) None of the above

Answers to MCQs

Correct answers as follows:

Q1 D	Q2 D	Q3 C	Q4 A	Q5 D

42 My Child Looks Pale!

Pallor – Back to Basics

What is Pallor?

Pallor refers to paleness or whitish (mild yellowish) hue instead of pinkish hue to skin and is at times a complaint of the patient. It is not equivalent of anemia. It results most commonly due to reduced hemoglobin – anemia but it may also be caused by peripheral vasoconstriction as happens in rising fever or due to sudden stress or shock. At times, stretched skin due to severe edema also looks pale to simulate anemia and is referred to as waxy pallor. Carotenemia (due to excess of consumption of carrots) also gives a pale-yellow hue to skin due to its pigment. Occasionally, severe pallor is mistaken for mild jaundice because of pale yellow hue to skin.

What is Anemia?

Anemia refers to decreased red blood cell mass lower than age-appropriate standard norms that is accompanied with reduced hemoglobin. It results in decreased oxygen carrying capacity. It is important to note that hemoglobin in normal newborn is as high as 16-17 Gm%, at 3 months of age it comes down to as low as 10 Gm% and then slowly rises to adult level over next few years. So, 10 Gm% hemoglobin in newborn is anemia and at 3 months it is normal because it is physiological dip as a result of decreased erythropoiesis due to increased tissue oxygenation and reduced production of erythropoietin.

How to Make Sure that Pallor is Due to Anemia

It is easy to note that paleness due to rising fever or shock is restricted only to periphery and also skin looks cold with child looking sick. Severe edema is obvious not to miss. Besides skin looking pale, mucous membranes are also pale due to anemia. However, conjunctiva may not appear pale in spite of anemia in case of conjunctivitis and so also mucous membrane in mouth not looking pale due to glossitis. Hence it is important to look for anemia in multiple sites for correct interpretation. All other conditions simulating pallor due to anemia reveal normal mucosal color.

Is it Possible to Assess Severity of Anemia on Clinical Examination?

It is difficult to assess degree of anemia in dark skinned individual. However, creases on the palm may offer some clue. Normally creases are well seen in normal individuals while they are not much visible in anemic person as they also become pale. It is best to compare your own palm with that of the patient to get fair idea of anemia and also to some extent degree of anemia. Though one must note that such a clinical sign is not very sensitive and not a substitute to hemoglobin estimation.

Is it Possible to Judge Duration of Existing Anemia on Clinical Examination?

Acute severe anemia presents with cardiac decompensation in terms of signs of cardiac failure. Chronic anemia rarely shows such signs because nature has time to compensate for poor hemoglobin and patient restricts his activities.

Physiology of Anemia

It is important to know basic physiology that would help in the diagnosis of type of anemia. Stem cell in bone marrow go through several maturation phases (progenitor cell to erythroblast to normoblast to reticulocyte to mature RBC). Hemoglobin is incorporated in late stages of normoblast and continues to be present in reticulocytes and RBCs. Life of reticulocyte in peripheral circulation is just one day while life of RBC is about 120 days. Naturally there are many RBCs in peripheral blood smear but very few reticulocytes. Routinely there are no normoblasts in peripheral circulation. When RBCs are lysed at the end of their life, hemoglobin is released and broken down to heme and globin. Globin a protein is stored in body and heme is further broken down to iron and biliverdin, iron is also stored in the body and biliverdin forms bilirubin that needs to be conjugated by liver enzyme to make it water soluble and excreted via urine and stool.

Clinical Relevance of Physiology of Anemia

It is obvious from physiology that increased hemolysis of RBCs will produce lots of unconjugated bilirubin that cannot be handled by liver and so result in jaundice. It is hemolytic jaundice in spite of liver being normal but can't handle excessive load of lysed RBCs. This being unconjugated bilirubin is not water soluble and so can't be excreted in urine. Thus, urine is not high colored in hemolytic anemia and physical findings include enlarged spleen and liver – a result of increased work on the part of these organs. Increased number of reticulocytes or presence of normoblasts in peripheral blood smear suggests increased bone marrow production to compensate for increased RBCs destruction as happens in hemolytic anemia. Thus, jaundice is not always a liver disease. On the other hand, if there are small number of RBCs along with decreased number of WBCs and platelets, it would suggest bone marrow suppression as happens in aplastic anemia. Presence of blast cells in peripheral blood smear would suggest leukemia.

Types of Hemoglobin

There are three types of hemoglobin – HbA (98-99% of total hemoglobin in adults) seen in normal individuals beyond the age of 2-4 months, consisting of alpha and beta chains., HbA2 consisting of alpha and delta chains that is also present in normal individuals beyond 2-4 months but is in small amount just 1-2% of total hemoglobin. HbF (fetal hemoglobin) found up to the age of 2-4 months of age, consisting of alpha and gamma chains and it disappears thereafter in normal individuals. Persistence of fetal hemoglobin beyond 4 months of age or increased amount of HbA2 (beyond 2% of total hemoglobin) suggest abnormality.

Nutrients Necessary to form Hemoglobin

Iron, vitamin B12 and folate are major nutrients required to form hemoglobin, deficiency of which leads to significant anemia. Less than 10% Iron in food is absorbed through intestines in iron-sufficient individuals as process of absorption is hindered by presence of calcium and phytates in diet. However, nature maintains balance by increased iron absorption to an extent, in iron-deficient individuals. Heme iron (from non-vegetarian food) is better absorbed than non-heme iron. Vegetarian food lacks in Vitamin B12 unless person consumes adequate amount of dairy products. It is absorbed in ileum and not jejunum (most other nutrients are absorbed through jejunum). Other factors contribute to smaller extent and include vitamin C, few micronutrients and thyroxin, deficiency of which cause mild degree of anemia.

Types of Anemia and their Clinical Correlates

1. **Deficiency anemia** is most common type of anemia. It is mainly caused by diet deficient in iron, B12 or folate. At times it may also be a result of deficient digestion and/or absorption in spite of adequate intake as happens in intestinal diseases. It may also be due to loss of blood as happens in hook work infestation or intestinal bleeding as in local intestinal pathology. Thus, mere supplementation may not suffice in case of intestinal pathological conditions. Such patients present with refractory anemia. Iron deficiency anemia presents with platynychia or koilonychia while B12 deficiency has knuckle pigmentation. There is no hepatosplenomegaly and patient does not look so sick.

2. **Bone marrow disorders** result either from marrow suppression as in aplastic anemia or due to infiltration of marrow as in leukemia or other similar disorders. Such patients present with purpuric spots or other bleeding manifestations and are sick looking. Infiltrative marrow disorders present with hepatosplenomegaly while aplasia without organomegaly.

3. **Hemolytic anemia** is either due to congenital abnormality as in thalassemia, other hemoglobinopathies or spherocytosis while it may be acquired due to antibody mediated destruction as in autoimmune hemolytic anemia. Such patients present with mild jaundice besides severe anemia and have hepatosplenomegaly (thalassemia major is an exception as it does not present with jaundice in spite of excessive hemolysis. This is because red blood cells are destroyed in bone marrow before hemoglobin is added into them). Those with congenital disorder are not sick looking, short with abnormal facial characteristics due to extramedullary erythropoiesis necessary to compensate excessive hemolysis.

Following table summarizes above findings

	Liver	**Spleen**	**Jaundice**	**Sick**	**others**
Iron deficiency	-	-	-	no	nail signs
B12 deficiency	-	-	-	no	knuckle sign
Congnital hemolytic	++	++	+	no	facial signs
Aquired hemolytic	++	++	+	mild	-
Aplastic	-	-	-	sick	-
Leukemia	++	++	-	sick	purpura
Blood basic investigations					
	WBC	**Platelets**	**MCV**	**RDW**	**Others**
Iron deficiency	N	N	low	high	micro-hypo
B12 deficiency	low	low	high	high	macro
Hemolytic	N	N	variable	N	micro-hypo
Bone marrow	low	low	variable	variable	blasts

Treatment

Deficiency anemia needs relevant supplementation. Oral iron therapy works well as iron absorption is enhanced in deficient state. Parenteral therapy is not indicated and packed cell blood transfusion is not necessary unless child presents in cardiac failure that is rare. B12 deficiency often needs parenteral therapy as absorption depends on intrinsic gastric factor. However oral treatment may be tried first. Folate deficiency is treated with oral supplements. Diet modification is important to prevent recurrence. Other types of anemia need specialized care and should be left to specialists.

Take Home Message

Pallor is not equivalent of anemia. Subjective assessment in mild or moderate anemia is not dependable, especially in dark skinned individuals. Creases on palms offer clue to severity of anemia to some extent. Simple algorithm depicted above helps in clinical diagnosis of type of anemia. CBC and peripheral blood smear almost confirms type of anemia and may need further specialized tests to fine-tune diagnosis. Oral supplementation in deficiency anemia is adequate and in case of refractory deficiency anemia, one must rule out intestinal disorders. Specialized care is necessary for other types of anemia.

MCQs

1. Anemia with hepatosplenomegaly is feature of

A) Iron deficiency anemia
B) Thalassemia
C) Aplastic anemia
D) Vitamin B12 deficiency anemia

2. Anemia with jaundice is feature of

A) Leukemia
B) Thalassemia
C) Autoimmune hemolytic anemia
D) Iron deficiency anemia

3. Which of the following cells ARE NOT seen in blood peripheral smear in normal individual?

A) Reticulocyte
B) Platelet
C) Normoblast
D) Monocyte

4. Which of the following condition shows microcytosis (small size RBCs) besides iron deficiency anemia?

A) Vitamin B12 deficiency
B) Aplastic anemia
C) Thalassemia
D) Leukemia

5. RDW (red cell width) is increased in this conditions

A) Aplastic anemia

B) Leukemia

C) Vitamin B12 deficiency

D) Hemolytic anemia

Answers to MCQs

Correct answers as follows:

Q1 B	Q2 C	Q3 C	Q4 C	Q5 C

43 Bedside Diagnosis of Anemia Possible!

Clinical Application of Basic Concepts of Pallor

Pallor is not equivalent to anemia, though in routine practice, pallor is mostly due to anemia. Acute severe anemia presents as shock as happens in case of large amount of blood loss while chronic severe anemia may present as congestive cardiac failure. Slowly progressive anemia may be well compensated without cardiac dysfunction.

Three major groups of diseases present with anemia – deficiency, hemolysis and bone marrow dysfunction. It is possible to differentiate these groups by history and physical examination. CBC and peripheral blood smear are excellent screening tests that nearly confirm group diagnosis. Further specialized tests may be necessary to define subgroup final diagnosis. This approach helps to minimize laboratory tests instead of ordering battery of tests.

Case Based Study

Case 1

One year old child presented with pallor noticed by mother over last few weeks. There were no other significant symptoms. He was exclusively breast-fed for first 6 months and thereafter mother introduced diluted cow milk while continuing breast feeds and occasional cereal.

As there are no symptoms of cardiac decompensation, it appears to be chronic severe anemia. Absence of jaundice mostly rules out hemolytic anemia (though thalassemia major has no jaundice). In absence of purpura (indicating low platelets) and any significant sickness, bone marrow disease is not possible. This leaves us with deficiency anemia. This child consumes milk only that is poor in iron and so this is mostly iron deficiency anemia.

Physical examination showed not sick looking, pallor ++, koilonychias +, wt 8.5 kg, length 74 cms (both normal meaning that this is getting enough calories and proteins), temp normal, HR 120 RR 28 (mild proportionate increase in heart and respiratory rate in absence of fever suggesting mild strain on heart), liver 3F +, firm, not tender, liver span 8 cms, spleen not palpable, signs of rickets +.

This child has signs of iron deficiency anemia as suggested by koilonychias and also had rickets. Milk is poor source of both iron and vitamin D and hence it is compatible with our thinking. However deficiency anemia does not present with hepatomegaly. Considering mild increase in HR and RR, it denotes congested liver though without congestive cardiac failure as yet. This child would present with cardiac failure, if not treated.

Thus, clinical diagnosis is **iron deficiency anemia on the brink of cardiac failure.** Blood smear showed microcytic hypochromic anemia with low MCV and high RDW, characteristic of iron deficiency anemia. There is no need to further confirm with serum iron studies. Oral iron supplement with ferrous sulphate is ideal (choice depends on tolerance in individual child) and will show rise of one gram of Hb in one week.

Iron deficiency anemia is most common in the community, especially in children and women. Iron and vitamin D deficiency go together in a child on predominant milk diet. It is due to poor intake of iron but also due to poor absorption of iron from food due to calcium and phytates in the diet. At times, persistent intestinal microscopic bleeding would cause iron deficiency, which is resistant to treatment because of continued loss of blood.

Case 2

Two year old child presented with severe pallor and no other symptoms. Six months ago, he was seen for severe pallor for which blood transfusion was given without arriving at any definite diagnosis. He was exclusively breast-fed for first 5 months and then mother started complementary feeds gradually increasing to family vegetarian diet over next 6 months. After the age of one year, he was on family food with small amount of cow milk. He has grown well over last two years. No family history of similar disease. No history of consanguinity.

This child has recurrent anemia in spite of one blood transfusion 6 months ago for similar complaints. Analyzing present episode, it suggests deficiency anemia because of absence of any other symptoms suggestive of either hemolytic anemia or bone marrow involvement. He is consuming very little milk after first 6 months of life though he is on full family diet. Lack of dairy products in a vegetarian diet runs a risk of vitamin B12 deficiency. So, this may be B12 deficiency anemia. However odd point is recurrence of anemia within 6 months. This is explained on the basis of absence of B12 supplementation during last episode wherein blood transfusion improved his hemoglobin temporarily only to go down again.

Physical examination showed comfortable child not sick looking, wt 11 kg, length 87 cms, pallor ++, pigmented knuckles, mild icterus, no abnormal facies, liver and spleen not enlarged and other systems normal. Severe anemia without hepatosplenomegaly in a comfortable child with pigmented knuckles suggests B12 deficiency anemia. However odd point is presence of icterus that is normally seen in hemolytic anemia. Absence of enlarged liver and spleen and abnormal facies (due to extra-medullary hemopoiesis) ruled out hemolytic anemia. 5% of B12 deficiency anemia patients may have mild jaundice. So, diagnosis stays to be **vitamin B12 deficiency anemia.** This is suggested by macrocytic anemia with increased MCV and RDW and further confirmed by serum Vitamin B12 level. Ideal treatment consists of parenteral Vitamin B12 as oral absorption may be erratic due to insufficient intrinsic factor in stomach. As this child was not treated with Vitamin B12 last time, anemia recurred.

Vitamin B12 deficiency is typically seen after the age of one year as milk intake goes down. It is often missed as iron deficiency is far more common. At times, intestinal malabsorption or diseases of ileum in particular lead to vitamin B12 deficiency. (Most nutrients are absorbed through jejunum but vitamin B12 is absorbed in ileum).

Case 3

Two month old infant presented with pallor noticed since last one month and focal seizure involving left upper limb one hour prior to hospitalization. There was no jaundice or purpura or bleeding. He was born after full term with forceps delivery. Baby cried immediately and was on breast feeds throughout.

Anemia in two months old infant is not a deficiency anemia as fetus derives all the nutrients from mother that last for few months after birth and continued exclusive breast feeds will nourish the infant ideally. This was a full term born infant and not preterm who may present with anemia so early in life due to short period of nutrient transfer from mother to fetus. It is also unlikely a hemolytic anemia as it would present with jaundice. It may be therefore bone marrow problem, however there is no clue in absence of purpura or bleeding (due to thrombocytopenia). With this discussion, one is not sure about type of anemia on history alone. Focal seizure suggests space occupying lesion in motor cortex. Brain tumors are rare at this age and so correlating with anemia, this may be a hematoma – could be attributed to trauma caused by forceps delivery. Such a hematoma may account for loss of blood and hence anemia. Typical subdural hematoma may accumulate blood over time to lead to anemia as well as focal seizure.

Physical examination showed conscious infant, weight 3.5 kg (birth weight 2.5 kg), length 55 cms, head O 40 cms, pallor ++, no icterus, liver 2F +, soft, spleen not palpable, mild weakness of left upper limb, anterior fontannel mildly boggy suggesting mile increased intracranial tension. Anemia without hepatosplenomegaly or purpura and comfortable infant suggested deficiency anemia a result of slow progressive subdural bleed. Hence diagnosis of **subdural hematoma** with significant anemia is certain. It can be proved by USG of skull (CT scan may not be necessary) and deficiency anemia by CBC and peripheral smear. It is worth noting that deficiency anemia may result from slow bleeding anywhere in the body, at times bleeding is hidden – commonly in intestines as in hook work infestation or any other bleeder such as polyposis. Treatment may need evacuation of hematoma and antiepileptic drug such as phenobarbitone for about 6 months and iron supplements.

Case 4

Two month old infant presented with pallor noticed since last few days and irritable since then, reluctant to feed. Born after full term normal delivery and has been on exclusive breast feeds.

This infant has been sick as evident by loss of appetite and irritability and has presented with recent onset of anemia. It is obviously not a deficient anemia at this age and also unlikely to be congenital hemolytic anemia as infant is sick. So most likely this is bone marrow disease – either aplastic anemia or any other infiltrative disorder such as leukemia. Physical examination showed sick looking infant, weight 4.3 kg, length 53 cms, head O 39 cms, pallor++, liver 2 F+, soft, spleen just palpable, deformity of left forearm. This anemia is without hepatosplenomegaly (liver 2 f+ and spleen just palpable at this age is within normal limits) in a sick irritable infant with congenital malformed limb suggests congenital aplastic anemia. Presence of any congenital malformation seen on physical examination demands search for any other malformations that may as well be hidden. So clinical diagnosis is **congenital aplastic anemia.** CBC will show pancytopenia and diagnosis can be confirmed by bone marrow aspiration. There is no specific drug treatment and marrow transplant is indicated.

Case 5

Six year old child presented with lump in left upper quadrant of abdomen noticed and feeling fatigue since last few months. Past history of one episode of severe abdominal pain lasting for a day and settled down by itself without definite diagnosis. There is history of consanguinity. Lump in left upper quadrant of abdomen suggests enlarged spleen and feeling fatigue over few months indicates chronic anemia. Chronic anemia with splenomegaly is either due to hemolytic anemia or bone marrow disease such as leukemia or storage disorder. One episode of severe abdominal pain that lasted for a day does not suggest a colic. Abdominal pain may be inflammatory, vasogenic, neurogenic, referred or psychogenic. Inflammatory pain is not possible as there are no symptoms of inflammation and neurogenic pain is ruled out as it is localized to direction of a nerve. So, this may be vasogenic pain. Bone marrow disease would not cause vasogenic pain while hemolytic anemia that may cause vasogenic pain is sickle cell disease. Thus, diagnosis of sickle cell anemia is most likely. History of consanguinity favors such a diagnosis.

Physical examination showed weight 18 kg, height 102 cms, pallor +, liver 3F+, not tender, spleen 4F+, firm, no icterus, no ascites, rest of the systems are normal. It supports diagnosis of hemolytic anemia in view of hepatosplenomegaly with anemia but without jaundice. (Jaundice in hemolytic anemia is classically seen in congenital spherocytosis and acquired autoimmune hemolytic anemia. Jaundice is absent in thalassemia. However sickle cell disease may affect liver and cause jaundice that is not hemolytic but due to affection of liver). Thus diagnosis in this child is **sickle cell anemia.** Diagnosis can be confirmed by hemoglobin electrophoresis that would show hemoglobin S. It is called sickle cell anemia because RBCs are sickle shaped instead of spherical that impedes smooth flow of blood in capillaries. Treatment is symptomatic.

Sickle cell anemia rarely presents with severe anemia but manifests with vascular obstruction (occlusion of blood vessels) in the form of dactylitis, hemiplegia due to middle cerebral artery occlusion or abdominal or chest pain. Such events get aggravated by dehydration.

Case 6

Four year old child presented with fever and irritability for one week and pallor noticed since last two days. There are no other complaints. Child was well prior to onset of symptoms. Fever suggests either infection or inflammation. Viral infection presents with cold, cough and most often self-limiting., so it is unlikely. Bacterial infection usually has localizing symptoms which this child does not have. So, it may be non-infective illness. Pallor indicates hematological illness and irritability may suggest pain that has not been localized and hence likely to be generalized. Generalized pain may be either muscle or bony pain. Pallor with bony pain may indicate possibility of leukemia.

Physical examination showed sick looking child, irritable, pallor++, liver 4F +, soft, not tender, spleen 2F +, large cervical lymph nodes on both sides, firm, not tender. In view of hepatosplenomegaly and lymphadenopathy with pallor, **acute lymphoblastic leukemia** is most likely. Diagnosis is confirmed by peripheral blood smear showing blast cells along with low hemoglobin and platelet count with lymphocytosis and if necessary, by bone marrow examination. Further studies are necessary to define more details for which specialized tests are necessary. These specialized studies can tailor-made chemotherapy and also help in prognostication.

Early diagnosis of leukemia is important. However, steroid therapy and/or blood transfusion given for severe anemia without proper diagnosis can not only result in delayed diagnosis but also be the cause of poor outcome in case of leukemia. In fact, steroid therapy without proper diagnosis and justification is always frought with danger.

Case 7

Two year old child presented with gradually increasing pallor over last 4 months and deviation of angle of mouth noticed over last two days. He had been otherwise well. Pallor in this child may be due to deficiency anemia, hemolytic anemia (without jaundice) or chronic bone marrow disease due to storage. Deviation of angle of mouth suggests facial nerve palsy. In absence of any other neurological symptoms, facial nerve must be involved at its exit from the skull or beyond. If it is at the exit, it must be due to compression of enlarged bone while if it is due to lesion beyond exit, it may be unrelated to anemia. General rule is to ascribe all symptoms to a single disease and hence it may be safe to assume that facial nerve is caught at its exit from skull due to enlarged bone. Bone may be enlarged due to abnormal storage in the bone as happens in osteopetrosis.

Physical examination showed comfortable child not sick looking but stunted, pallor ++, liver 4F+, not tender, spleen 2F +, lower motor neuron facial palsy. Anemia with hepatosplenomegaly in absence of icterus and abnormal facies rules out hemolytic anemia and favors bone marrow storage disease, such as **osteopetrosis** in which bone is thickened that leads to compression of cranial nerves leaving skull bone.

Diagnosis can be confirmed by X-rays showing dense bony structure without differentiation between cortex and marrow cavity. There is no specific treatment and transplant is the only possibility.

This case illustrates a type of problem that involves not only anemia but also involved neurological system that would make a search for unusual cause of anemia. Similar problem of anemia with neurological affection has been discussed in one of the earlier cases - subdural hematoma presenting as anemia and a focal seizure.

Case 8

Eight year old child presented with gradually progressive abdominal distension, loss of appetite and weight over last 6 months and pallor noticed over last two months. Progressive abdominal distension over long period suggests enlarged liver with or without enlarged spleen. Any other space occupying lesion is also possible such as tumor or cyst. Loss of appetite and weight denotes catabolic state often representing generalized disease. Absence of fever rules out infective or inflammatory disease. Pallor indicates anemia that has developed over last two months and so suggests complication of generalized disease now affecting bone marrow. Thus, this is most likely to be storage disorder due to abnormal metabolism. Exact nature of storage is not possible to define on history or physical examination.

Physical examination showed weight 18 kg, height 105 cms, pallor ++, no icterus, liver 5F

+, firm, not tender, spleen 5F +. Firm. This child is undernourished and stunted suggesting chronic catabolic disease involving liver and spleen and lately affecting bone marrow as well. It favors **storage disorder.** Further specialized tests can prove exact metabolic defect. One of the common storage disorder at this age is Gaucher's disease result of specific enzyme deficiency. It can be treated with enzyme replacement.

Storage disorder due to accumulation of abnormal metabolite results in organomegaly without functional disturbance in the affecting organ till late in the course of disease. It is only when bone marrow is involved that hematological manifestations point out to the diagnosis.

Take Home Message

It is important to make sure that pallor is due to anemia though it is almost always true. Few pointers in the history such as sickness, short stature, malnutrition, abnormal facies, abdominal distension, jaundice, purpura and affection of other systems in the body can easily suggest group diagnosis of anemia – deficiency, hemolytic or bone marrow disease. Physical examination can nearly support diagnosis inferred by the analysis of history and further confirmed with specific tests instead of battery of tests.

MCQs

1. Jaundice is not seen in this hemolytic anemia

A) Autoimmune hemolytic anemia

B) Thalassemia

C) Congenital spherocytosis

D) G6PD deficiency

2. Jaundice is rarely seen in

A) Iron deficiency anemia

B) Vitamin B12 deficiency anemia

C) Aplastic anemia

D) Leukemia

3. Hepatosplenomegaly is not a feature of

A) Congenital spherocytosis

B) Thalassemia

C) Vitamin B12 deficiency anemia

D) Leukemia

4. Pancytopenia is seen in

A) Aplastic anemia

B) Leukemia

C) Vitamin B12 deficiency anemia

D) All of them

5. X-ray of bones nearly confirms diagnosis of this condition

A) Thalassemia

B) Leukemia

C) Osteopetrosis

D) Iron deficiency anemia

Answers to MCQs

Correct answers as follows:

Q1 B	Q2 B	Q3 C	Q4 D	Q5 C

44 Every Yellow Is Not Jaundice

Back to Basics – Jaundice

What is Jaundice?

It is yellow discoloration of sclera, skin and mucous membranes. It is visible in sclera as icterus, only when serum bilirubin exceeds 2 mg%. (Icterus is a bird with yellow beak) Normal serum bilirubin level varies between 0.2 and 1 mg and hence jaundice is not visible early in the course of rising bilirubin till it crosses 2 mg%.

Clinical Correlate of Jaundice

Patients report yellow colored urine before icterus is visible in eyes. However, urine is high colored in many other conditions such as concentrated urine due to dehydration, hematuria and drug induced urine color. Though shade of high colored urine is different in all these conditions, urine is dark yellow in jaundice. Yellow color of urine is due to excretion of water-soluble conjugated bilirubin while unconjugated bilirubin being not water soluble, cannot be excreted in urine and so, urine is not yellow in hemolytic jaundice even when sclera is yellow. Thus, urine color differentiates hemolytic jaundice from hepatobiliary jaundice. Mild icterus is not easy to make out as sclera may appear muddy due to environmental exposure in non-jaundiced individuals or also in case of vitamin A deficiency and is often confused with icterus. Skin and mucous membranes appear yellow only when jaundice becomes severe. In fact, common cause of yellow skin is carotenemia (due to consumption of carrots in normal individuals) wherein eyes are not yellow and so it cannot be confused with jaundice. Mild yellowish hue is also seen in anemia.

Physiology of Jaundice

Natural breakdown of RBCs at the end of their life span of about 120 days, hemoglobin is released. Hemoglobin consists of heme and globin, heme is iron and biliverdin. Globin a protein and iron are stored in the body while biliverdin is converted to bilirubin that is bound to albumin and transported to liver where it is conjugated to water soluble form. It is excreted in duodenum via bile and then excreted in stools and urine.

On and average, 1% of RBCs break down each day and amount of bilirubin formed can be easily handled by metabolic processes in the liver. In fact, liver has lots of functional reserve but to a limit. So, when this limit is exceeded, jaundice develops due to accumulated bilirubin.

Types of Jaundice

1. **Hemolytic jaundice**

   Excessive breakdown of RBCs results in large amount of bilirubin that cannot be handled by normal liver. Hence unconjugated bilirubin accumulates in the body. Unconjugated bilirubin is not water soluble and so cannot be excreted. Thus, urine is not high colored in hemolytic jaundice. Unconjugated bilirubin may accumulate in brain leading to dysfunction (bilirubin encephalopathy due to immature blood-brain barrier) especially in a newborn baby or if large amount is produced as in case of rare disorder – Crigler-Najjar syndrome. It typically happens in severe hemolysis due to Rh blood group incompatibility in a neonate. Besides blood group incompatibility in a neonate, increased hemolysis occurs due to congenital defects as in case of Thalassemia, sickle cell disease, spherocytosis and G6PD deficiency (jaundice occurs with exposure of some of the drugs) and also in acquired autoimmune hemolysis.

2. **Hepatocellular jaundice due to liver cell damage**

   It is a result of hepatic cell damage. Liver has lots of reserve and only 15% of liver cells are enough to handle normal amount of bilirubin. Thus, when more than 85% of liver cells are involved, even small amount of unconjugated bilirubin produced by normal RBCs breakdown cannot be handled resulting in jaundice. Depending upon degree of conjugation defect, part of bilirubin that gets conjugated is excreted in urine and so urine is high colored. As liver cells are damaged, other liver functions (production and metabolism) are also affected.

3. **Hepatocellular jaundice due to isolated functional defect**

   Deficient enzyme responsible for conjugation fails to convert normal amount of unconjugated bilirubin that accumulates in the body (simulating hemolytic jaundice) and as it is not water soluble, urine is not high colored. (Crigler-Najjar or Gilbert syndrome) Deficient enzyme responsible for bilirubin excretion results in accumulation of conjugated bilirubin that colors urine yellow (Dubin-Johnson and Rotor syndrome).

4. **Biliary jaundice**

   Normal amount of bilirubin produced is conjugated by liver but due to obstruction to excretion into the intestines, conjugated bilirubin accumulates in the body. However as conjugated bilirubin is water-soluble, it is excreted in urine and so urine is high colored. As bilirubin cannot enter intestines, stool is clay colored. (Normal stool is brownish or yellowish in color due to presence of stercobilin – excretory form of conjugated bilirubin in intestines). Biliary obstruction may be due to congenital defect such as biliary atresia or acquired conditions such as biliary calculus, cholangitis or due to external compression of biliary tract as in malignancy.

5. **Hepatobiliary or biliaryhepatic jaundice**

   Liver cell – hepatocyte disease if not controlled in time spreads to biliary tract (compression of biliary radicals due to edema of inflamed hepatocytes) and often patients present as hepatobiliary disease – meaning both the components of liver – hepatocyte and biliary tract are involved. Similar situation arises when primary biliary tract disease spreads to hepatocytes (as happens in intrahepatic biliary obstruction) thus involving both the structure. It is important to assess primary disease in such hepatobiliary disorders. Thus, it is clear that timely intervention of hepatocyte or biliary tract disease may prevent spread of disease to other parts of the liver and complicate the problem.

Clinical Approach to Jaundice

Confirm jaundice

Mild degree of jaundice may not be easily discernible unless one examines eyes against natural sunlight. At times, muddy sclera may be mistaken for jaundice. Mild jaundice does not give yellow hue to skin or mucous membranes. Yellowish skin without yellow eyes suggest carotenemia and not jaundice. High colored urine may also be due to other causes. Urine is not high colored in hemolytic jaundice. Similarly, clay-colored stools may be due to fat malabsorption or giardiasis besides obstructive jaundice. Once clinical jaundice is confirmed, high colored urine suggests either hepatocyte or biliary tract disease. Clay colored stools and itching favor biliary obstruction though may also be seen in severe hepatocyte disease. Normal urine color indicates hemolytic jaundice that is also characterized by pallor. However, pallor and yellowish tinge may look similar and may be mistaken for one another. In hemolytic jaundice, pallor is more prominent than jaundice which is mild. Hepatocyte or biliary tract disease may also look pale due to co-morbid conditions but jaundice is presenting finding. In a short duration of jaundice, (hepatitis A or E infection) sickness disproportionate to degree of jaundice favors hepatocyte disease while high degree of jaundice with reasonably maintained health status indicates biliary disease. In a long duration jaundice as in case of hepatitis B or C infection, metabolic liver diseases (Wilson's disease) and cirrhosis, nutrition and growth are affected. Hepatomegaly with or without splenomegaly are seen in almost all of these cases of jaundice. In chronic hepatocyte disease such as cirrhosis, there may not be jaundice until late stages, at which time ascites is also often present. However, absence of hepatosplenomegaly in presence of jaundice suggests specific enzyme deficiency and such patients are otherwise healthy without any liver dysfunction or pallor.

Complications

Portal hypertension is seen in chronic liver diseases and manifests as hepatosplenomegaly with ascites. Liver cell failure is characterized by encephalopathy and bleeding.

Investigations

Serum bilirubin – direct (conjugated) and indirect (unconjugated) components.

Direct bilirubin more than 2 mg% is considered as conjugated bilirubinemia irrespective of total and indirect bilirubin levels. When total bilirubin is less than 5 mg%, direct component more than 20% of total is also considered as conjugated bilirubinemia. For example, when total bilirubin is 2 mg% and direct component is 0.5 mg%, it denotes direct bilirubinemia even when indirect bilirubin is higher than direct bilirubin.

SGPT (ALT) and SGOT (AST)

These are intracellular enzymes and so liver cell destruction leads to increase in enzymes level in blood. SGPT is more specific to liver pathology as SGOT also increases in other diseases such as heart or skeletal muscle affection. SGPT is higher than SGOT in primary liver disease while SGOT is more than SGPT in systemic diseases with liver involvement. Hence it is ideal to order both enzymes in assessment of liver disease. SGPT is very high in acute destruction of liver cells as seen in acute viral A hepatitis, in which SGPT may be in thousands. Per se, it does not suggest any serious illness but indicates acute disease.

Serum proteins – albumin and globulin

Serum albumin level goes down in chronic liver cell disease but not in acute liver cell disease as half-life of albumin is three weeks and takes time to go down. Serum globulins are often increased in immune mediated disorders.

Alkaline phosphatase

Serum levels of alkaline phosphatase increase in biliary obstruction. However it is not specific to biliary disease as it is also increased in muscle diseases.

Gamma GT

Gamma glutamyl transferase: High level of this enzyme is more specific in biliary obstruction as it is not increased in muscle disease.

Prothrombin time

As hepatocyte produces coagulation factors, prothrombin time is increased in severe liver disease and hence it is a measure of severity of disease. It indicates liver cell failure.

Viral markers

In suspected viral hepatitis (A,B,C,E), viral markers may help in confirming diagnosis. Hepatitis B virus has surface, core and e antigen and host responds with antibodies to surface and e antigen. Core antigen is present only in liver cells and so no antibodies are seen in blood. Other viruses may also affect liver such as CMV or HIV.

Urinalysis

Presence of bile salts and pigments confirms diagnosis of conjugated bilirubinemia. CBC is not much useful except in cases where one suspects acute bacterial infection as in acute cholangitis.

Imaging

USG helps in delineating patency of bile ducts and presence of bile in gall bladder. It also may suggest echo-structure of liver that may be corroborative.

Histopathology of liver

Liver biopsy is reserved for diagnosis of cirrhosis and chronic hepatitis.

Management

Most of liver diseases are treated with symptomatic therapy and have no specific therapy except hepatitis B and C can be treated with drugs but should be best managed by specialists. Autoimmune hepatitis is treated with steroids. Biliary tract disorders may be surgically treatable. Liver transplant is now possible for many diseases.

Take Home Message

Jaunice may be due to conjugated bilirubinemia (high colored urine) or unconjugated bilirubinemia (normal urine color). Jaundice is mild in proportion to sickness in hepatocyte disease while jaundice is severe in an apparently normal child in an extra-hepatic biliary obstruction. Absence of hepato-splenomegaly with jaundice suggests enzyme disorders. Laboratory tests in primary liver diseases offer specific interpretation – serum bilirubin denotes extent of the disease, ALT (SGPT) the acuity, serum albumin the chronicity and prothrombin time the seriousness, GGT the biliary tract obstruction.

MCQs

1. Icterus is visible only when serum bilirubin level increases beyond

A) 0.5 mg%
B) 1 mg%
C) 1.5 mg%
D) 2 mg%

2. Which of the following levels suggest direct bilirubinemia?

A) Total bilirubin 3 mg% - direct 0.5 mg%
B) Total bilirubin 1.6 mg% - direct 0.8 mg%
C) Total bilirubin 1 mg% - direct 0.2 mg%
D) Total bilirubin 10 mg% - direct 1.5 mg%

3. Liver is not enlarged in this jaundice

A) Hepatitis
B) Cirrhosis
C) Enzyme disease – Gilbert disease
D) Hemolytic jaundice

4. Which of the following statement is wrong?

A) High colored urine in hepatitis
B) Urine may not be high colored in cirrhosis
C) High colored urine in autoimmune hemolytic anemia
D) High colored urine in biliary obstruction

5. Very high levels of SGPT are common in

A) Severe liver disease
B) Chronic liver disease
C) Acute liver disease
D) Liver cell failure

Answers to MCQs

Correct answers as follows:

Q1 D	Q2 B	Q3 C	Q4 C	Q5 C

45 Jaundice without Liver Disease, Liver Disease Without Jaundice

Clinical Application of Basic Concepts

Icterus in sclera is evident in most cases except in early phase of the disease. High colored urine is easily noticeable though seen only in conjugated bilirubinemia. Once jaundice is suspected, color of urine and stool offer clue to type of jaundice. High colored urine is characteristic of hepatocyte disease while clay-colored stools of biliary obstruction. However, severe hepatocyte disease also may have clay-colored stools. Sick look in spite of mild jaundice favors hepatocyte disease while deep jaundice in apparently healthy individual suggests biliary obstruction. Normal urine color indicates indirect bilirubinemia and if due to hemolysis, pallor is the main symptom with milder jaundice. Thus, history alone can diagnose probable group of disorder. Physical examination nearly can confirm diagnosis. General appearance – sick or not sick, enlarged liver and/or spleen, other signs of liver disease such as edema or ascites, significant pallor offer clues to diagnosis. Thus, history and physical examination can help order specific tests to confirm diagnosis and avoid battery of test that may not be necessary.

Case-Based Discussion

Case 1

8 year old child presented with moderate degree of fever for two days followed by high fever for next 3 days without any other symptoms. On D5, mother noticed high colored urine and mild icterus.

Onset with moderate fever followed by high degree of fever suggests bacteremic bacterial infection that has not localized so far until D5. Non-localizing bacteremic infection typically is typhoid fever. Now that child develops jaundice, it is mostly a complication of typhoid fever. Viral A hepatitis classically starts with prodrome of nausea, vomiting and anorexia followed in a day or two with jaundice and so it is not viral hepatitis. Had it been irregular pattern of fever, one may have considered malarial hepatitis.

Physical examination showed sick looking child, febrile, mild icterus, tumid abdomen, liver 3F+, span of 9 cms, spleen just palpable.

CBC showed Hb 11 Gm%, WBC 3000 P 30 L 60 M10 E0, pl 80000, total bilirubin 4.3 mg% Direct 3.4 mg% SGPT 170 SGOT 250 Alk phos normal

CBC is typical of typhoid fever – leukopenia, lymphocytosis, monocytosis, thrombocytopenia. SGOT > SGPT indicates systemic extra-hepatic infection with secondary liver involvement and not primary liver disease. Blood culture grew S Typhi.

Typhoid fever with hepatitis was confirmed. Jaundice appearing few days after onset of fever indicates extra-hepatic infection with subsequent involvement of the liver. It could be a result of direct extension of primary infection (typhoid or malaria) or immune complication of primary infection (leptospirosis or different viral infection including Covid– part of multisystem inflammatory disease). Jaundice presenting early in the course of a disease is usually due to primary liver disease.

Case 2

6 year old child's mother accidentally noticed yellow tinge in the eyes but child was quite normal without any complaints. On direct questioning, urine color was normal.

Normal urine color rules out hepatocyte and biliary disease. It may be hemolytic jaundice but pallor was not noticed. Physical examination showed mild icterus but no pallor or hepatosplenomegaly. Growth and nutrition were normal. It rules out hemolytic jaundice. This is a normal child with mild unconjugated (indirect) bilirubinemia. It suggests enzyme deficiency – **Gilbert disease.**

Diagnosis may be confirmed by liver biopsy but it is not indicated as clinical diagnosis strongly suggests a benign disease and so invasive investigation may be avoided. This is a specific enzyme deficiency but all other liver functions are normal. It is a benign condition and child will lead normal life without any problem but with jaundice. This case illustrates an example of jaundice without any evidence of liver or hemolytic disease in a healthy asymptomatic child. Such a presentation is typical of an enzyme defect that is benign though persistent and has no treatment. However Crigler-Najjar syndrome is another enzyme defect causing indirect bilirubinemia but is severe and has a risk of brain damage (typically basal ganglia).

Case 3

8 year old child was accidentally noticed to have yellow eyes while he was getting ready to go to school. As he was fine, he insisted to go to school. On his return, his doctor diagnosed it as viral A hepatitis and suggested no specific treatment. Viral A hepatitis presents with a prodrome of nausea, vomiting and severe anorexia before developing jaundice and child does feel weak. So, this is most unlikely to be viral A hepatitis. At this point we need to follow the child closely for further progression. Next morning when he got up to brush teeth, he suddenly fainted and mother noticed severe jaundice. He was rushed to the hospital.

It is evident that this child has developed fulminant liver disease that has worsened just over a day. Sudden fainting may suggest severe anemia or syncope. So, this child seems to be suffering from acutely worsening liver disease with or without anemia.

Physical examination showed a sick child, deep icterus, severely pale, liver 5F+ firm, spleen not palpable, no ascites. This child has combination of acutely worsening jaundice with severe anemia. Acute onset of severe anemia may be due to hemolysis or occult hemorrhage. Sudden onset of any symptoms may be either immune mediated or metabolic. Autoimmune hemolytic anemia and autoimmune hepatitis don't go together and child in either of these two conditions is not very sick. So, this may be metabolic disorder. Most common metabolic liver disorder > 5 years of age **is Wilson's disease.** It was confirmed by low serum ceruloplasmin. Wilson's disease is a genetic disorder and presents with a wide spectrum of symptoms of varied duration. It is treated with chelating agents such as D-penicillamine and zinc. This child had developed acute fulminant liver disease and so had no time for drugs to act. He underwent urgent liver transplant and survived.

Case 4

8 year old child presented with high fever, severe body ache and headache for last 4 days. Fever would respond poorly to paracetamol and he would look sick throughout the illness. Body ache was so severe that he could not walk because of pain. On D6, he developed high colored urine and jaundice. Analyzing fever before onset of jaundice, these symptoms are common to viral infections, malaria and also typhoid or any other severe bacterial infection. Severe body ache – myalgia – to an extent of inability to walk is unusual feature in this child. Typical viral infection would often have cold, cough etc and usually settle within 3-4 days. Malaria presents generally with erratic fever pattern and typhoid typically starts with moderate degree of fever that rises over next few days. Hence it may be evolving bacterial infection that has not yet produced any localizing symptom. Such infections include bacterial endocarditis, leptospirosis, rickettsia or brucellosis. Development of jaundice suggests hepatic complication of extra-hepatic disease and leptospirosis is one of such diseases presenting with liver and kidney affection. Physical examination showed sick looking child, highly febrile, congested eyes, oral mucosa and throat, icterus +, liver 3F+, soft, not tender, spleen not palpable, other systems normal. Jaundice developing few days after high fever with severe myalgia and headache favors diagnosis of leptospirosis. One may have to look for involvement of other organs, if not clinically visible, by relevant laboratory tests.

Investigations showed Hb 9 Gm%, WBC 18000 P 72 L 25 M 3 E 0 Pl 2.5 Serum bilirubin total 4 mg% Direct 3.2 mg%, SGPT 250 SGOT 375 Alk Phos 85 Serum proteins 5.7 Gm% Alb 3.4 Gm%, serum creatinine 1.8 mg%

Laboratory tests demonstrate neutrophilic leukocytosis favoring acute infection, conjugated bilirubinemia with increased enzymes suggestive of hepatocyte disease and high serum creatinine indicates nephritis.

Leptospirosis with liver and kidney involvement was considered. It was confirmed with IgM antibody to leptospira. Amoxycillin or Doxycycline are drugs of choice. Leptospirosis is a bacterial infection contracted through injured skin exposed to contaminated urine of rodents or other animals while walking in a water-logged area. It presents with high fever with severe myalgia and congested mucosa and few patients develop immune mediated complications affecting commonly liver and kidney but also any other organ may be involved.

Case 5

One month old infant presented with jaundice that started on D3 of life and was considered to be physiological jaundice that would settle down by itself. However, it persisted over next four weeks and hence child was brought to a doctor. Infant had normal delivery and had been on exclusive breast feeds. He had gained one kg of weight in last one month and was happy in spite of jaundice. Urine color was normal. Normal urine color rules out conjugated bilirubinemia and hence hepatocyte and biliary tract diseases are unlikely. It may be hemolytic jaundice but pallor would have been a major complaint that is not so in this infant. Thus, it is unconjugated bilirubinemia but without hemolysis; it could be an enzyme deficiency such Crigler-Najjar syndrome that presents with severe progressive jaundice or Gilbert syndrome that presents with mild jaundice later in childhood. Physical examination was normal.

Serum bilirubin was 3.2 mg% direct 0.4 mg%, other tests N. So by exclusion, we need to look at other causes. Other causes of such jaundice are breast milk jaundice or breast feeding jaundice. Breast feeding jaundice is due to inadequate breast milk intake resulting in decrease in enterohepatic circulation. Such an infant would not gain adequate weight. Breast milk jaundice is due to a chemical substance present in breast milk that leads to jaundice that is self-limiting. As this infant had grown well, **breast milk jaundice** is the diagnosis.

There is no need to stop breast feeding as in spite of continuing breast milk, jaundice is known to disappear over next few weeks. One may prove diagnosis of breast milk jaundice by withdrawing breast milk for few days and demonstrating clearing of jaundice. However, it is not necessary as transient withdrawal may disrupt breast milk secretions besides mother gets wrong impression that her breast milk is not suiting the infant.

Case 6

One month old infant presented with jaundice since D 3 of life and was considered to be physiological jaundice. However, jaundice persisted over next four weeks. Urine color was normal. Baby was born after full term normal delivery with birth weight of 2.5 kg, infant was on exclusive breast feeds. Mother complained about lethargy as baby would not cry for a feed and had to be coaxed to feed. Jaundice with normal urine color suggests unconjugated bilirubinemia. It is unlikely to be hemolytic jaundice as pallor would have been a major symptom. So, it is non-hemolytic indirect bilirubinemia. Infant with enzyme deficiency would not have been lethargic unless jaundice went on increasing fast. In which case, it would have resulted in convulsions or refusal of feeds. So, we need to think beyond common causes. This infant is lethargic that may suggest brain involvement that is likely to be slowly evolving disease as there are no acute symptoms of brain disease such as convulsions or refusal of feeds.

Physical examination showed lethargic infant, weight 3.4 kg, length 49 cms, head O 36 cm, heart rate 70/minute, no pallor, no hepatosplenomegaly, no other abnormality. This infant has gained weight well but has bradycardia and his length is short for his age. This suggests delayed bone growth characteristic of **congenital hypothyroidism**. Lethargy and bradycardia are other typical features of hypothyroidism. Diagnosis can be confirmed by serum T3, T4 and TSH levels. Treatment with thyroid hormone supplement would be necessary for life.

It is important to diagnose congenital hypothyroidism right at birth to avoid permanent brain damage. It is ideal to order TSH level on cord blood on every infant at birth to suspect hypothyroidism even before symptoms develop. Prevalence of congenital hypothyroidism is one in 3500 live births and so quite high to justify routine screening for hypothyroidism at birth. Most obstetric centers in India now screen for congenital hypothyroidism. Bone age depicts bone maturation and is estimated on X-ray by special charts (Grulich-Pyle chart). Absence of lower femoral and upper tibial epiphysis at birth suggests delayed bone maturation that is the hallmark of congenital hypothyroidism.

Case 7

8 year old child presented with fever for two days followed by jaundice. Urine color was normal. Child had been healthy without any prior illness.

Jaundice with normal urine color is due to unconjugated bilirubin. So, this is likely to be either hemolytic jaundice or due to enzyme deficiency. Enzyme deficiency is not triggered by fever but hemolysis may and so it may be acute hemolytic jaundice. Presence of pallor may favor hemolysis and absence of pallor enzyme deficiency.

Physical examination showed healthy child, well grown, pallor++, mild icterus, liver 1F +, soft, spleen 2F +, no other abnormality.

Pallor with splenomegaly suggests hemolysis and so this is hemolytic jaundice. As onset of this illness was with fever, it is likely to be acquired autoimmune hemolytic anemia and jaundice.

Investigations showed Hb 8 Gm%, normal total and differential WBC and platelets, serum bilirubin 3 mg% with direct 0.4 mg%.

This confirms anemia with unconjugated bilirubinemia. Coomb's test is positive indicating antibody related hemolysis.

This condition may be self-limiting and if not, need to be treated with steroids and if necessary, with packed cell transfusion. Blood transfusion may itself aggravate further antibody destruction and so reserved only if necessary. In such a case, there has to be proper match between donor's and recipient's rare blood groups.

Case 8

8 year old child presented with jaundice and abdominal distension for last one week. On direct questioning, he was not well over last 6 months. He had poor appetite, loose stools at times, feeling weak and had lost 2 kg weight. This suggests chronic progressive illness. Prior to developing jaundice and abdominal distension, his past history would have made us search for chronic evolving disease. As only localizing symptom of loose stools relate to gastrointestinal tract, one would think of GI disease. However loose stools are not frequent and there are no other symptoms of GI disturbances such as vomiting, flatulence or abdominal pain. Such a disturbance may denote indigestion which may be due to liver, biliary system or pancreatic disorders. Biliary or pancreatic disorders would present with pain. Absence of pain in this child may therefore suggest evolving hepatocyte disease. Abdominal distension noticed over just a week suggests ascites and in ascites in chronic liver disease indicates decompensation with portal hypertension.

Physical examination showed weight 16 kg, height 110 cms, icterus +, liver 4F +,firm, liver span 10 cms, spleen 3 F+, firm, ascites +, other systems normal

Investigations showed Hb 10 Gm%, serum bilirubin 5.2 mg, Direct 4.1 mg%, SGPT 100, SGOT 60 Serum proteins 4.2 Gm%, Albumin 2.3 Gm%, INR 1.8

Laboratory tests prove chronic liver disease (low serum albumin) that has recently decompensated (bilirubinemia with mild raised enzymes but raised INR). Diagnosis of **cirrhosis** can be confirmed by liver biopsy that may be dangerous at this stage with liver beginning to fail. It may not offer much more information and so may be deferred. Etiology may not be apparent with liver biopsy. Treatment is symptomatic.

Cirrhosis is different from fibrosis. In cirrhosis, besides fibrosis, there is an attempt at regeneration of liver tissue. This is the end result of chronic hepatocyte damage caused by various disorders such as hepatitis B or C infection, autoimmune hepatitis, metabolic disorders such as Wilson disease and also by toxins.

Take Home Message

Detailed history can initially differentiate between conjugated bilirubinemia (high colored urine) and unconjugated bilirubinemia (normal urine color) and further between hepatocyte (sickness in spite of mild jaundice) and biliary tract disease (normal health in spite of deep jaundice). Ultimately both hepatocyte and biliary tract disease involve other areas and present as hepatobiliary disease. Pallor is the major feature of hemolytic jaundice. Jaundice without hepatosplenomegaly denotes enzyme defect.

MCQs

1. Which of the following statement is wrong?

A) High colored urine, clay colored stools is a biliary disease
B) High colored urine, and clay colored stools may be a hepatocyte disease
C) High colored urine and normal color stools may be hepatocyte disease
D) Normal urine and clay colored stools is a biliary disease

2. Which of the following statement is wrong?

A) Jaundice in malaria is unconjugated
B) Jaundice in malaria is conjugated
C) Jaundice may not occur in Malaria
D) None of the above

3. Nausea, vomiting and anorexia are features of

A) Chronic hepatitis
B) Cirrhosis
C) Typhoid hepatitis
D) Viral A hepatitis

4. Jaundice without enlarged liver suggests

A) Wilson's disease
B) Biliary tract obstruction
C) Chronic hepatitis
D) Malarial hepatitis

5. Jaundice without splenomegaly is seen in this condition

A) Malaria hepatitis
B) Cirrhosis
C) Enzyme deficiency
D) Typhoid hepatitis

Answers to MCQs

Correct answers as follows:

Q1 D	Q2 A	Q3 D	Q4 B	Q5 C

46 Edema – Fluid in Wrong Sites!

Back to Basics

Edema refers to increased collection of fluids in interstitial spaces including third space (pleural and peritoneal). It results from imbalance between pressures in intravascular and extravascular compartments. In health, two thirds of total body fluid is intracellular (part of extravascular compartment) and remaining is divided into intravascular (plasma and lymph), interstitial and small amount in transcellular space (ocular, cerebrospinal fluid, fluid in pleura, peritoneum and joint space). Transcellular fluid is static and not in balance with other compartments.

Pressure Between Compartments

Intravascular pressure pushes fluid out of vessels. Mean arterial pressure is 70-90 mm Hg, at arterial capillary end 30 mm Hg and at venous end. Intravascular osmotic pressure pulls fluid into vessels. 19 mm Hg pressure is exerted by albumin and 9 mm Hg by cations in plasma. Interstitial osmotic pressure of 8 mm Hg is contributed by interstitial albumin. Interstitial fluid also exerts negative pressure of 3 mm Hg also helps in pulling the fluid into vessels.

Net Effect

Pressure at arterial capillary end (pushing out) is more than at venous end (pulling in). This difference results in leaking of fluid at arterial capillary end. However, 90% of leaked fluid is reabsorbed at venous end because of large venous surface and big pores and remaining 10% is absorbed through lymphatics back into circulation. This is the way balance is maintained in health and no edema results.

Genesis of Edema

It is clear from above mentioned physiology that edema results when there is imbalance in pressures. Increase in hydrostatic pressure and decrease in osmotic pressure pushes fluid out of intravascular compartment. Edema also results in case of capillary leak (as happens in dengue fever) and also due to lymphatic block (lymphedema). In renal conditions, fluid retention and excess of sodium leads to leakage into interstitial spaces and hence edema results. In case of protein malnutrition, decrease in albumin causes edema and so also in liver disease in which excess fluid accumulates in peritoneal cavity due to portal hypertension. In congestive cardiac failure, edema results due to increase in hydrostatic pressure. Capillary leak besides edema, also results in fluid collection in pleural or peritoneal cavity. Lymphatic obstruction as well as venous obstruction leads to localized edema related to site of obstruction. In angiedema, allergic inflammation leaks out fluid locally out of capillaries resulting in local edema (sudden swelling of eyes or lips).

Common Causes of Edema

Renal – acute nephritis and nephrotic syndrome presents with sudden onset of periorbital edema. Patient typically complains of eyelid edema noticed on waking up in the morning. This is because of acute onset edema is first visible in loose connective tissue around eyes and venous congestion around face during sleep makes it appear typically on waking up in the morning.

Angiedema – this is another condition where onset of edema is sudden and so again noticed around eyes in addition to swelling of lips with redness and itching.

Chronic liver disease – presents with edema feet and collection of fluid in peritoneal cavity due to portal hypertension. As onset of edema in liver disease is slow, it manifests on dependent parts on feet. In acute liver disease such as acute hepatitis, there is no edema as half-life of albumin is 2-3 weeks and hence it takes that much long time before edema manifests.

Congestive cardiac failure presents with edema feet as edema develops slowly and so seen on dependent parts over feet in an ambulant patient. In non-ambulant patient, it may be seen on sacral area – dependent part of the body in lying down position. Though sacral edema is not noticed by patient

Protein malnutrition (PEM) presents as edema feet often of acute onset. This is because subclinical hypoproteinemia exists over time but a trigger such as acute diarrhea manifests edema simulating acute onset. Unlike acute onset edema in an apparently normal individual in a renal disease, acute onset edema in PEM manifests in a chronically sick individual.

Capillary leak syndrome presents with edema in dependent parts but spread fast to serous cavities.

Lymphatic or venous obstruction at a particular site presents with localized edema (say of one leg only) as against generalized edema (both legs).

Myxedema is seen in hypothyroidism and **lipedema** in morbid obese patient. Edema is non-pitting in these conditions and so also in chronic lymphatic obstruction due to thickening of accumulated lymph (as in chronic filariasis).

Clinical Approach

Detailed history – Assess whether edema is generalized or localized. Obviously causes would vary.

Onset of edema – acute onset edema noticed around eyes is mostly due to acute renal disease and also may be seen in angiedema (it is localized and with itching, redness). Capillary leak syndrome may also develop edema in a short time including in serous cavities. Slow onset of edema is classical in other conditions such as liver, cardiac diseases and PEM (latter condition seem to manifest acute edema but in reality, it is subclinical edema triggered by an event such as diarrhea)

Degree of edema – severe sudden onset edema is typical of nephrotic syndrome referred to as anasarca. Rarely it may be seen in late stages of other disorders in young children.

Urine output – oliguria is seen in acute nephritis along with high colored urine due to hematuria. Oliguria may also appear in dehydrated state due to poor intake or loss of fluids as in diarrhea and also seen in cardiac failure due to poor renal perfusion and in severe intravascular constriction due to massive edema in liver disease or capillary leak.

High colored urine may be due to hematuria, jaundice and also concentrated urine due to dehydration.

Accompanying symptoms would pinpoint to a specific organ involvement such as jaundice in liver disease, breathlessness and palpitation in cardiac disease and irritability or lethargy in PEM.

Physical examination: It is necessary to confirm pitting edema by transient pressure over bony surface such as shin of tibia. Edema is pitting in most conditions though it may be non-pitting in hypothyroidism and chronic lymphatic obstruction.

State of health offers clue. Comfortable child with massive edema is typical of nephrotic syndrome. Child is acutely sick looking in capillary leak syndrome while chronic sick look is seen in liver, cardiac diseases or in PEM. Ascites is typical of chronic liver disease and may be seen in nephrotic syndrome and capillary leak along with pleural effusion.

Other signs such as systemic hypertension would suggest a renal disease, jaundice and hepatomegaly a chronic liver disease, enlarged liver also in cardiac disorder due to congestive cardiac failure, cardiomegaly and heart murmur indicative of cardiac disease and signs of PEM such as skin, hair and mental changes denoting severe protein malnutrition.

Investigations

Provisional diagnosis would help in ordering specific investigations. Urinalysis and biochemistry in renal disease, urine for bile salts and pigments and liver function tests in liver disease, chest X-ray, ECG and 2D echo cardiogram in cardiac disease are main investigations. Other tests would depend on primary conditions.

Management

Edema per se rarely needs drug therapy and so management is focused on primary organ disease. Diuretics should not be routine prescription for every edema and choice of diuretic may also depend on type of disease. In severe edema due to nephrotic syndrome, diuretic is rarely required as it may lead to intravascular constriction with further damage to kidneys and hence cautious approach is necessary. Diuretics may be useful in cardiac failure and certainly not in PEM.

Take Home Message

Edema is a presenting symptom of a renal disease, angioneurotic edema or localized venous or lymphatic obstruction. Edema is not a presenting symptom in liver or heart disease and protein malnutrition as these diseases present with other symptoms in which edema is often noticed by the doctor. Sudden weight gain may be due to edema that is missed on physical examination. It is not difficult to find the cause of edema clinically.

MCQa

1. This fluid is not in balance with fluid in other sites

A) Interstitial
B) Intracellular
C) Transcellular
D) Intravascular

2. Which of the following statement is WRONG? Edema results from

A) Increased capillary pressure
B) Increased capillary permeability
C) lymphatic obstruction
D) None of the above

3. Which of the following statement is WRONG? Ascites in case of generalized edema is seen in

A) Cirrhosis of liver
B) Protein malnutrition
C) Nephrotic syndrome
D) Capillary leak

4. Which of the following statement is WRONG? Oliguria may be present in

A) Nephrotic syndrome
B) Cardiac failure
C) Capillary leak
D) Myxedema

5. This patient is well and happy in spite of edema

A) Capillary leak
B) Nephrotic syndrome
C) Protein malnutrition
D) Angiedema

Answers to MCQs

Correct answers as follows:

Q1 C	Q2 D	Q3 B	Q4 D	Q5 B

47 Edema – Timely Intervention a Need!

Clinical Application of Basic Concepts

Edema results from various factors such as increased hydrostatic pressure, reduced osmotic pressure, increased permeability of capillaries and lymphatic or venous obstruction. Fluid collects in interstitial spaces and serous cavities. Understanding pathogenesis helps in defining probable cause of edema and relevant timely intervention. Acute onset edema in a normal individual is first perceived in loose connective tissue around eyes before it is noticed elsewhere as happens typically in acute renal disease and angiedema. Chronic cardiac disorders present with edema on dependent parts – legs in an ambulatory persons while chronic liver disease has localizing fluid collection in peritoneal cavity – ascites besides edema of legs. Protein-calorie malnutrition may manifest edema suddenly, triggered by minor illness such as diarrhea. Edema in an acutely sick child may represent capillary leak as seen in dengue fever. Localized edema is due to venous or lymphatic obstruction.

Case-Based Discussion

Case 1

Eight year old child presented with acute onset of edema of eyelids noticed one morning on waking up. On next day, he developed breathlessness. On direct questioning, he had oliguria and cola colored urine.

Acute onset of periorbital edema with oliguria and cola colored urine suggestive of hematuria is in favor of acute glomerulonephritis - AGN. Breathlessness in this child may be due to hypertension a result of AGN.

Physical examination showed mild edema feet and around eyes, HR 140/min, RR 35/min, BP 150/100 mm Hg, systemic examination normal. It is diagnostic of **Acute glomerulonephritis**. Investigations – urinalysis RBCs ++, granular casts +, proteins +, serum creatinine 1.8 mg%, ASO high titer.

In children > 5 year of age, it is most likely due to post-streptococcal infection and if so, prognosis is very good. Improvement is quick with symptomatic treatment though microscopic hematuria may continue for few weeks. To confirm improving situation, serum C3 level should be ordered. It is low at the peak of illness, starts rising during recovery. If

C3 level continues to be low, it may indicate chronicity of the disease and needs referral to a specialist. If AGN presents in younger child, it may be due to other infections and prognosis may be guarded.

Case 2

Four year old child presented with acute onset of edema around eyes. There were no other symptoms. On direct questioning, urine output was normal and urine was colorless. However, child had itching and redness around the swelling that also spread to lips.

This suggests **angiedema** – allergic process and not renal disease.

Physical examination showed edema around both lower eyelids looking pink. There was no edema anywhere else, Blood pressure was normal and so also heart and respiratory rate, systemic examination was normal.

There is no need for any investigations or any drug therapy. It settles down by itself. Antihistamines and steroids are not necessary unless child presents with laryngeal edema causing inspiratory obstruction, it is rare.

Case 3

One year old infant presented with loose stools for two days followed by acute onset edema of face and feet. He was born after full term and normal delivery with birth weight of 2.6 kg. He was on exclusive breast feeding for first 6 months and thereafter mother started dilute cow milk and occasional watery mixture of rice and dal.

Diet history clearly suggest inadequate intake of calories and proteins for last 6 months and hence edema is likely to be due to nutritional deficiency – PEM. His subclinical deficiency must have been precipitated by episode of loose stools and thus edema developed acutely though he must have had low serum proteins even before episode of loose stools. Physical examination showed wt 9 kg, length 70 cms, head O 45 cms, lethargic but irritable on disturbance, edema feet ++, abdomen distended, liver 3F +, firm, liver span 7 cms, spleen not palpable, no ascites, other systems normal, Diagnosis of **protein energy malnutrition** is evident. There is no need of investigations to prove the diagnosis, however one may look for other deficiencies such as anemia and also evidence of any occult infection such as tuberculosis or urinary tract infection.

Treatment revolves around resuscitation in case of severe PEM, restoration of deficiencies, rehabilitation and prevention by proper counselling.

It is important to note that acute onset edema in this child occurred in a poorly growing child and hence, it suggests occult hypoproteinemia that became manifest with acute diarrhea. Thus, this is a chronic disease manifesting acute edema as against a renal disease with acute onset edema in a healthy child.

Case 4

Ten year old child presented with oliguria and cola colored urine for last few days. Physical examination showed minimal edema feet and investigations suggested diagnosis of glomerulonephritis.

While diagnosis of glomerulonephritis is acceptable, it seems to be different than classical post-streptococcal acute glomerulonephritis. Hence it was decided follow this child clinically and also with repeat serum C3 level.

Physical examination showed persistent mild edema feet, oliguria and hematuria. Also, his blood pressure revealed increasing though on 95th centile for age. It suggests development of hypertension.

C3 level continued to be low even at the end of 6 weeks of persistent glomerulonephritis. It suggested diagnosis of **chronic glomerulonephritis**.

This child should be referred to a specialist for further management that may need renal biopsy to define probable cause and prognosticate the disease.

This case illustrates the need for clinical suspicion of unusual type of glomerulonephritis and value of serum C3 level in follow-up of acute glomerulonephritis. Besides clinical abnormality, persistent low C3 level is a marker for need for referral. This case represents the way a generalist should pick-up an atypical course of a disease with timely referral to a specialist. If missed, patient often presents with chronic persistent disease which is obvious but too late.

Case 5

Two year old child presented with acute onset edema noticed first around eyelids that was followed 12 hours later with generalized edema all over the body. There was no history of oliguria, high colored urine or any other symptoms. Sudden development of generalized edema without any prior symptoms and edema starting around eyes suggests renal glomerular pathology. In view of absence of oliguria or high colored urine and massive edema favor glomerular epithelial pathology such as nephrotic syndrome.

Physical examination showed comfortable child, happy and active, blood pressure 90/50 mm Hg with massive generalized edema, abdominal distension with ascites but without hepatosplenomegaly. There were no other findings. These findings suggest severe hypoproteinemia that has led to massive generalized edema and also ascites but without endothelial glomerular involvement as evident by absence of oliguria, high colored urine or hypertension.

Investigations showed urine protein +++, urine – creatinine protein ratio of 3, serum proteins 4.2 Gm%, albumin 1 Gm%,, globulin 3.2 Gm%, serum cholesterol 320 mg and creatinine 0.5 mg.

Massive proteinuria and albuminuria, hypercholesterolemia and normal serum creatinine favor diagnosis of **minimal lesion nephrotic syndrome.**

Management consists of oral prednisolone 2 mg/kg/day for 4-6 weeks followed by two third total dose on alternate day for 4 weeks. Such a prolonged therapy during first attack offers better chance of complete remission without further relapse. However in case of relapse, similar therapy needs to be given but for shorter period.

Minimal lesion indicates pathology restricted to epithelium of glomerulus. It typically presents for the first time between 2 and 5 years of age and carries usually good prognosis in spite of relapses. If this child develops diarrhea, there may also be oliguria due to dehydration and urine color also may be high colored. Diarrhea in such a child may be due to edema of intestinal mucosa that leads to malabsorption but may also be due to infection.

However, if such a child presents in later childhood (unusual age) or has oliguria and hypertension but with massive edema, it may suggest primary glomerular epithelial disease (because of massive edema) that has also involved glomerular endothelium (because of oliguria and hypertension). This is referred to as complicated nephrotic syndrome and needs referral to a specialist.

Case 6

Two year old child presented with history of fever and macular skin rash over last three days. Considering it to be viral infection, symptomatic treatment was given and fever abated. However very next day, child started vomiting and had severe abdominal pain. This was followed by edema feet and abdominal distension. On direct questioning, child had not passed urine for last 12 hours.

Initial symptoms do suggest viral infection but it did lead to unexpected symptoms of vomiting and abdominal pain. It indicates immune mediated complication and not extended viral infection as original symptoms had totally disappeared. Sudden abdominal pain along with vomiting suggests probable vascular complication involving intestines that is immune mediated. As child had not passed urine, it may denote shock and so abdominal pain is due to severe intestinal ischemia. This suggests capillary leak syndrome. Physical examination showed child in shock with cold extremities, pale skin, marked tachycardia, low blood pressure, mild edema feet, ascites and also mild pleural effusion. This is classical of **capillary leak syndrome** following probable dengue viral infection. Investigations confirmed dengue fever. Child was treated aggressively for shock and recovered in next two days. This case illustrates how primary infection may get better but lead to immune mediated complications within a day or two of apparent cure of primary infection. Such a situation cannot be anticipated but every child should be observed for 2-3 days after apparent cure for such a possible complication. If diagnosed in time, child can be saved. Rarely, such immune mediated complications may manifest even after few weeks of primary viral infection (Covid 19 pandemic is an example).

Case 7

8 year old child presented with history of progressive abdominal distension over last 6 months and edema of feet noticed over last two months. He had lost 3 kg weight and had poor appetite.

This looks to be chronic progressive disorder as evident by loss of weight over few months. Abdominal distension could be due to organomegaly (commonly enlarged liver with or without spleen) or ascites. Further development of edema feet in this case indicates chronic liver disease. In absence of jaundice, it may be well compensated liver disease (means liver has not failed though poorly functioning).

Physical examination showed chronically sick looking child, edema feet +, abdominal distension, liver 3 cms +, firm, liver span 9 cms +, spleen 2 cms +, no ascites, no jaundice, other systems normal

Firm and enlarged liver with splenomegaly favors chronic liver disease with portal hypertension. Absence of ascites, bleeding or encephalopathy suggests well compensated chronic liver disease such as **cirrhosis.**

Investigations – Hb 9 Gm%, serum proteins 5.2 Gm%, albumin 2.4 Gm%, globulin 2.8 Gm%, ALT (SGPT) 210, AST (SGOT) 160, Serum bilirubin 0.9 mg.

There is marked hypoalbuminemia with mild rise in liver enzymes with normal bilirubin. (Bilirubin is increased only when more than 85% of liver cells are damaged and so in chronic liver disease, increased bilirubin or jaundice suggests liver gradually failing. However in acute hepatitis, increased bilirubin does not mean failing liver).

Diagnosis of cirrhosis can be confirmed by liver biopsy. Management is palliative.

Hypoalbuminemia in a patient with enlarged liver is a marker of chronic liver disease and should be picked up even before edema manifests. It is rare to find hypoalbuminemia in acute liver disease unless such an acute liver disease occurs in an individual with occult asymptomatic liver pathology such as obesity, undernutrition and hepatitis B infection carrier state.

Case 8

10 year old child presented with history of breathlessness and edema feet over last few days. On direct questioning, he used to feel breathless on exertion but had ignored the same. There was no past history of any major disease. This child seems to be having slowly progressive cardiac disease and now presenting with failure as evident by breathlessness and edema feet.

Physical examination showed sick child, HR 120/min, RR 27/min, BP 120/60 mm Hg, mild edema feet, engorged neck veins with positive hepatojugular reflex, apex beat on 6th intercostal space outside midclavicular line, systolic murmur at mitral area conducted to axilla.

These findings suggest **mitral regurgitation with CCF**. It is mostly due to Rheumatic disease though there is no past history of throat infection or arthritis. (Throat infection may often be mild or even asymptomatic and so not reported). Diagnosis can be confirmed by chest X-ray, ECG and 2D echocardiogram (showing active valvulitis) and etiology indicated by high anti-streptolysin O titer.

If this is active carditis, it is treated with steroids followed by aspirin and further long acting penicillin to prevent relapses. Besides, symptomatic therapy for CCF is necessary.

Edema in cardiac failure denotes right sided failure. It is not a common finding in congenital heart disease but may be seen in chronic acquired heart disease due to rheumatic fever. Most other cardiac conditions present with either left ventricular or biventricular failure. Isolated right sided failure is nature's way to avoid left sided failure and is possible only in chronic disorders where nature has time to compensate.

Take Home Message

Analysis of edema illustrates importance of chief complaint. If edema is a chief complaint, it is mostly renal in origin whereas most other conditions present with other symptoms in which edema is often noticed by the doctor. Angiedema is an exception and presents acutely in a healthy child. Final diagnosis is easy in terms of system affected and further can be confirmed by physical examination and necessary investigations.

MCQs

1. Which of the following statements is wrong related to classical post-streptococcal acute glomerulonephritis?

A) Typical age group is beyond 5 years
B) Microscopic hematuria may persist for weeks
C) Edema and oliguria improve quickly
D) Prognosis is guarded

2. Urinalysis is completely normal in spite of edema

A) Acute nephritis
B) Cardiac failure
C) Angiedema
D) Liver disease

3. Child with edema may be breathless in

A) Acute nephritis
B) Nephrotic syndrome
C) Angiedema
D) All of the above

4. Which of the following statement is wrong? Relapse is possible in

A) Nephrotic syndrome
B) Cardiac failure
C) Cirrhosis
D) Protein malnutrition

5. Blood pressure may be abnormal in this child with edema

A) Nephrotic syndrome
B) Capillary leak
C) Cardiac failure
D) All of the above

Answers to MCQs

Correct answers as follows:

Q1 D	Q2 C	Q3 D	Q4 C	Q5 D

48 Bulging Abdomen –Sign of Ill-Health!

Back to Basics – Abdominal Distension

What is Abdominal Distension?

Distension refers to enlargement, dilation or ballooning effect and when applied to abdominal distension, it commonly relates to intra-abdominal space occupation or swelling but also may be related to abdominal wall. It is a subjective observation by the patient or a doctor but abdominal girth can be measured, specially to monitor progress in generalized abdominal distension. Patients often complain of bloating – a sensation of fullness and tightness attributed to "gas". Localized abdominal distension usually presents as swelling in a part of abdomen. Abdomen of normal young infant is protuberant due to liver and spleen being accommodated in the abdomen unlike in an adult in whom these organs are mostly in the chest.

Causes of Abdominal Distension

There are several causes of abdominal distension that can be grouped – most of the words describing these groups start from alphabet F – feces, flatus, fat, fetus, fluid, flab (flabby abdominal muscles), food and functional. Other causes include organomegaly (enlarged liver and/or spleen) and any other space occupying lesions such as tumor or cyst. Each of these disorders may result from varied causes.

Defining Causes in Each Group

Feces (often along with accumulation of flatus) leading to abdominal distension may be acute as in intestinal obstruction or paralytic ileus due to sepsis or hypokalemia and also may be chronic as in case of subacute intestinal obstruction due to congenital megacolon or intestinal tuberculosis. One of the most common causes is habitual constipation due to low fiber in the diet and poor bowel habits. It may also be caused by inadequate food intake or intestinal disorders such as irritable bowel syndrome or inflammatory bowel disease, dyspepsia (indigestion) or systemic disorders such as diabetes and hypothyroidism.

Flatus (retained gas) may also be caused by all above mentioned disorders besides lactose intolerance and aerophagy.

Fluid in abdomen may lie free in peritoneal cavity (ascites) or may be localized (mesenteric or ovarian cyst). Ascites fluid may be transudate (non-inflammatory) as in case of portal hypertension and nephrotic syndrome or exudate (inflammatory) as in case of peritonitis or malignancy.

Organomegaly (enlarged liver with or without splenomegaly) may be due to primary liver or hematological diseases, systemic infections or storage disorders.

Flab (flabby abdominal muscles) may result from malnutrition due to loss of muscle mass or generalized poor muscle tone. Stretched abdominal muscles for longer period as in pregnancy may also result in flabby abdominal muscles.

Food may lead to abdominal distension due to indigestion, constipation, food intolerance or allergy.

Functional disorders may result in abdominal distension due to gut-brain interaction. This is a result of mental stress or anxiety in a susceptible individual who cannot cope up with it. It is now clear that emotions are controlled by gut while brain is responsible for action. During anticipated stress situation (student appearing for examination), one may get urge to pass stool or urine once more. If one sees something frightful, intestines cramp, it is a result of gut-brain interaction. And in colloquial English language, we say "it is my gut feeling". This is how gut-brain interaction results in various intestinal disorders. Bloating – a sensation of fullness in abdomen may not be due to accumulation of gas (flatus) but even without gas. This is due to contraction of diaphragm (result of gut-brain interaction) that pushes liver and spleen into abdomen resulting in abdominal distension. Fat and fetus are easy to make out.

Localized swelling if very large, especially retroperitoneal, may present as abdominal distension but if lies anteriorly in the abdomen, it is complained of as lump in abdomen. Typically enlarged spleen presents as lump in left hypochondrium.

Clinical Approach

Detailed history analysis and focused physical examination can offer provisional diagnosis.

Onset may be acute in surgical or metabolic diseases while gradual in many other conditions.

Progression helps to define probable cause, Waxing and waning abdominal distension suggests either constipation or gaseous distension. Progressive generalized distension for few days but remaining stable thereafter indicates probable ascites while organomegaly or other tumors/cysts may present as slowly progressive localized abdominal distension over several weeks.

Accompanying symptoms such as vomiting, constipation, diarrhea, abdominal pain, pallor, jaundice help to localize the disease to a specific organ and also define probable pathology.

Personal history of loss of appetite or weight, sleep and behavior disturbances offer clue to diagnosis and so also past, family and drug therapy history.

Site of abdominal distension – generalized or localized.

Shape of distended abdomen in case of generalized abdominal distension, flank fullness suggests fluid (ascites) while distension mainly in upper part of abdomen as depicted by downward displacement of umbilicus indicates enlarged liver (distance between xiphisternum and umbilicus is much more than distance between umbilicus and symphysis pubis – normally umbilicus is placed midway between xiphisternum and symphysis pubis).

Percussion can differentiate between gaseous distension (tympanic note) and fluid (dull note) and further ascites is confirmed by demonstration of shifting dullness whereas absence of shifting dullness suggests encysted fluid as in case of mesenteric or ovarian cyst.

Localized distension in a particular quadrant of abdomen is related to organs in that quadrant. Thus, enlarged spleen presents as lump in abdomen in left hypochondrium and swelling increasing across to right iliac fossa. Enlarged kidney presents as lump in lumbar region and appendicular lump in right iliac fossa.(Neuroblastoma and Wilms tumor are other causes of localizes swelling). Wilms tumor does not cross midline while neuroblastoma often spreads across the abdomen. (Tumor due to neuroblastoma may not be palpable and at times even not picked up on routine imaging). Large lymph node mass present in the middle of abdomen. Enlarged liver may not present as localized abdominal distension unless large enough, especially in older children and adults.

Consistency relates to duration and pathology of disease. Firm hepatomegaly suggests chronic process while hard liver or any mass indicates probable malignancy. Soft swelling may suggest cyst or softening lymph nodes.

Pain and Tenderness indicate inflammatory process or stretching of capsule as in case of enlarged liver or lymph nodes. Congested liver as in congestive cardiac failure is also tender, though chronic congestion may not cause pain.

Other systems affection may offer clue to probable cause. Hematological diseases may present with pallor, purpura, bony tenderness or generalized lymphadenopathy. Tender enlarged liver with engorgement of neck veins and hepatojugular reflex suggests congestive cardiac failure while congested liver due to constrictive pericarditis is often missed as it presents as enlarged liver without hepatojugular reflex and obvious cardiac symptoms.

Neurological manifestation may suggest neurometabolic disorders that present with hepatosplenomegaly and abdominal distension as in case of Gaucher or Nimman-Pick disease.

Investigations

Provisional diagnosis is a prerequisite to planning investigations that would help in minimizing tests. Acute abdominal distension demands abdominal X-ray in erect position to rule out intestinal obstruction. USG of abdomen is useful in variety of conditions causing abdominal distension. Biochemical tests are reserved for specific organ involvement. Ascites tap can help in differentiating exudate from transudate by serum ascites albumin gradient. Histopathological diagnosis is important in chronic liver disease as well as tumors.

Treatment

It is possible only when final diagnosis has been reached. Few conditions may be amenable to surgery or drugs while palliative therapy is possible for some other conditions.

Take Home Message

Acute onset of abdominal distension is usually a surgical disease in a sick individual while one that presents over few days (may be in a sick person) or weeks (often in non-sick individual) is usually due to medical disorders. Localized swelling relates to the organs occupying in a particular quadrant while generalized distension is due to accumulation of gas (tympanic note on percussion) or fluid (dull note on percussion and shifting dullness). Occasionally, very large mass may present as generalized abdominal distension.

MCQs

1. Which of the following statement is WRONG? Abdominal distension exists without intra-abdominal pathology in

A) Normal infant
B) Malnourished child
C) Obese child
D) None of the above

2. Which of the following statement is WRONG? Abdominal distension waxes and wanes over short time in

A) Aerophagia
B) Malnutrition
C) Subacute intestinal obstruction
D) Habitual constipation

3. This condition presents with chronic abdominal distension due to constipation

A) Congenital megacolon
B) Acute intestinal obstruction
C) Paralytic ileus
D) Intestinal tuberculosis

4. Ascites is a feature of

A) Abdominal tuberculosis
B) Capillary leak syndrome
C) Portal hypertension
D) All of the above

5. Most useful parameter in examination of ascites fluid is

A) Cell count
B) Protein content
C) Serum ascites albumin gradient
D) Sugar content

Answers to MCQs

Correct answers as follows:

Q1 D	Q2 C	Q3 A	Q4 D	Q5 C

49 Abdominal Distension – Don't Ignore

Clinical Application of Basic Concepts

Abdominal distension may be generalized due to accumulation of gas, collection of fluid or chronic constipation with accumulation of feces. Distension caused by flatus or feces wax and wane while there is no variation in other conditions. Typically, enlarged liver presents as upper abdominal distension that displaces umbilicus downwards from its usual mid-position. Enlarged spleen or any other mass in abdomen presents as lump in a specific quadrant of abdomen. Surgical conditions leading to abdominal distension are usually acute while medical conditions are often chronic. Of course, there are exceptions on both side such as, congenital megacolon a chronic surgical problem and paralytic ileus following diarrhea as acute medical problem. Hypotonia of abdominal muscles and excess of abdominal fat may also lead to abdominal distension though it is not a primary presentation.

Case-Based Discussion

Case 1

8 year old child presented with periumbilical pain and generalized abdominal distension for 2 days. It was accompanied with mild fever, occasional vomit and loose stool. Vomitus contained food particles and not bile stained. Sudden onset of abdominal pain and abdominal distension suggest acute inflammatory pathology and occasional vomit and loose stool rules out primary intestinal disease but related to structure near to intestine. Had it been a primary intestinal disease, loose stools and/or vomit would have been prominent symptoms. Acute infection in a healthy child generally presents with high fever, though low grade infection may cause low grade fever. It may also be non-infective inflammatory disease.

Physical examination on D2 showed a sick looking child and generalized abdominal distension, tenderness all over and guarding. It denotes oncoming acute inflammatory condition. Next day pain shifted to right iliac fossa and became severe. Diagnosis of **acute appendicitis** was considered and proved on USG.

Parents refuse surgery and next day, pain disappeared. Does it suggest sudden natural recovery?

On physical examination, child looked much more sick, HR 140, BP 80/50 mmHg, CRT > 4 seconds, child was in shock. This suggests appendix had developed **gangrene** and so pain disappeared but child went into shock endangering life. This case illustrates a fact that symptom relief may not be all well and we should go by overall condition.

Visceral abdominal pain is diffuse, not severe and often accompanied with occasional vomiting or loose stools while parietal pain is severe and localized. This is why pain in appendicitis starts near umbilicus (appendix originates from midgut and hence initial location of pain) and then when peritoneum is involved, pain shifts to right iliac fossa and becomes severe. It is classic of acute appendicitis.

Case 2

One year old infant presented with gradually progressive abdominal distension. He was breast-fed for first 7 months and then also on semisolid food. On direct questioning, he was constipated from first month, had not gained weight over last few months. His development was normal. Breast-fed infant is never constipated unless there is something abnormal. Progressive abdominal distension and failure to gain weight are both a result of worsening constipation. This is likely to be chronic progressive lower intestinal obstruction, mostly congenital megacolon. Physical examination showed weight 7.2 kg, length 70 cm, moderate pallor, abdomen loaded with feces, per rectal examination revealed empty rectum and ribbon like stool coming out, suggesting colonic obstruction proximal to rectum. Diagnosis was conformed as **congenital megacolon** by barium enema and rectal biopsy showing absent ganglion cells. He was surgically treated.

Intestinal obstruction generally presents as an acute event but it may also be intermittent as in case of subacute intestinal obstruction due to intestinal tuberculosis. It is important to note that breast-fed infant is never constipated and this case is an example of chronic progressive intestinal obstruction in a breast-fed infant. Constipation in congenital megacolon may be initially considered to be due to habitual constipation though failure to thrive and persistent abdominal distension are the clues to a pathological problem.

Case 3

One year old infant presented with loose stools and abdominal distension for 2 days. Loose stools stopped suddenly but abdominal distension worsened. There was no vomiting or any other symptom.

When any symptom suddenly and unexpectedly gets better, it is often indicative of a complication. In this child, loose stools suddenly stopped, which may suggest either intussusception or paralytic ileus. Intussusception presents as abdominal pain and vomiting and so not likely in this child. Paralytic ileus may be a manifestation of sepsis or hypokalemia. As this child has had no fever, sepsis is not likely and so it may be hypokalemia.

Physical examination on D3 showed a malnourished child, HR 120/min RR 25/min generalized abdominal distension, poor peristalsis, muscle hypotonia, deep tendon reflexes sluggish. Disproportionate tachycardia, muscle hypotonia and sluggish DTR suggest hypokalemia. Potassium is intracellular ion and so its deficiency affects skeletal and heart muscle besides intestinal muscle. That explains tachycardia and sluggish DTR. Serum potassium was low and the diagnosis of **hypokalemia** was confirmed. The child was treated with IV potassium – it is only an extreme situation that one needs to use IV potassium and that too with caution. Oral potassium supplements are ideal in the form of coconut water to prevent such hypokalemia, especially in malnourished children and elderly persons.

If a healthy child suffers from diarrhea, transient hypokalemia settles down by itself but as this child was malnourished having low potassium, hypokalemia after diarrhea may be life-threatening due to cardiac rhythm dysfunction or severe muscle paralysis affecting respiratory muscles. Such a complication may need potassium supplements urgently.

Potassium is excreted by the kidney only if it is in excess but it is also secreted continuously by renal tubules irrespective of potassium pool in the body. That is why person may feel tired even after short duration of illness such as viral fever or diarrhea. In a healthy individual, it settles down by itself in next 2-3 days.

Case 4

Two years old child presented with fever and skin rash for 2 days. Fever abated but child developed abdominal distension and became sicker.

Fever and skin rash suggests viral infection that seemed to settle by itself as expected. Whenever new symptoms appear unexpectedly while original symptoms get better, this is likely to be either metabolic or immune mediated complication. As this child also got sicker, it is likely to be immune reaction to viral infection. Sudden development of abdominal distension denotes fluid collection – ascites due to capillary leak. Sickness in such a case is due to development of shock. Physical examination showed signs of shock, mild edema of feet and ascites. It suggests diagnosis of **capillary leak syndrome** following dengue viral infection that can be confirmed with NS1 antigen and IgM antibodies.

Such a complication must be diagnosed in its early stage of compensation as denoted by poor urine output and change in behavior of the child in spite of fever abating. At this stage, there are no obvious signs of shock and child can recover with IV fluids maintaining intravascular volume till capillary leak stops naturally. However once uncompensated shock develops with low blood pressure, it may be irreversible.

Any infection may trigger excessive immune response that may appear few days after fever disappears or even may occur with continuation of fever. Any unexpected course of events in a given infection should alert a physician about such a complication.

Case 5

8 year old child presented with abdominal distension for a week. There were no other symptoms.

Acute onset of abdominal distension would have other symptoms such as vomiting/ constipation in case of intestinal obstruction or fever, skin rash in case of capillary leak syndrome or diarrhea preceding abdominal distension. As this child did not report any such symptoms, on direct questioning, it was revealed that he was not well for the past 5 months with loss of appetite and weight as well as mild abdominal distension. So, it is clear now that this child has a chronic disease that seems to have developed worsening abdominal distension over the last week. It suggests ascites in a child with chronic liver disease.

Physical examination showed weight 23 kg, height 120 cm, mild pallor, edema feet, no jaundice, liver 4F +, firm, not tender, span 9 cm, spleen 2F +, ascites +.

These findings are in favor of chronic liver disease – cirrhosis with ascites. The cause may be either exposure to poisons such as alcohol or previous infections such as HBV or HCV. Laboratory investigations showed serum bilirubin 1.2 mg D 0.6 mg ALT 230 AST 180 Alk phos normal Serum proteins 5.3 Gm%, Albumin 2.1 Gm%.

Diagnosis of **cirrhosis** is made that can be proved by liver biopsy and further tests to assess the probable cause. Treatment is merely symptomatic.

This case illustrates the importance of detailed history that should always begin with assessing whether the patient was genuinely normal prior to the onset of a recent problem. This is because minor symptoms existing before the onset of major symptoms are often ignored by patients or relatives and not reported unless asked for it specifically. The best way to ensure that a patient was completely well prior to the onset of present problem is to inquire about activity, energy, appetite, sleep, behavior, bowel and urination – in short detailed personal history. Minor symptom does present with change in one or more of these factors.

Case 6

10 year old child presented with gradually increasing generalized abdominal distension over last 6 months. There were no other symptoms. He remained healthy during this time.

This child seems to have slowly progressive space occupying lesion in abdomen that has not caused any organ dysfunction. So, it must be a benign condition. As abdominal distension was generalized, it may be either ascites or very large mass. Ascites would have presented with other symptoms as generalized edema in nephrotic syndrome or other symptoms as in chronic liver disease. Both are unlikely in this child. Very large benign mass is possible though it could have produced pressure on some organs with some symptoms. So at this stage, history clearly suggests benign intra-abdominal mass.

Physical examination showed healthy normal child with generalized abdominal distension with dullness all over but without shifting dullness. Though rarely, shifting dullness may be absent in case of very large ascites. So, this child has fluid containing mass that means cyst. Abdominal USG confirmed it to be a **mesenteric cyst.** It was removed surgically.

This case illustrates a fact that patient or in this case, mother of a child was giving a clue by stating that there was slowly progressive abdominal distension over last six months. Ascites does not present in this way over such a long period. It is always right to believe what patient says as it is rarely proved wrong. It is especially true when mother reports about her child.

Case 7

8 year old child presented with gradually progressive abdominal distension over last one year, loss of appetite and weight over last 6 months and feeling tired over last 3 months.

This is slowly progressive disease with probable hepatosplenomegaly and lately has developed severe anemia as suggested by feeling of tiredness. So disease must have started in liver and/or spleen and now spread to bone marrow. Such a disease is likely to be due to storage of abnormal metabolites – metabolic disorder.

Physical examination showed wasted and stunted child with severe pallor, liver 3F +, firm, span 10 cm, spleen 5F +, no ascites or jaundice.

Such a massive enlargement of liver and spleen without any liver dysfunction is typical of storage disorder that has spread to bone marrow and hence severe anemia.

Laboratory tests showed Hb 5 Gm%, WBC 2300 Pl 0.4 lakhs, LFT normal, USG showed large liver and spleen, no evidence of portal hypertension.

Further specific enzyme studies confirmed diagnosis of **Gaucher disease.**

If diagnosed early before significant damage, enzyme replacement is possible though such a therapy is very costly. Once disease spread to brain, there would be no use of enzyme replacement therapy.

Progressive abdominal distension over months are broadly of three types – present without disturbed health as in case of mesenteric cyst/benign tumor or with hepatosplenomegaly and growth failure but without liver dysfunction as in storage disorder or with abnormal liver functions as in cirrhosis with portal hypertension and ascites.

Case 8

8 year old child presented with abdominal distension off and on for last 6 months. Abdominal distension would be waxing and waning and he also had occasional loose stools. He had not lost weight or appetite.

Waxing and waning abdominal distension is either due to flatus or constipation. As this child is not constipated, it must be flatus. It is necessary to find out cause of excessive flatus. As he has remained healthy, it is unlikely to be any significant pathology. It could be due to irregular food habits, life style or due to stress or anxiety – **functional disorder.**

Physical examination did not reveal any abnormality except moderate abdominal distension with tympanic note on percussion suggestive of gas.

This child does not need any tests but needs counseling. It is well known that intestines sense the stress first and sends message to brain to execute appropriate action. Hence, functional disorders are often related to gastrointestinal system and may present as dyspepsia, abdominal pain or distension, change in bowel habits such as diarrhea or constipation, anorexia, nausea and vomiting. Diagnosis of such disorders depend on high index of suspicion in a typical situation aided by exclusion of other pathological conditions. Irritable bowel syndrome is one such example, diagnosis of which is based on standard criteria.

Take Home Message

Acute onset of abdominal distension represents mostly a serious problem unless it is waxing and waning. Chronic persistent abdominal distension is caused by either fluid, organomegaly or tumor. Accompanying symptoms guide to a probable cause and physical examination can finetune the diagnosis with relevant specific tests. Non-specific abdominal USG findings such as lymph nodes, free fluid, gaseous distension of intestines, calcification in the liver or thickened urinary bladder need cautious clinical correlation.

MCQs

1. This surgical condition is not chronic

A) Appendicitis
B) Intestinal obstruction due to TB
C) Congenital megacolon
D) Obstructed hernia

2. This condition with abdominal distension does not present with pain

A) Inflammatory bowel disease
B) Intestinal TB
C) Storage disorder
D) Functional problem

3. Which of the following statement is WRONG?

A) Ascites may be due to liver disease
B) Ascites may not be due to liver disease
C) Ascites may occur without liver disease
D) None of the above

4. Paralytic ileus may result from

A) Acute diarrhea
B) Sepsis
C) Electrolyte disturbance
D) All of the above

5. Which test may be abnormal in abdominal distension due to functional disorder?

A) Stool microscopy
B) Abdominal USG
C) Colonoscopy
D) None of the above

Answers to MCQs

Correct answers as follows:

Q1 D	Q2 C	Q3 D	Q4 D	Q5 B

50 My Child Suddenly Became Stiff!

Back to Basics – Seizure

What is Seizure?

Brain is like an electrical network in which neurons (nerve cells) communicate with each other through electrical signals to generate multiple functions. Disturbance in this electrical circuit leads to a sudden abnormal event that is referred to as seizure. It is different than a convulsion. Convulsion is a seizure affecting motor cortex with tonic (stiffness) or clonic (jerky movements).

What Goes Wrong in Electrical Circuit?

Biochemically, it is the ionic imbalance that leads to either too much of excitatory transmission response or too little of inhibitory response and results in a seizure. Most often ionic balance is restored by nature itself and so seizure stops by itself within 1-2 minutes. Nature rarely fails, but if does happen then seizure continues for longer time and it would need a drug to stop it.

What is the Difference Between Seizure and Convulsion?

Convulsion is a type of seizure which manifests as jerking movements or stiffness of some parts of the body. However, seizure may present without such movements or stiffness because manifestations depend upon which part of the brain is responsible for sudden electrical discharge. Convulsion results when part of the brain that controls voluntary body movements (motor system) is involved. Involvement of other parts of the cerebral cortex do not manifest with convulsion but presents as sudden attack of emotional disturbances if temporal lobe is the site of abnormal electrical discharge or when parietal lobe is involved, result is sensory manifestations. Thus, seizure may not present with convulsion though convulsion is most common type of a seizure and many times, both terms are used interchangeably, though not scientifically correct.

Types of Seizures

They are classified into two major groups – generalized and localized (focal) depending on extent of involvement. Each group is further divided into motor (presents as movements - convulsion) and non-motor (without movements). Generlized seizure always present with loss of consciousness even for a brief period while localized seizure may or may not lose consciousness (focal with impaired awareness or focal aware). At times, localized seizure may spread to other parts and become generalized. Hence it is the onset of seizure that decides focal or generalized. At times it is difficult to classify seizure type as it may be mixed and also may change.

Presentation of Seizure Types

Generalized motor seizure may present as stiffness (tonic), jerky movements (clonic) or both (tonic-clonic), atonic (sudden loss of muscle strength) and myoclonic (muscle spasm). In tonic seizure, spasm of respiratory muscles leads to apnea and cyanosis. In-built neural mechanism breaks this phase, breathing starts and clonic phase begins. Generalized non-motor seizure (absence seizure) presents with very transient lapse of awareness when person stops momentarily and in few seconds. resume what he was doing. Localized (focal) motor seizure presents as abnormal movements of a part of the body with or without loss of consciousness. Focal non-motor presents as emotional change without loss of consciousness.

What is Epilepsy?

Unprovoked recurrent seizures are referred to as epilepsy. Unprovoked means seizure occurs without any apparent trigger factor. It may be idiopathic (cause not known), often genetic or at times secondary to previous brain damage.

Etiology of Seizure

It is classified into acute symptomatic (due to present existing disease), remote symptomatic (due to brain damage resulting from previous disease) or idiopathic (cause not known).

Acute symptomatic seizure – Most common cause is simple febrile seizure. It occurs due to sudden rise in body temperature in a genetically susceptible child. Around 5% of normal children suffer from simple febrile seizure. First episode usually presents between age of 6 months and 2 years though such a seizure may recur even up to the age of 6 years. Seizure typically occurs during first 24 hours of onset of fever, lasts for a minute or less, is self-limiting and child becomes normal without any sequelae. There is no need for treatment though recurrence can be prevented by use of clonazepam (2.5 mg twice a day for 3 doses orally) only during first 24-36 hours of onset of fever along with an antipyretic. (Though control of fever may not prevent a simple febrile seizure and at times, seizure may present before fever is noticed).

Intracranial infection may occur at any age and is accompanied with persistent fever, vomiting and change in sensorium. Such a child needs hospitalization.

Hypocalcemia is another cause that may present in an infant or young toddler having active vitamin D deficiency rickets. This is a seizure that does not end with post-ictal (at the end of seizure) drowsiness. Neonate born with low birth weight may also suffer from hypocalcemia.

Remote symptomatic seizure – It is a result of brain damage caused by previous illness that may have resolved completely though leaving behind epileptogenic focus. Obviously one clue to such remote symptomatic seizure is a child with developmental delay. Birth injury, significant serious head injury, severe brain infections and congenital brain malformations are common causes of remote symptomatic seizure. Treatment consists of using anti-epileptic drugs.

Idiopathic seizure – It occurs in normal brain and may be triggered by subtle event such as minor illness. Often such a seizure may not recur. If recurs, it is termed as idiopathic epilepsy. Modern science may find specific cause for such idiopathic seizure or epilepsy in the form of genetic or biochemical defect. Hence, what has been referred to as idiopathic epilepsy is now being proved to be a genetic disorder.

Seizure mimics – There are several conditions that mimic a seizure and it is important to differentiate them. Such conditions include movement disorders (dystonia) or benign sleep myoclonus, sudden fall (syncope, vertigo), breath-holding spasm. Each of these conditions have typical presentation that is different from a seizure. Most of them retain consciousness.

Clinical Approach

Detailed history of the event is most important. It should be obtained from one who has actually observed the event. Ideally it could be captured on video that helps a lot. This is because onset of seizure is vital to understand nature of seizure. If onset is missed, vital information is lacking. Besides onset, duration, progress and accompanying symptoms offer a clue to probable diagnosis. Seizure preceded by fever may be simple febrile seizure or fever triggered hypocalcemic seizure (both of them recover quickly) or intracranial infection (that is accompanied with vomiting and change in sensorium). Seizure without fever may be remote symptomatic (abnormal brain function) or idiopathic (cause unkown).

Physical examination can detect abnormal neurological findings if any and whether these findings denote active disease or old disease. Normal neurological status suggests either simple febrile convulsion or hypocalcemia that leaves no sequelae. Child with active meningitis is sick besides neck rigidity and drowsiness whereas those with remote symptomatic seizures also have abnormal neurological findings but child is not sick and has delayed development.

Investigations

Probable diagnosis decides whether tests are required or not. Simple febrile seizure does not need any test, it is a clinical diagnosis based on characteristic presentation and exclusion of other causes. Meningitis is proved by CSF examination, hypocalcemia due to vitamin D deficiency by serum calcium, phosphorus and alkaline phosphatase and bone X-ray. Brain damage due to previous disease may need neuro-imaging. EEG is required only in case of epilepsy.

Management

Most often seizure stops on its own before any intervention. Only when patient presents during active seizure, one may use diazepam or midazolam to control the event. However, as one can't anticipate how long the seizure may last, it is best to attempt to control the seizure. Nasal puff of midazolam is easy to administer even by parents that aborts the attack quickly. Long term anti-convulsant drugs are not necessary except in case of epilepsy or when active symptomatic seizure has a risk of recurrence. Simple febrile seizure needs no treatment but recurrence can be prevented by clobazam given at the onset of fever along with antipyretic drug. Three doses at 12 hours interval suffice as chance of seizure is only in first 24 hours of onset of fever.

Take Home Message

Occurrence of a seizure is frightening to parents and a challenge to a doctor. However, only action doctor needs to undertake is to stop a seizure and a decision about the need of immediate hospitalization (meningitis, severe head injury or uncontrolled seizure) and subsequent need for investigations (in case of recurrent seizures). Most of the times, a seizure stops by itself but if patient presents with active seizure, diazepam or midazolam may be required.

MCQs

1. Which of the following statement is wrong?

A) Seizure may not present with movements
B) Seizure may occur without loss of consciousness
C) Seizure is always preceded by some symptoms
D) Seizure may not recover by itself

2. This type of generalized seizure is not associated with movements

A) Clonic
B) Tonic/Clonic
C) Myoclonic
D) Absence

3. Which of the following statement is wrong
A) Focal motor seizure presents without loss of consciousness
B) Focal motor seizure presents with loss of consciousness
C) Focal non-motor seizure presents with loss of consciousness
D) None of the above

4. These seizures end with sleepiness except
A) Simple febrile seizure
B) Seizure due to hypocalcemia
C) Seizure due to meningitis
D) Idiopathic epilepsy

5. Transient loss of consciousness may be seen in this condition even when it is not a seizure
A) Vertigo
B) Breath holding spasm
C) Syncope
D) Benign sleep myoclonus

Answers to MCQs

Correct answers as follows:

Q1 C	Q2 D	Q3 C	Q4 B	Q5 B

51 Seizure – Must Act Fast!

Clinical Application of Basic Concepts

Must Find Out

Is it a seizure or seizure-mimic? If seizure, is it generalized or focal? If generalized, is it motor or non-motor? is it tonic, clonic, tonic-clonic, atonic or myoclonic? If focal, is it focal aware or focal with impaired awareness? Is it acute symptomatic seizure, remote symptomatic seizure or idiopathic seizure? Is it epilepsy, if so is it epileptic syndrome?

Seizure is a paroxysmal event that may mimic non-seizure disorder. Hence one must confirm an event to be a seizure before embarking on its cause. Most seizures are recognized by jerky movements of the limbs and transient loss of consciousness with staring spell. However, seizure also can present without loss of consciousness and it needs to be recognized. Movement disorders present with typical pattern without change in sensorium. Syncope occurs mostly in standing position and recovers in seconds. Breath-holding spasm is typically triggered by emotional stress as child holds breath in expiration and may turn blue or pale. One must inquire about sequence of events from a witness and if possible, captured video record. It helps to define nature of the event. Feeling giddy or rotational movements may suggest vertigo.

Once we know it is a seizure, next is to find out its cause. Preceding events, type of seizure and post-seizure events offer clue to diagnosis. Thus, detailed history is important. Age group helps to define common causes, simple febrile seizure is common in early childhood and so also hypocalcemia due to rickets. Idiopathic epilepsy is diagnosed in children > 5 years of age. Physical examination may be totally normal as in case of simple febrile convulsion, idiopathic epilepsy or hypocalcemia. Localizing neurological signs may represent either recent or old brain lesion responsible for seizure. Thus, it is important to consider whether it is acute or remote symptomatic seizure.

Case-Based Discussion

Case 1

One year old infant presented with high fever followed in next 18 hours with a generalized seizure that lasted for a minute. Child remained bit dazed thereafter for few minutes and then recovered completely without any neurological sequelae. He had no prior illness.

He had grown well and had achieved normal milestones. There was no family history of similar or any other neurological disorders.

This child has had normal brain development and has remained neurologically normal after the seizure that was self-limiting and triggered by high fever.

Physical examination showed no neurological abnormality and cause of fever was considered to be viral infection that settled within next two days without any specific therapy. It supported diagnosis of **simple febrile seizure.**

This child does not need any drug therapy and this being the first seizure, there is no need for prophylactic therapy. Parents were counselled about possible recurrence during first 24 hours of onset of fever. However, in case of recurrence, one may suggest midazolam nasal spray as an immediate rescue drug to stop a seizure. It can be used by parents at home and seizure stops immediately.

Simple febrile seizure never occurs beyond age of 5-6 years and has no relation to future epilepsy.

It is important not to prescribe an antibiotic for suspected simple febrile seizure as acute bacterial meningitis may be masked. If antibiotic is considered for whatever reason, CSF examination is a must before starting antibiotic.

Case 2

One year old infant presented with high fever followed in next 18 hours with generalized seizure that lasted for few minutes and stopped on its own. It was not followed by any post-ictal event in the form of drowsiness and he remained totally normal. However, within next two hours, he had another similar episode that lasted just for few seconds. He was fine thereafter. Fever disappeared over next two days. He had normal growth and development. There was no family history of similar disorder. On direct questioning, he was bottle fed and consumed about a liter of milk each day with very little solid food – he was bottle addicted.

This seizure did not result in post-ictal events and it is a clue to probable diagnosis of hypocalcemic seizure. As he was mainly on milk diet, he had a risk of developing vitamin D deficiency as milk is poor source of vitamin D and this infant would not have been exposed to sunlight. So rickets may have contributed to hypocalcemia triggered by viral infection. Physical examination showed signs of rickets without any neurological abnormality. It supported diagnosis of **hypocalcemia** as a cause of seizure.

Vitamin D deficiency rickets can be confirmed by bone X-ray and high serum alkaline phosphatase with either low or normal serum calcium and low phosphorus level. Serum calcium may be normal in this child because nature moves available calcium from bone to blood and thereafter to tissues. However, it takes few hours to replenish calcium at tissue level and that is the reason that this child had another seizure though it was for shorter duration. But once calcium is replenished in neurological tissues, seizure stops.

If one saw this child during a seizure, IV calcium could have been administered for quick replenishment. However, if one saw this child after second seizure, one may consider oral replacement of calcium along with vitamin D. It is ideal to delay starting vitamin D supplement for few days before administration of oral calcium because vitamin D is likely to deposit calcium into bone from whatever is available in tissues and it may precipitate a seizure. Once rickets is fully cured, there is no risk of hypocalcemia.

Case 3

One year old infant presented with high fever followed by irritability and vomiting for two days. On D3, he developed a generalized seizure that lasted for few minutes and was followed by drowsiness for few minutes. Fever and irritability continued with occasional vomiting.

This child has developed a seizure on D 3 of onset of fever and so this is certainly not a simple febrile seizure or fever triggered hypocalcemia. Irritability and vomiting suggest probable increased intracranial pressure. It favors diagnosis of bacterial meningitis. Initially the disease is localized only to meninges but subsequently cortex is affected, if not treated in time and presents as seizure.

Physical examination showed highly febrile sick looking child. He was drowsy but when disturbed was irritable. He had meningeal signs in the form of neck stiffness. There were no localizing signs. Anterior fontannel was open and bulging. It favors the diagnosis of **bacterial meningitis**.

It was confirmed by CSF showing 400 cells 90% polymorphs, proteins 250 mg% and sugar 20 mg%. Culture showed pneumococcus sensitive to all antibiotics. This child was treated with IV Ceftriaxone and luckily recovered completely. Older child with acute bacterial meningitis rarely presents with seizures as disease remains localized to meninges for a long period. On the other extreme of age, neonate presents with generalized seizure in acute bacterial meningitis as disease spreads quickly from meninges to brain cortex. Neuroimaging is justified in acute bacterial meningitis only in presence of focal signs that may suggest brain abscess or subdural empyema.

Case 4

Two year old child presented with high fever and drowsiness followed a day later with generalized seizure. On direct questioning, he was not keeping well over last two months with recurrent episodes of fever that were treated each time with antibiotic but without diagnosis and would get temporarily better. He had lost 2 kg of weight and felt sick. There were no other significant illnesses prior to onset of this problem two months ago. There was no significant family history and he denied contact with any contagious disease. This child has subacute onset of disease with recurrent fever. It suggests continuous disease with recurrent illness as evident by his progressive loss of weight and sickness. So, it is same disease that suddenly developed high fever, drowsiness and seizure. Such a neurological manifestation came up suddenly that suggests immune reaction to existing infection and in the background of subacute disease. It favors probable diagnosis of TB meningitis. Unlike bacterial meningitis, this child has had brain cell affection early in the course of the disease – encephalopathy without much increased intracranial pressure.

Physical examination showed malnourished child, drowsy, mild neck stiffness, positive Macewan's sign – cracked pot sound suggestive of raised intracranial tension, left sided hemiparesis with left sided facial palsy with spasticity, brisk deep tendon reflexes and extensor plantar reflex.

Pathologically these signs represent meningeal inflammation with hydrocephalus, vasculitis affecting middle cerebral artery as evident by hemiparesis with facial palsy and brain cell edema as shown by drowsiness. These pathological findings are typical of TB meningitis.

CSF showed 120 cells, mostly lymphocytes, 120 mg% proteins and 35 mg% sugar. CT scan showed meningeal enhancement with hydrocephalus and brain edema. CSF culture for TB was negative and so also GeneXpert. Chest X-ray was normal. Even in absence of proof, **TB meningitis** was diagnosed on circumstantial evidence. This child was treated with anti-TB drugs and steroids and made a recovery but was left behind with brain damage.

Family screening for tuberculosis with a chest X-ray is ideal to suspect tuberculosis in young children as tuberculosis is a paucibacillary disease in children (bacilli are small in number) that makes confirmation difficult. This child presented in late stage of the disease with drowsiness and convulsion and hence was left with brain damage. In fact, at such a stage, disease is often fatal If picked up before developing any change in sensorium or convulsion, there could be complete recovery without damage. Thus, it is vital to diagnose tubercular meningitis in early stage for better outcome. Theoretically, fungal infection can also present in the same way but it is usually seen in immune-compromised patients.

Case 5

Two year old child presented with high fever and drowsiness that worsened over next 8 hours followed by generalized seizure that lasted for 10 minutes that came under control with drugs. He was apparently well prior to onset of present illness. He maintained normal growth and development. There was no significant past or family history or contact with any contagious disease.

This history denotes fast progression of neurological disease with brain cell affection in the form of progressive brain cell edema with deepening consciousness and seizure. It could be viral encephalitis or autoimmune encephalopathy. Both conditions look similar with very small difference that may not be discernible. Autoimmune encephalitis generally precedes with febrile illness by at least 2-3 days with an interval of apparently normal period before onset of neurological disease. As this child did not have any recent illness, it may favor viral encephalitis.

Physical examination showed febrile child, unconscious responding to painful stimuli with no localizing signs. It suggests generalized brain cell edema of probably due to viral infection. However, any other cause such as toxic encephalitis or fever triggered metabolic encephalopathy cannot be ruled out.

Investigations – Hb 11 Gm%, WBC 4000 P 55 L 43 M 2 E 0 Pl 1.8 lakhs, malarial parasites not detected, CSF cells 80 mostly lymphocytes, 60 mg% proteins, normal sugar, culture –ve, MRI scan of brain showed diffuse brain edema.

Diagnosis of **viral encephalitis** was made and treated with IV acyclovir –antiviral antibiotic mainly acting against herpes viral infection, though administered empirically. Child also received anti-edema measures. Including anti-convulsant drugs. He improved luckily though etiology could not be proved.

Diagnosis of viral encephalitis is often made without a final proof though modern technology can help to diagnose the type of viral infection. Not all viral infections can be treated with anti-viral drugs but herpes virus can be successfully treated only if therapy is started in first two days. Hence the need for early definitive diagnosis. In absence of such a facility, empirical treatment with acyclovir is justified.

Case 6

Ten year old child presented with jerky movements of left upper limb that lasted for 5 minutes and stopped by itself. There was no loss of consciousness. He was well prior to onset of this event and remained normal thereafter as well. There was no significant past or family history.

This history suggests focal seizure (focal aware). It is not a movement disorder as it occurred suddenly and also stopped by itself. Cause of this seizure cannot be assessed on history, except a fact that there must be local lesion in motor cortex. Physical examination showed no abnormality. It meant an apparently silent lesion that must have manifested suddenly without any obvious trigger factor. Such a lesion may be any local structural malformation that must have existed since birth or it may have resulted from focal swelling that may have resulted from local inflammation or infection. But its exact cause cannot be guessed at this stage and needs investigations.

CT scan of brain showed ring enhancing lesion in right motor cortex that had surrounding edema suggestive of inflammatory origin and not a congenital malformation. Such a local inflammatory lesion is commonly due to chronic infection such as tuberculosis or neurocysticercosis – a parasitic infection that gets transmitted from consuming uncooked meat. CT scan often fails to differentiate between these two lesions. Based on presence of multiple lesions on CT scan, diagnosis of tuberculosis – **tuberculoma** was made. Child was treated with standard anti-TB therapy with steroids. On follow-up, this child showed disappearance of lesion on repeat CT scan.

Diagnosis of tuberculoma is often circumstantial. If CT scan finds a scolex of the parasite, diagnosis of neurocysticercosis can be confirmed. In absence of such clues, spectroscopy may be useful to differentiate these two conditions. Without definitive diagnosis in such a situation, management is debatable. This child certainly needs anti-convulsant drug – carbamazepine is the drug of choice and one may decide to observe further course. However, there is always a risk of tuberculosis spreading to affect brain cell with dire consequences. On the other hand, treatment of neurocysticercosis is short for few weeks as against minimum 6 months for tuberculosis. So, decision should be taken after discussing with parents and explaining pros and cons of all options. If this child is purely vegetarian, chances of cysticercosis is very low unless he consumed vegetarian food contaminated by uncooked meat without knowing. Thus, many such patients end up with anti-TB treatment with steroids.

Case 7

Ten year old child presented with sudden onset of generalized seizure that lasted for few minutes and stopped on its own. He was healthy child with normal brain development and had no symptoms prior to onset of this event. History suggests unprovoked generalized seizure. Physical examination was normal and so diagnosis of **probable idiopathic epilepsy** was considered though not labelled at this stage as very definition of epilepsy is recurrent seizures. One may have to wait for further course. As it is the first episode, one may consider clinical follow-up without any tests. EEG at this stage may not be interpretive as normal EEG does not rule out epilepsy and abnormal EEG may be found in small number of normal children. There is no risk even if there was another similar seizure. Though one can be prepared with nasal midazolam spray to control seizure. Most of such seizures are short lasting and self-limiting without causing any brain damage.

EEG may help to rule out focal epilepsy with generalization as many times, no one else has observed onset of a seizure that may have been focal which spread to all the areas resulting in generalized seizure as the presentation. EEG was normal in this child, confirming it to be generalized seizure. CT scan of brain is not justified in this child. Parents were counselled and no treatment was advised.

Case 8

Thirteen year old child suddenly fell down while standing for morning prayers in school. He was well till this event happened. He had arrived at school as usual after normal breakfast. No one had noticed onset of this event as it was only when he fell down that everyone around him noticed. By the time his friends offered help, he had got up, was bit dazed for a few minutes but became normal quickly. One cannot be sure whether this was a seizure that made him fall down or whether it was pseudo-seizure – syncope. However, fact that he got up within few seconds would go in favor of syncope. Though difference between the two is evident only if one knows the onset of this event.

Physical examination was normal as expected and so diagnosis of **syncope** was considered.

As this event occurred without any known provocation, it may be a result of neurogenic syncope – vasovagal attack due to unknown stress, such as fear, starving or lack of sleep, the event that typically occurs in standing position. It is a clinical diagnosis and does not justify any tests such as tilt-table test where sudden tilt of position may induce the attack. However, if such an event occurred while exercising or during sport activities, one may have to take a serious note of it as it may represent cardiogenic syncope. It may be fatal if not diagnosed properly unlike vasovagal attack. If cardiogenic syncope is suspected, one must order ECG and echo-cardiogram to pick up any functional or structural abnormality – one must rule out long QT – it is often familial and so history of sudden death in the family should arouse suspicion of cardiogenic syncope.

Take Home Message

Seizure must be differentiated from seizure-mimic (pseudo-seizure). Detailed history from an observer helps to confirm a seizure. Seizure may manifest without a convulsion. Non-convulsive seizure is not easy to pick-up. What presents as a generalized seizure may have a focal origin that is easily missed unless there is an observer around when a child develops a seizure. As drug of choice is different, in case of doubt, EEG helps to rule out a focal seizure. Acute symptomatic seizure is triggered by an active disease such as an intracranial infection, metabolic disorder or severe head injury. Remote symptomatic seizure results from pre-existing brain damage and idiopathic seizure is unprovoked, cause is not evident but may be genetic in origin. Most often, a seizure stops by itself but brain damage is likely if it continues for more than five minutes. Hence it is ideal to control a seizure by midazolam, if possible. Parents or care-takers can be trained to administer the drug via a nasal puff that is easily available.

MCQs

1. Which of the following statement related to simple febrile seizure is WRONG?
A) It may occur with any degree of fever
B) It may occur anytime up to 6 years of age
C) It may recur many times
D) None of the above

2. This seizure is not accompanied with any post-ictal drowsiness
A) Simple febrile seizure
B) Idiopathic epilepsy
C) Hypocalcemia
D) TB meningitis

3. This seizure is preceded by fever and irritability
A) Simple febrile seizure
B) Bacterial meningitis
C) TB meningitis
D) Fever triggered hypocalcemia

4. Which of the following seizure needs EEG?
A) Simple febrile seizure
B) TB meningitis
C) Focal seizure
D) Hypocalcemia

5. Which of the following statement related to neurogenic syncope is TRUE?
A) It may occur in any position
B) It may occur at any age
C) It recovers within seconds
D) It may end with drowsiness

Answers to MCQs

Correct answers as follows:

Q1 D	Q2 C	Q3 B	Q4 C	Q5 C

52 Headache - An Invisible Problem

Back to Basics

Pathogenesis of Pain in General

Most commonly, pain is a result of inflammation that is accompanied with swelling, warmth and redness besides pain or tenderness – not all the features are always present. However non-inflammatory types of pain may be neurogenic, vascular, psychogenic or referred. They are not accompanied with symptoms and signs of inflammation and so present without swelling, warmth or redness. Neurogenic and vasogenic type of pain is localized to their respective areas of supply. Psychogenic pain is not due to any physical disease but patient does feel it genuinely. It is a pain of convenience that does not disturb health, sleep or activities of choice. Pain at one site may originate from the other site because these two sites share same nerve connections – it is a referred pain. So, one may have to be careful to assess origin of pain that may have either no signs or hidden signs.

What is Headache?

Pain or discomfort arising from any part inside or around the head (skull) is referred to as headache. What makes it worrisome is the fact that it is mostly invisible to an outsider including a doctor as it is not accompanied with swelling. And if there is a swelling, it needs to be carefully detected as it is at obscure places. It poses a challenge though luckily most causes of headache are not serious. It is important to note that infants and toddlers up to the age of around 4 years are not able to localize pain and they present with excessive crying or irritability, depending on severity of pain. In general, headache is a complaint of older children and adults.

Brain does not Feel Pain

Brain cells are devoid of sensory nerve supply and so also lung parenchyma. These are the only two structures in the body without sensory nerve endings. Though brain does help to perceive and localize the pain. Pain is carried by sensory nerve endings from the site of affection up to thalamus – the receiving center that in turn relays the information to somatosensory cortex. It is the cortex that would take appropriate action to guard against pain.

How does Intracranial Pathology Cause Pain?

It is the surrounding structures in the intracranial cavity that have sensory nerve endings and pain arises from them and not the brain cell. Thus, meningeal irritation or inflammation leads to headache and so also due to increased intracranial pressure as happens in progressive hydrocephalus or brain tumor.

Other Areas in or Around Skull that Cause Headache

Temporomandibular joint, ear, paranasal sinuses and teeth are parts included in skull that may cause a person to report headache. Eye resides in the socket in the skull and so eye strain can be mistaken for headache. Though it is not strictly pain but just discomfort due to strain of extra-ocular muscles. It is common to ascribe headache to refractive error but that is not true. Cervical neck pathology with muscle spasm and also tightness of facial muscles (tension headache) lead to headache. It may also be caused by temporomandibular joint or dental pathology. Pain may also arise from the mind itself – psychogenic headache.

Causes of Headache

Acute onset of high fever is associated with headache that can be severe in **dengue, influenza or other viral infections** as well as in Typhoid and malaria. In such cases, headache is temporarily relieved with reduction of fever though may increase again with rising fever. This is important as it rules out intracranial infection such as meningitis that also starts with high fever followed by headache that continues even if fever is temporarily controlled. So, always inquire about relation between fever and headache. Obviously, there are no neurological signs in non-neurological febrile patients with headache, though subtle signs during initial stage of meningitis may be easily missed.

Intracranial infection such as **bacterial meningitis** must be ruled out in case of fever with headache. Typically, such a child presents also with irritability and vomiting, headache persists in spite of temporary reduction of fever. This fact must be assessed carefully so that diagnosis of meningitis can be suspected even before clinical signs appear such as neck stiffness and other signs of meningeal irritation.

Acute **sinusitis** is not common in children and chronic sinusitis is difficult to diagnose but certainly is a cause of headache. It may be suspected in case of persistent nasal discharge in spite of proper treatment. Maxillary sinuses appear by the age of 3 years and frontal sinuses by 7 years. Ethmoidal and sphenoidal sinuses are present at birth but rarely involved. Child under the age of 4-5 years, cannot localize pain and hence sinusitis is considered only in older children.

Migraine is another common cause of headache in older children and is suspected by recurrent attacks of headache with strong family history.

Intracranial space occupying lesions is always at the back of mind especially when headache is progressive and often presents on getting up in the morning with natural relief thereafter through the day in early stage of the disease. Thereafter ofcourse, headache is continuous and accompanied with vomiting.

Hypertension is another cause of headache as it contributes to increased intracranial pressure.

Trauma as a result of head injury may be superficial in the scalp or deep intracranially. Blood-shot eyes or bleeding through nose or ear are warning signs of brain injury, besides change in behavior and vomiting. However, vomiting occurring immediately after head injury is due to fright and crying and not indicative of brain injury. Superficial injury presents with swelling on the scalp and may not be visible but palpable.

Tension headache is due to tightness of facial muscles as a result of inability to relax as may happen due to stress or anxiety.

Psychogenic headache is pain of convenience as it disappears completely during happy hours and does not anyway affect health and well-being. Rarely, **TM joint, ear or dental pathology** may also present with headache and easily overlooked.

Clinical Approach to Headache

Site and type of headache may offer some clues. Patient often complains of bitemporal headache while localized headache may be due to disease at underlying site. Dull continuous pain is more common though throbbing pain may be of vascular origin.

Onset – fever associated with headache is easy to differentiate between presence or absence of intracranial infection as mentioned above by simple question – does fever and headache are relieved temporarily with antipyretic or whether headache continues in spite of fever control. Of course, headache in intracranial infection is preceded by irritability and vomiting. Headache without associated fever may be due to migraine that is often recurrent with positive family history and also due to hypertension, often secondary to renal disease.

Duration and progress – short duration headache with fever disappears once disease is controlled. Migraine typically lasts for some hours and settles by itself to recur again after few days. At the height of headache, vomiting along with intolerance to sound and light are other manifestations before headache resolves by itself or after an analgesic. Slowly progressive headache over few days to weeks often accompanied with vomiting suggests probable brain tumor that may begin with morning headache on getting up and relieved after an hour or so. This is because intracranial pressure is temporarily increased to a small extent in normal persons due to venous congestion during sleep. In normal individual, such an increase in intracranial pressure is small enough not to manifest but in presence of developing brain tumor, small increase of intracranial pressure in the morning is good enough to manifest headache only to be relieved on its own as venous congestion disappears with increasing activity. However once brain tumor enlarges, it would manifest with headache for increasing periods and not restricted only to mornings.

Tension headache is also chronic but at steady level with mild exacerbations and remissions. Psychogenic headache is of convenience and does not disturb sleep or play and growth and well-being is well maintained.

Physical examination reveals abnormal neurological findings in case of meningitis and brain tumor. In other conditions causing headache, there are no clinical abnormalities except in case of hypertension and subtle signs of chronic sinusitis.

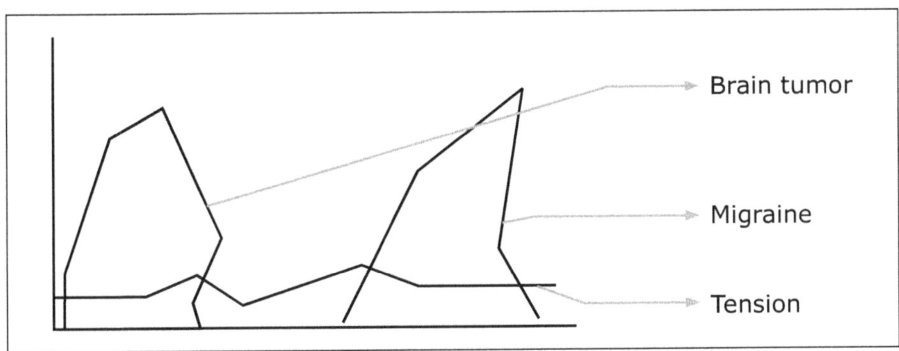

For simplification, chronic headache progression is represented by the graph above that easily can differentiate between brain tumor, migraine and tension headache. Of course, brain tumor would also present with neurological signs. It is ideal to examine other areas around skull – TM joint, teeth/gums and ear as well as neck.

Investigations

Acute bacterial meningitis is confirmed by CSF showing high number of WBCs – mostly neutrophils and high proteins with low sugar and culture can detect organism responsible for meningitis, provided test is ordered prior to starting an antibiotics. Antigen can still be detected in patients who are already on antibiotics.

Neuroimaging – CT scan is diagnostic of brain tumor though etiology needs to be assessed. Brain tumors are also caused by infections such as tuberculosis or cysticercosis besides benign and malignant diseases. Etiology can be assessed only by biopsy or usually diagnosis is considered with circumstantial evidence in case of tuberculosis or neurocysticercosis, supported by spectroscopy. X-ray of paranasal sinuses has low sensitivity to demonstrate changes in sinusitis and ideally CT scan is necessary. However, in view of radiation exposure, diagnosis of chronic sinusitis can be made on clinical basis and treated. Diagnosis of migraine and tension headache is entirely clinical and it is important to rule out other conditions in case of doubt.

Management

Analgesics are mainstay of symptomatic treatment. Besides, several drugs are tried in Migraine but there is no single drug therapy that can be strongly recommended. Flunarizine, cyproheptadine and beta-blockers are tried with variable success and are reserved for those patients who suffer frequent severe attacks difficult to alleviate with analgesics. One should search for offending trigger factors that also vary in individual patients such as coffee, nuts or sleep deprivation. Infections are treated by specific antibiotics.

Take Home Message

Headache presenting with fever does not pose a diagnostic challenge and so also chronic progressive headache due to intracranial space-occupying lesion. However chronic persistent or recurrent headache needs proper evaluation. Chronic sinusitis presents without fever and is easily overlooked, though persistent nasal purulent discharge and generalized vague ill-health offer clue to the diagnosis of chronic sinusitis. Tension headache and psychogenic headache are not easy to differentiate from one another. Migraine may present with atypical pattern with transient paresis. It is ideal to seek help of a specialist in such cases.

MCQs

1. Localized headache may be a feature of

A) Meningitis
B) Brain tumor
C) Migraine
D) Tension headache

2. Headache should not be ascribed to this organ

A) Teeth
B) TM Joint
C) Neck
D) Eyes

3. Which of the following statements related to sinusitis is RIGHT?

A) Diagnosis is based on the history of persistent nasal discharge > 2 weeks
B) Sinusitis occurs only in older children
C) Localized tenderness is not easy to demonstrate
D) All of the above

4. Headache due to severe head injury is often caused by

A) Subarachnoid hemorrhage
B) Subdural hemorrhage
C) Extradural hemorrhage
D) All of the above

5. Hypertension in children may present as headache and may result from

A) Renal disease
B) Adrenal disease
C) Vascular disease
D) All of the above

Answers to MCQs

Correct answers as follows:

Q1 C	Q2 D	Q3 D	Q4 B	Q5 D

53 Headache – Think Beyond the Brain!

Clinical Application of Basic Concepts

Onset, duration and progress of headache in addition to site and type offer enough clues to come to a reasonable diagnosis. Accompanying symptoms add to making correct decisions. Acute onset headache is usually due to infection or migraine and rarely due to acute onset of hypertension as in the case of acute glomerulonephritis. Headache due to meningitis starts with fever and irritability before headache and vomiting appear and headache continues in spite of temporary control of fever with paracetamol. Headache accompanied by general extra-cranial infections such as influenza, malaria, typhoid etc. are related to high fever and so headache disappears along with fever only to recur again as fever comes up. Chronic headache is usually due to tension headache or psychological – the pain of convenience but also may be due to chronic sinusitis that is difficult to diagnose. Seen only in older children after frontal sinuses appear by 7-8 years of age and persistent nasal discharge in spite of usual treatment is the clue to diagnose chronic sinusitis. Recurrent headache is classically an attack of migraine with an intervening period absolutely normal. It is the progressive headache and headache associated with vomiting that needs proper evaluation. Headache due to brain tumor starts often as morning headache on waking up that gets better by itself within next couple hours and rest of the day goes fine. This is the beginning of the problem that may get worst over time. It is important to recognize it in time to take proper action. It is easy to note that investigations are often not required to find out the cause of the headache and so a CT scan should be reserved only for suspected raised intracranial pressure and should not be considered just to allay anxiety keeping in mind radiation exposure. There is no clarity about the safe limit of radiation exposure in children and it is best avoided, if possible.

Case 1

6 year old child presented with high fever and headache for the last two days. There were no other symptoms. He was normal prior to the onset of this illness and had no significant past illnesses. Another sibling had a similar illness.

Physical examination showed no localizing signs and the child did look better when his fever was temporarily controlled with paracetamol. It favors the diagnosis of **viral infection.**

The child got well within the next two days without specific therapy. As fever and headache appeared together on the very first day of illness, meningitis is unlikely. One may decide to observe further trend of fever as it may resolve by itself if it is a viral infection or it may get worse. Specific investigations may be necessary to diagnose the cause of fever but not for headache.

Case 2

Six year old child presented with high fever for two days followed by irritability, headache and vomiting over next 24 hours. He was reported to be sick with poor intake of fluids and was lethargic. Irritability followed by headache and vomiting two days after onset of fever clearly suggests intracranial infection.

Physical examination showed sick looking child, lethargic with mild neck stiffness but no other localizing neurological signs. This suggests bacterial meningitis. CSF showed 130 cells most of them neutrophils with 100 mg of protein and 35 mg of sugar – consistent with the diagnosis of **bacterial meningitis**. CSF culture was negative. The child was treated with IV ceftriaxone and recovered completely without any sequelae.

The first two days of fever denote the bacteremic phase and thereafter as bacteria settle in the meninges, localizing symptoms appear such as irritability, headache and vomiting. Another disease such as viral meningitis (often termed aseptic meningitis) may present in a similar way though, the child is not sick and shows improving trend over two days. CSF examination is a must to prove diagnosis of meningitis and CSF culture often would identify bacteria causing meningitis. In absence of positive CSF culture, one should choose antibiotic based on age-related epidemiology.

Case 3

Eight year old child presented with puffiness of eyelids and reduced amount of urine that was high colored over last 24 hours followed by severe headache. There was no fever. Two weeks ago, he had suffered from throat infection that was treated with antibiotics and got well. Puffiness of eyelids and oliguria with probable hematuria indicates acute onset of glomerulonephritis. Headache following this episode is likely to be due to acute onset hypertension – accompaniment of glomerulonephritis.

Physical examination revealed puffy eyelids, mild edema of feet and blood pressure of 160/100 mm Hg. There were no neurological or cardiac findings – so there were no other complications of hypertension. Fundus examination was also normal. Urinalysis showed RBCs, granular casts and proteins, serum creatinine and urea were raised. This confirmed diagnosis of **acute glomerulonephritis**. Child was treated with anti-hypertensive drug and other symptomatic measures and he improved over next two days. Mostly, such a disease runs a favorable course especially if it has followed streptococcal throat infection.

However other infections also cause similar illness that may not share good prognosis. Hence it is ideal to order serum C3 level that is low at the peak of illness and gets back to normal as disease improves. Persistence of low C3 level after 2-3 months of apparent cure suggests incomplete improvement and needs referral to a specialist. Thus, serum C3 level is important to monitor every patient of acute glomerulonephritis

Case 4

Ten year old child presented with acute onset of severe throbbing headache that got worse over next few hours to an extent that he could not tolerate light or sound. He vomited twice at the peak of headache. He did not find much relief with analgesic but headache gradually subsided and he was back to normal. He never had headache in the past though his mother often had episodes of severe headache for which she always took analgesics as all investigations ordered by her doctor were negative. This history is classical of **migraine** with positive family history. It is a bed-side diagnosis but based on classical history of an episode and supported by family history.

Physical examination was completely normal. Investigations were not ordered as there was no suspicion of any other disease and analgesic was prescribed on SOS basis. Patient suffering from migraine should be advised to watch for any obvious trigger factors that could be avoided to prevent an attack. Though it is not easy to pinpoint to trigger factors. It is important to counsel about possible recurrences and symptomatic management with analgesics. Frequent attacks may justify trial with some drugs like flunarizine or cyproheptadine or betablocker given for few months to assess, if they would help. It is important to note that migraine can present in different ways such as transient paresis or severe abdominal pain. Diagnosis of migraine in such presentations is difficult and all other conditions need to be ruled out before labelling it. Migraine is considered to be of vascular origin and hence such a bizarre presentation. But in all such presentations, a common factor is self-limiting episode within few hours with complete recovery but often recurrent.

Case 5

Ten year old child presented with low grade fever and running nose with mild to moderate headache off and on for two weeks. He reported poor appetite and had lost 1 kg weight over last two weeks. There was no vomiting or lethargy. He always suffered from repeated cold and cough at times with fever and he was diagnosed as allergic rhinitis with at times secondary infection needing antibiotic therapy. He was not on any long-term treatment for allergy.

Superficially to look at, low grade fever with loss of appetite and weight may suggest probable tuberculosis but cold has been a predominant symptom that is against tuberculosis. Headache in this child is another clue that is obviously not a neurological symptom as it is not accompanied with lethargy or vomiting. Thus, this looks to be chronic sinusitis.

Physical examination showed congested nasal mucosa with mucopurulent discharge in a chronically sick looking child. Tenderness over frontal or maxillary sinuses could not be demonstrated as such finding is often difficult to assess, especially it being chronic disease. In acute sinusitis, it could be possible to detect sinus tenderness. Diagnosis of **chronic sinusitis** is again based on interpretation of history. This child was treated with a course of antibiotics for 10 days along with long term therapy for allergic rhinitis in the form of intranasal steroids.

Routine investigations are not helpful to prove the diagnosis of chronic sinusitis. CBC, ESR and X-ray of paranasal sinuses are mostly inconclusive. CT scan of paranasal sinuses may prove the diagnosis though radiation exposure may be a consideration and so one can depend on bed-side clinical diagnosis unless patient does not improve as expected. In such a case, further management is best left to a specialist.

Case 6

Eight year old child presented with a headache every morning on waking up that lasted for an hour but over the next few days, the headache was increasing in duration as well as intensity though getting better with an analgesic. He also had occasional vomiting along with headache on some days. He was advised to take an analgesic as and when necessary, considering the probability of migraine as his mother suffered from migraine. And it was ascribed to his habit of going to be pretty late at night. However, when the headache started worsening, he was advised for further tests. This symptom is classical of gradually increasing intracranial pressure, due to space-occupying lesion, either tumor or hydrocephalus.

Physical examination showed mild intentional tremors. These findings in the background of a history of gradually worsening headache suggest a **cerebellar tumor.** CT scan confirmed the presence of a tumor and luckily it turned out to be a benign mass that could be removed.

Supratentorial brain tumor presents with localizing symptom such as a focal seizure in the initial stage, much before it can lead to headache due to increased intracranial pressure while infratentorial tumor presents with raised intracranial pressure and headache along with many other symptoms because the infratentorial area is a small space crowded by multiple structures.

Case 7

Twelve year old child complained of low-grade headache off and on for the last two months. It was nearly constant though severity fluctuated to some extent but it was never severe. There were no other accompanying symptoms like vomiting or fever. There were hardly any days without a headache. It disturbed the child and parents as no cause was found even after investigations including a CT scan of the brain. This symptom of chronic headache has never been severe or worsening over weeks and without any other symptoms.

Physical examination was normal. This is typical of **tension headache.** It is due to tense muscles of the face and neck, often a result of stress and inability to relax. Tension headache is a diagnosis of exclusion and based on history analysis and normal physical examination as well as the absence of any impact on general health. There is no need for any investigations though most patients have had even CT scan – just to make sure that one is not missing anything. There is no drug treatment though an analgesic may relieve headache for a while but frequent use should be avoided as all analgesics produce side effects, especially on kidneys. Prolonged use of analgesics is the most common cause of chronic renal failure in adults. Counseling is an important aspect of management and parents must participate in destressing the child in every way possible.

Case 8

Twelve year old child presented with headache off and on for the last four months. It was sporadic, at times severe but without any other symptoms. His health status was well maintained and so also his food intake, play activities and sleep. On a detailed analysis of history, there was no clue to the causation of headache.

Physical examination was completely normal. There was no need for any tests though they already had done CT scan of the brain that ruled out any brain pathology. Parents were told to document the timing, duration and severity of headache episodes as well as aggravating and relieving factors, if any and assured that there was no major cause to worry. It was clear that headache never came in the way of those activities but headache surfaced when he was made to undertake any act that he hated to do so. So, this was the headache of convenience – **psychogenic headache.** Parents were counseled. Placebo was prescribed and the child improved over time.

It is worth noting that headache is genuinely felt by such a patient though there is no organic cause and this is not malingering. Diagnosis is made with the exclusion of other causes and only in case of suspicion, neuro-imaging may be necessary though routinely should be avoided for the fear of radiation exposure. Counseling is an important part of management and help of an expert may be necessary.

Take Home Message

Headache is a common symptom in the general population including older children. Even when benign conditions are among the most common causes, patients always worry about headache if it is severe, recurrent or long-lasting. Refractive error is commonly blamed for headache though it is not true but most patients undergo eye check and many opt for CT scan to allay their anxiety. Detailed history and physical examination almost always can define probable cause and investigations should be reserved only for a few conditions. However, treating benign persistent or recurrent headache such as tension headache, psychogenic headache or migraine is often a challenge and need a referral to a specialist.

MCQs

1. This symptom can differentiate headache caused by meningitis from extra-cranial infections such as viral infection

A) Degree of fever
B) Occasional vomiting
C) Irritability
D) Interferbile period

2. Which of the following statements related to neck stiffness are RIGHT?

A) It suggests meningitis
B) It may not suggest meningitis
C) It may be seen in typhoid fever
D) All of the above

3. Which of the following statement related to cause of hypertension is WRONG?

A) Renal glomerular disease
B) Renal tubular disease
C) Coarctation of aorta
D) Adrenal disease

4. Chronic sinusitis in children is best suspected by

A) Tenderness over sinuses
B) High fever
C) Persistence of mucopurulent nasal discharge > 2 weeks
D) None of the above

5. Migraine can present as

A) Headache

B) Abdominal pain

C) Transient brain stroke

D) All of the above

Answers to MCQs

Correct answers as follows:

Q1 D	Q2 D	Q3 B	Q4 C	Q5 D

54 My Legs Ache!

Back to Basics

Introduction

Leg ache is the most common complaint of localized limb pain. It is so because we use legs more than upper limbs and hence leg ache may be a part of generalized body pain though maximally felt in legs. However, pain may arise from any extremity. There are multiple layers of tissues in a limb and pain may arise from any of these structures.

Pathogenesis of Pain – A Revision

Pain is commonly a result of inflammation but also may be vasogenic, neurogenic, psychogenic or even referred to a distant site other than the site of a disease. Inflammation is easy to make out as it is accompanied by swelling, redness, tenderness and warmth besides pain. Vasogenic pain in the limb may arise from the affection of draining veins. Neurogenic limb pain may be shooting or burning. Both vasogenic and neurogenic pain are localized to the area of supply. Tired muscles accumulate metabolites that cause pain while sustained contraction of muscles causes severe cramps.

Anatomical Parts of a Limb

It consists of skin, soft tissue, muscles, bones, tendons, ligaments, joints, blood vessels and nerves. Obviously, pain may arise from any of these parts or may involve more than one part. It is important to define the anatomy of the disease as pathology and etiology are different in the affection of each part.

Common Causes of Pain in Limbs

Trauma – impacted foreign body or splinter, injection site, sports injuries to muscle, tendon, bone or joint

Infection – bacterial cellulitis, abscess, osteomyelitis and arthritis, as well as myositis, viral myositis, syphilis

Non-infective inflammation – rheumatic fever, Juvenile idiopathic arthritis and other rheumatological disorders, dermatomyositis, bone malignancy

Vitamin deficiency – rickets, osteomalacia, scurvy

Vascular – vasculitis, sickle cell disease, deep vein thrombosis, aseptic necrosis of bone, osteochondrosis

Hematological – leukemia, hemophilia

Neurogenic – herpes, peripheral neuritis

Idiopathic – growing pain, restless leg syndrome

Psychogenic or functional – pain amplification syndrome

Referred pain – hip joint pain from psoas abscess

Clinical Approach to Pain in limbs History

Age group – children are at risk of injuries. Young infants present with an accidental birth injury or one caused by vigorous massage or pulled elbow while lifting the child. Children under the age of 4-5 years cannot localize pain and may be difficult to assess.

Localized or generalized – trauma, bacterial infection, herpes, and arthritis are causes of local pain while viral infection with myositis, vitamin C and D deficiency, and leukemia are conditions that result in more widespread pain in all the limbs.

Origin – Acute onset is typical of trauma or at times vascular or neurogenic pathology. Infection and inflammation are never very acute, they manifest over 2-3 days or even longer.

Duration and progress – traumatic and infective conditions are usually short-lasting as they get diagnosed and treated early. Other conditions may have a prolonged course. Most conditions result in continuous pain but growing pain manifests in the later part of the evening. Hemophilia may cause recurrent arthritis.

Relation to rest and activity – morning stiffness or pain is typical of inflammatory arthritis while pain in the evening after daily activity suggests degenerative arthritis (not seen in children). Arthritis may present with arthralgia in the initial stages and so pain may be the only factor. Similarly, growing pain manifests after a day's activity and is relieved by massage and rest. (Inflammatory pain is aggravated by touching or pressing but if it is relieved by massage, it denotes pain arising from tired muscles as in case of growing pain). Pain caused by muscle cramps is relieved by trying to relax the affected muscle by suitably changing position.

Degree and type of pain – severe pain suggests severe inflammation as in fracture or acute cellulitis or osteomyelitis. (In fact, in children, cellulitis should be viewed as probable osteomyelitis). Burning pain is characteristic of herpes zoster while dull ache may suggest mild inflammation or non-inflammatory disorders. Shooting pain down the leg may suggest a pinched nerve due to a vertebral disease.

Accompanying symptoms – swelling suggests inflammatory disease – either trauma, infection or non-infective disorders. Fever indicates wide spread disease as viral myositis or severe localized inflammation as in osteomyelitis or abscess. Significant pallor or purpura denote hematological disorder.

Past history – similar illness is seen in few rheumatological disorders and hemophilia

Family history – may guide to genetic or familial disorders such as hemophilia, sickle cell disease or some of the rheumatological disorders.

Physical Examination

Sick or not sick – Child is sick looking in cases of Infection and non-infective inflammation while trauma, hemophilia, growing pain etc do not present with significant sick look.

Local swelling denotes local inflammation. Generalized pain is not accompanied with swelling except in polyarticular disease. Localized bony swelling is seen in osteochondrosis and also in bone tumors.

Local warmth and tenderness signifies severe inflammation as in case of septic arthritis or osteomyelitis.

Restriction of movement – Severe painful conditions do not permit any movement of affected limb. Pain due to periarticular disease is evident on active movement of the affected joint but not on passive movement. It differentiates articular from periarticular disease. Pain in arthritis is aggravated by active as well as passive movement.

Localized muscle wasting signifies chronic pathology as seen in wasting of quadriceps in chronic arthritis of knee. Similarly, deformities and contractures are seen in chronic arthritis.

Hematological signs such as pallor or purpura denotes probable leukemia. It often presents as vague limb pain but sickness and other signs including hepatosplenomegaly and lymphadenopathy would suggest correct diagnosis. It is often missed as rheumatological disorder and wrongly prescribed steroids – it is a fatal mistake. In fact, steroids are rarely necessary in management of limb pain. Bleeding gums suggest scurvy though it may also be a manifestation of other hematological disorders such as leukemia. However, scurvy presents as pseudoparalysis (severe pain resembling paralysis).

Cardiac signs may be seen in rheumatic fever and at times in other rheumatological disorders.

Absence of any abnormal signs may suggest diagnosis of growing pain, pain amplification syndrome or functional pain.

Investigations

CBC helps in suspected acute osteomyelitis or arthritis as well as hematological disorders such as leukemia or sickle cell disease. ESR/CRP detects degree of inflammation but not the cause. Suspected rheumatological diseases need specific tests and it is not rational to ask for ANA (it is specific for SLE with positive dsDNA) or RA factor (positive in older female child with polyarticular disease) in every case of arthritis. Such tests are better reserved for specialists. X-ray detects signs of rickets, scurvy and also bone injury.

Management

Specific treatment depends on final diagnosis. However symptomatic treatment with analgesic may be tried till then. Neurogenic pain such as in case of herpes zoster is not easy to control with analgesics. Steroids should never be used in undiagnosed limb pain lest leukemia is missed with dire consequences of poor outcome.

Take Home Message

Lower limb pain is a common complaint in most benign conditions such as growing pain or one caused by hypermobility of joints or restless leg syndrome but they pose a challenge in treatment. Diseases presenting with pain can be simply treatable as in case of vitamin D or C deficiency. Limb pain can be a part of generalized body pain as in case of viral myositis that is self-limiting. However, limb pain may be an initial symptom of a serious disease such as leukemia or chronic persisting rheumatological disorder. In these cases, steroids should never be used without proper diagnosis and referral to a specialist is ideal.

MCQs

1. This condition presents with pain without swelling

A) Neurogenic pain
B) Growing pain
C) Functional pain
D) All of the above

2. Infection causing limb pain is often associated with swelling but not in this condition

A) Cellulitis
B) Herpes zoster
C) Syphilis
D) Osteomyelitis

3. This rheumatological disorder presents with severe pain with minimal or no swelling

A) Juvenile idiopathic arthritis
B) Vasculitis
C) Rheumatic fever with arthritis
D) Juvenile dermatomyositis

4. Pain associated with bleeding disorder is seen in

A) Leukemia
B) Scurvy
C) Vasculitis
D) All of the above

5. Which of the following statement is RIGHT?

A) Pain and swelling are severe in septic arthritis
B) Swelling is much more than pain in juvenile idiopathic arthritis
C) Pain is more than swelling in juvenile dermatomyositis
D) All of the above

Answers to MCQs

Correct answers as follows:

Q1 D	Q2 B	Q3 C	Q4 D	Q5 D

55 Leg Pain – May be a Sinister Symptom!

Clinical Application of Basic Concepts

Pain in both lower limbs represents a generalized disease while pain in one limb may be due to local pathology. Pain without swelling denotes non-inflammatory disease. Generalized pain in the limbs with fever may be due to myalgia caused by a viral infection, malaria, leptospirosis or typhoid fever or due to bony pain as in leukemia. Pain as the only symptom without swelling or fever may be due to physical as well as functional disorders that pose a diagnostic challenge. Etiology is not known in a few of these conditions such as growing pains, fibromyalgia or restless leg syndrome. A non-organic functional disorder is diagnosed by analysis of detailed history but only after ruling out other conditions.

Case Based Study

Case 1

Six year old child presented with generalized limb pain and headache for a day followed by high fever. There were no other symptoms. He was temporarily better for a few hours after paracetamol but pain and fever would recur. Three days later, he became well without any specific treatment.

Physical examination showed no localizing signs and as the child got better without any specific treatment, it was labeled as **viral infection with myalgia.** There is no need for any investigations in such a case. On the first day when pain in the limbs is the only symptom, one may not be sure of further evolution of the disease though it is often a forerunner of fever. One should wait for fever to appear in such situations. Once fever comes up, one is still not sure about the cause of fever. However, if the child looks better during the inter-febrile period, it is mostly a viral infection and one would expect quick improvement.

Case 2

Six year old child presented with fever and severe leg ache along with headache for the last two days. The pain was so severe that he could not walk and had to be lifted to reach the doctor. There were no other symptoms. On detailed questioning, this boy had waded through knee-deep water during heavy rains a few days prior to the onset of this illness.

Physical examination showed severe congestion in conjunctiva – almost red eye – characteristic of leptospirosis. Diagnosis of **leptospirosis** was confirmed by the presence of IgM leptospira antibodies. It is important to order liver and renal function tests as these two organs are often involved in the immune phase of the disease and one may find biochemical abnormality before symptoms may ensue.

He was treated with doxycycline and recovered completely. Leptospirosis presents with symptoms similar to many other infections. Severe myalgia with conjunctival congestion is also common to many diseases. This case illustrates the fact that history taking is an art of asking questions based on rational thinking and if the history of wading through knee-deep water is missed, one may not consider the diagnosis of leptospirosis. Such a history is unlikely to come forth from parents. The etiology of febrile illness during the rainy season should consider specific diseases such as malaria and typhoid besides common viral infections and leptospirosis.

One must watch carefully for the immune phase involving the liver and kidney besides other organs such as the brain that may overlap with fever or follow after a short afebrile period.

Case 3

Three year old child presented with fever and excessive irritability for last three days. There were no other specific symptoms. He was apparently well prior to this illness. Fever suggests probable infection or inflammation and excessive irritability denotes pain; the site of pain is not clear as a child at this age can't localize the pain. In absence of any other localizing symptoms, it is likely to be a generalized pain. It may be either myalgia or bony pain. It can be decided easily on physical examination.

Physical examination showed significant pallor without any other signs such as lymphadenopathy or hepatosplenomegaly. It may suggest the possibility of leukemia as marrow aplasia does not cause pain. Diagnosis of **acute lymphoblastic leukemia** was confirmed by blood tests and further referred to a specialist for management.

Acute leukemia in an early stage may present with fever as the only symptom and physical examination may elicit pallor, purpura or bony tenderness. It is not easy to document bony tenderness in a crying child. A high index of suspicion can help the diagnosis of acute leukemia in the early stage. Further immunological tests are necessary for a complete diagnosis.

Case 4

Three year old female child presented with pain on standing and walking for last four days. Initially it was thought to be due to an unnoticed fall or injury though child denied any such accident. There were no other symptoms. As pain persisted, parents noticed that child resisted movements of right leg and there was fullness of right knee joint. This seems to be pain arising from either knee joint or periarticular tissues around the joint or bone. As there was no significant fever, acute infection is unlikely. So, it may be non-infective inflammation and leukemia should also be kept in mind.

Physical examination showed knee joint swelling with restricted active and passive movements. This confirms articular involvement. Periarticular disease presents with free passive movements though active movements are restricted. So, diagnosis of arthritis is made though etiology is not evident. One may have to wait to see further progress over days or weeks. Till then clinical follow-up is the most rational way forward. On detailed physical examination, few small joints of hand were also affected though minimally. So, this was not monoarthritis as thought of initially but it was pauciarthritis with three other joints involved. This pointed strongly to **Juvenile idiopathic arthritis.**

Investigations – CBC was within normal limits though ESR was 75 mm that indicated inflammation. It pointed to a probable juvenile idiopathic arthritis. Child was treated with non-steroidal anti-inflammatory drugs and weekly methotrexate.

It is important to note that patient may complain of limb pain while walking, in the initial stage of developing arthritis and subsequently, affection of small joints may be overlooked with a focus on a single large joint. Besides, examining all the joints, it is also important to look beyond the joints as other organs are also often involved in JIA such as iridocyclitis.

Case 5

One year old severely malnourished infant presented with excessive irritability and paucity of limb movements for last two days. There was no fever or any other significant symptoms. This child was fed with dilute milk without any solid food till date. He had past history of two episodes of loose stools. Paucity of movements may suggest neurological disease but excessive irritability may denote possibility of severe painful conditions affecting all limbs that has resulted in pseudo-paralysis. So, it may represent generalized limb pain. In absence of fever, it is less likely to be infection or non-infective inflammation, though severely malnourished infant may not respond with fever in spite of serious infection or inflammation. Leukemia is a possibility and so also scurvy as this child is severely malnourished.

Physical examination showed severe malnutrition – weight 4.5 kg, length 65 cms, head O 43 cms, significant pallor, painful movements of all limbs, no purpura or bleeding gums, no hepatosplenomegaly or lymphadenopathy. Other systems were normal including nervous system. Absence of enlargement of liver, spleen or lymph nodes favor diagnosis of scurvy in this child. Bleeding gums are seen only when many teeth erupt and as this child had only two teeth, this sign may not appear so early. Bony tenderness is seen in both scurvy and leukemia but is difficult to note in a crying infant and so not dependable.

Investigations ruled out leukemia and so diagnosis of scurvy was made. It can be proved by low serum vitamin C levels though such a test is not routinely available. So best diagnostic test is radiological demonstration of subperiosteal hemorrhage along with other epiphyseal changes. This child was confirmed to be suffering from **scurvy** besides multiple nutritional deficiencies. He was treated with 500 mg of Vitamin C per day and within three days, the pain had disappeared and he could move his limbs well and was no more irritable.

Scurvy manifests clinically only in absence of vitamin C in the diet for more than six months. Thus, it is seen beyond the age of six months and only in the severely malnourished child. Symptoms improve dramatically within a few days of oral administration of vitamin C and it is also a therapeutic test for scurvy. Vitamin C is not stored in the body and so the body depends on daily intake of vitamin C.

Case 6

Ten year old male child presented with pain and swelling of the left knee joint for two days. He was apparently well prior to the present problem. He started getting pain in the left knee region within half an hour after a trivial fall while walking. It was considered to be a sprain but got worst over the next two days. There was no fever.

Apparently, it would look like a traumatic injury but it is worth noting that fall was trivial though the outcome of the injury was much more severe. It suggests underlying pathology. Such preexisting pathology may be congenital malformation in the joint itself or functional disorder like hemophilia or an acquired condition like leukemia.

On detailed history, it was revealed that he would bleed easily after an injury that would take time to control. This in a male child suggested hemophilia and was further confirmed by a history of similar disease in the maternal uncle.

Physical examination showed significant swelling of the left knee joint with tenderness and restriction of movements – both active and passive – but without warmth or redness. This suggests the diagnosis of **hemophilia**. It was confirmed by blood tests showing very low levels of factor 8. Management consists of factor 8 replacement to stop further bleeding. Physiotherapy is necessary to prevent contractures but only when the risk of bleeding is minimized and even then, one needs to exercise caution while doing physiotherapy. Such a child is prone to trivial injury and so should be advised not to participate in physical sports.

Case 7

Eight year old child presented with a history of pain and paucity of movements of both legs for the last four days. There were no other significant symptoms. He had suffered from a simple viral infection a few days prior to this illness but had recovered completely without any specific drugs. It is important to decide whether this is true paresis or pseudoparesis due to severe pain. On direct questioning, it was revealed that he could not move his limbs at all and so it was true paresis. A neurological condition that presents with pain may be due to affection of nerve roots or also due to spasm of affected muscles as a result of anterior horn cell irritation as in the case of polio or polio-like viral infection.

Physical examination showed lower motor neuron involvement with symmetrical affection of both lower limbs without the involvement of upper limbs or other areas. Further on raising the leg straight, the pain was exaggerated suggesting root involvement. This favored diagnosis of ascending polyneuritis – Guillain Barre syndrome. He was treated with IV gamma globulin and recovered completely over the next few days. It is an autoimmune disease that may worsen over the next few days and involve respiratory muscles requiring mechanical ventilation or also involve cranial nerves and autonomic nervous system. Most of the patients recover though few may remain with residual paresis.

Case 8

Ten year old child presented with a history of pain in both legs mainly in the evenings for the last two months. Throughout the day, he would remain active without pain but by late evening especially just before going to bed, he would complain of aches in both legs. The pain would get relieved with massage and he would fall asleep to get up and remain normal through the next entire day. There was no relief with pain killers though massage made him feel relieved. This history is classical of growing pain.

Physical examination of this child was totally normal. There is no need for any investigations in such a child. Parents were counseled about the diagnosis of **growing pain.** It suggests tired muscles with an accumulation of metabolic products that are absorbed following an increase in blood supply with massage or application of heat. The exact cause is not known though it is a benign condition and gets well by itself over time. One must avoid repeated use of analgesics that may lead to renal damage. Physical measures are good enough to offer relief.

Take Home Message

Pain in limbs may arise from many of the structures and it is important to determine the site of a lesion. Even a localized joint pain may begin with non-localizing pain in the limb and what looks like unilateral disease may also be a generalized disease. Pain cannot be localized by children under the age of 4-5 years and irritability may be the only presenting symptom. Generalized limb pain may arise from muscles or bones and differentiation is not easy, especially in young children. The cause of limb pain may vary from a very benign condition of unknown etiology to a very serious hematological vascular or neurological disease.

MCQs

1. Leptospirosis is suspected in the presence of

A) Severe myalgia
B) Conjunctival congestion
C) Increased serum creatinine
D) All of the above

2. This is the drug of choice in the treatment of leptospirosis

A) Gentamycin
B) Erythromycin
C) Doxycycline
D) None of the above

3. This factor differentiates generalized muscle pain from generalized bony pain

A) Severity of pain
B) High fever
C) Tenderness
D) None of the above

4. Pain may be so severe in this condition that it presents with pseudoparalysis

A) Leptospirosis
B) Scurvy
C) Both of them
D) None of them

5. This finding is classical of periarticular disease

A) Active and passive movements are painful
B) Active movements are painful but not passive
C) Passive movements are painful but not active
D) Both movements are not painful

Answers to MCQs

Correct answers as follows:

Q1 D	Q2 C	Q3 C	Q4 C	Q5 B

56 Breathlessness - It is Scary!

Introduction

Breathlessness refers to an increase in efforts of breathing. Normally air contains 20% oxygen and the volume of air inspired and expired in every breath without extra effort in a healthy individual at rest amounts to about 6-7 ml/kg body weight. It provides adequate oxygen and gets rid of carbon dioxide. Oxygen concentration is low at high altitudes where even a normal person feels breathless. When oxygen requirements are increased as in the case of physical exercise, a healthy individual can easily compensate to an extent by merely increasing respiratory rate. However, beyond a certain degree, a person has to make extra efforts by using accessory muscles of respiration that normally do not come into play. However, time may come when muscles of respiration get tired and cannot sustain efforts of breathing which may endanger life.

Body's Compensatory Mechanisms

Unfortunately, oxygen cannot be stored in the body and hence must be made available all the time. Nature has provided mechanisms that can compensate to an extent for increasing needs or disturbed respiratory function. The first step would be to increase the respiratory rate. There is a limit to increasing respiratory rate as there has to be enough time to exhale carbon dioxide as well. Normally, expiratory time is 2-3 times inspiratory time – IE ratio is 1:2 or 1:3. So when the respiratory rate cannot be further increased, nature tries the next step of using accessory muscles of respiration to push in more air with each breath. Intercostal muscles retract in the hope of sucking in air with more power and even smaller muscles contribute to such an effort. It reflects as an increased effort at breathing and the person feels uncomfortable and distressed. Concurrently, heart rate also increases and with increased respiratory and cardiac activity, oxygen demands also increase resulting in further imbalance. An increase in heart rate also has limitations as oxygen is supplied to the heart during diastole and there has to be enough time for diastole as well. In normal adults, systolic time is about 60% of the diastolic time though in young infants with faster heart rate, systolic and diastolic time may be equal or at times, even systolic time may be more than diastolic time. Initially, by increasing efforts of breathing, oxygen requirements are barely met but if the disease worsens by then or respiratory muscles get tired, tissues suffer from lack of oxygen and retained carbon dioxide. This stage demands urgent intervention as the body's available resources have failed.

Effects of Lack of Oxygen and Retained Carbon Dioxide

Effects of oxygen deficiency and/or retained carbon dioxide are felt by the brain the most as the brain needs a continuous supply of oxygen. Retention of carbon dioxide results in vasodilation of cerebral vessels that cause an increase in intracranial pressure and poor cerebral perfusion resulting in deficient oxygenation to brain cells, as also happens if oxygen is not available in an adequate amount from the lungs. It is how the brain gets affected. Next to suffer is the heart, followed by all other organs. Disturbed gas exchange results in a change in pH of blood resulting in acidosis which in turn affects heart function resulting in rhythm disturbances. Heart dysfunction adds to the trouble – typically heart and lungs work together – it is the cardiorespiratory system. The disease of one of them affects the other as well. Other systems have a functional reserve and so can tolerate abnormal respiratory functions to an extent but not the brain or heart.

Common Causes of Breathlessness

Though diseases of respiratory and cardiac systems predominate in leading to breathlessness, affection of other systems also may cause breathlessness though mediated through cardiorespiratory system. Neurological diseases that control breathing can also cause breathlessness. Metabolic acidosis results in tachypnea – deep and rapid breathing and may be mistaken for breathlessness though there is no increase in efforts of breathing. Cardiac disease may originate in the renal system as a result of hypertension and adrenal disease may also be the cause of hypertension. Similarly, severe anemia may cause cardiac dysfunction and thus, directly or indirectly, many systems may be involved and clinicians must be aware of it. Common respiratory causes include pneumonia, pleural effusion, asthma, chronic bronchitis with emphysema in adults, bronchiolitis in children, interstitial lung disease and upper airway obstruction as in the case of laryngitis. Common cardiac diseases in children are congenital heart defects and rheumatic heart disease (less common recently), myocardial diseases more in adults and so also hypertension. Neurological disorders presenting with breathlessness include lower motor neuron diseases such as ascending polyneuritis and polio-like illness. The central nervous disease may affect breathing rate, rhythm and depth but these are not presenting features. Diabetic ketoacidosis presents with tachypnea mimicking breathlessness.

Clinical Approach

Analysis of Detailed History

First step in the clinical approach is always to define the anatomy of the disease – which system is involved. It is often possible to define microanatomy. Thereafter one should find out pathology and etiology is often a guess based on anatomy and pathology.

Age – A young infant in the first three months has a high chance of cardiac disease but in later infancy and thereafter, pulmonary diseases are more prevalent.

Origin, duration, progress – respiratory diseases are often acute with exception of chronic interstitial lung disease while cardiac disorders are chronic with exception of acute myocarditis. Asthma is typically episodic and nocturnal. There is a difference between episodic and recurrent. Episode refers to similar presentation at similar time while recurrence may occur at any time.

Accompanying symptoms – Fever is common in respiratory diseases with exception of asthma while cardiac conditions are rarely accompanied with fever.

Cough followed by breathlessness is classical in respiratory disease though cough may be absent in bronchiolitis or interstitial lung disease while recurrent cough is feature of heart defect with pulmonary congestion such as left to right shunt in which presence of mild tachypnea is often overlooked.

Palpitation may be complained by older child suffering from heart disease and occasionally an observant mother may give a history of rapid precordial pulsations. Hypophonia or aphonia in a breathless child suggests paralysis of respiratory muscles. Often on direct questioning, one can get idea of abnormal audible respiratory sounds.

Stridor, wheeze or grunt denote upper airway inspiratory obstruction, lower airway expiratory obstruction and lung parenchymal disease respectively. Hissing sound suggests nasal obstruction.

Behavior of the child is an important early indicator of lack of oxygen or retained carbon dioxide. Confusion or irrelevant behavior denotes lack of oxygen while irritability is a feature of hypercarbia.

Physical examination – nutritional and growth parameters help in differentiating acute from chronic conditions. Degree of breathlessness is evident by presence or absence of chest retractions and accessory muscles in action. Respiratory and heart rate and blood pressure changes offer clue. Generally breathless child has tachypnea and tachycardia but if tachypnea is proportionately more as compared to tachycardia, it would suggest primary respiratory disease. While, if tachycardia is proportionately more as compared to tachypnea, it denotes cardiac disease. Hypertension may be due to renal or endocrinal disease and also due to coarctation of aorta. Behavior change, blood pressure and pallor, if any must be looked for.

Chest signs such as restricted movements, change in percussion note, diminished or abnormal breath sounds and foreign sounds denote pulmonary disease while enlarged heart and murmur indicate cardiac disease. Chest signs may be absent in interstitial lung disease as well as upper respiratory obstruction in laryngitis. Similarly, absence of murmur does not rule out cardiac disease.

Cyanosis is a late sign in respiratory diseases while it may be seen in an otherwise comfortable child with cyanotic heart defect. Paralysis of respiratory muscles are easy to note. Measurement of oxygen concentration by **pulse-oximeter** is now considered as part of physical examination as it can detect seriousness early enough to take proper corrective action. In most of the situations, clinical diagnosis is possible with analysis of detailed history and focused physical examination.

Investigations

Provisional diagnosis is a must before planning investigations. Tests are only to confirm or rule one or two similar diseases that are considered. Of course, test results must be interpreted in the light of clinical profile. CBC and chest X-ray are useful primary investigations in pulmonary diseases. While chest X-ray and ECG can give some clue to cardiac disease, echocardiogram is much more useful to get accurate information. One may need blood gas analysis in serious situations.

Management

Breathlessness is an emergency where patient needs hospitalization except an asthmatic who may be relieved of breathlessness in a short time with nebulized drugs. Specific treatment depends on final diagnosis but supportive therapy includes oxygenation, mechanical ventilation and hydration. Cardiac defects need surgical intervention for correction. Neurological disease such as ascending polyneuritis is treated with IV immunoglobulins and may need physiotherapy.

Take Home Message

Breathlessness (increase in work of breathing) and tachypnea are not synonymous though often used interchangeably. Tachypnea or increase in respiratory rate is the first compensatory mechanism by the body before breathlessness ensues and so it is important to pick up. While breathlessness is an emergency requiring immediate resuscitation by oxygenation and further action decided by probable diagnosis. Behavior change is the early manifestation of hypoxemia in acute respiratory diseases and irritability in case of retained carbon dioxide.

MCQs

1. Oxygen deficit may result from

A) Low oxygen concentration in the environment
B) In spite of normal oxygen concentration in environment
C) Pollution in the environment
D) All of the above

2. Which of the following statement is WRONG? Breathlessness may be the presenting symptom of

A) Renal disease
B) Endocrinal disease
C) Hematological disease
D) Vascular disease

3. Which of the following statement is WRONG? Hypoxic patient may have

A) Rapid and shallow respiration
B) Rapid and deep respiration
C) Slow and irregular respiration
D) All of the above

4. Which of the following statement is WRONG?

A) Pulse-ox may be abnormal in case of high fever
B) Pulse-ox may be abnormal in cardiac disease without breathlessness
C) Pulse-ox may be abnormal in a comfortable child
D) None of the above

5. Chest X-ray is not likely to be useful in this respiratory disease

A) Acute bronchiolitis
B) Chronic interstitial disease
C) Pleural effusion
D) Pneumonia

Answers to MCQs

Correct answers as follows:

Q1 D	Q2 C	Q3 B	Q4 D	Q5 B

57 Breathlessness – Need Early Recognition and Prompt Action

Clinical Application of Basic Concepts

Breathlessness is a symptom but much before it ensues, there are subtle clues for physicians to observe. A mild increase in respiratory rate is obvious especially in older children, only if carefully looked for. Mothers of young children often notice fast abdominal movements. Thus, tachypnea is the earliest sign and it is at this stage, that one can find out probable cause. An increase in heart rate is not evident to a patient unless an older child complains of palpitation. If this early phase is missed, respiratory distress manifests with chest retractions – evidence of increased work of breathing. By now effects of hypoxia and/or hypercarbia are seen and the earliest symptom of such abnormality is a change in behavior – a state of confusion, drowsiness or irritability. If this is missed, cyanosis develops a late sign indicating respiratory failure.

Case-Based Discussion

Case 1

Two year old healthy child presented with fever for a day followed by dry cough, noisy breathing and breathlessness that worsened over the next 12 hours and the fever continued. Dry cough suggests the involvement of upper airways and noisy breathing denotes obstruction to the passage of air that must have resulted in breathlessness. Fever indicates infection and as other symptoms have followed quickly after the onset of fever; it is most likely a viral infection.

Physical examination revealed not sick looking but uncomfortable child with stridor, RR 40/min, HR 115/min, mild fever, marked suprasternal retraction, normal breath sounds, no foreign sounds and other systems were normal. These findings are in favor of acute laryngeal obstruction due to viral infection – **viral laryngitis - croup**. This child was treated with oxygen and hydration and recovered within the next two days.

While this case is typical of croup, one must make sure that it is not a bacterial infection leading to upper airway obstruction as may happen in a retropharyngeal abscess or rarely bacterial tracheitis. Patients suffering from such diseases are sick and highly febrile. At times, upper airway obstruction may be caused by angioneurotic edema or laryngeal spasm due to tetany, in which case, there are other clues in the history and physical examination.

Case 2

Two year old healthy child presented with mild fever and cold followed a day later with breathlessness for which child required hospitalization. This history is almost similar to croup but this child has not reported any cough or noisy breathing. The absence of cough and noisy breathing rule out the affection of larger airways but smaller airways such as bronchioles do present without cough. It also may be a cardiac disease such as acute viral myocarditis. Further physical examination would differentiate between these two possibilities.

Physical examination revealed no sickness but discomfort, rapid shallow breathing, RR 60/min, HR 120/min, chest shows bilateral emphysema with diminished breath sounds without foreign sounds, liver 3F +, liver span 7 cms, not tender, hepato-jugular reflex absent, spleen just palpable, no cardiomegaly or murmur.

These findings favor the diagnosis of **acute bronchiolitis**. It is a clinical diagnosis and generally, no tests are necessary. Treatment is symptomatic with oxygenation and hydration. The prognosis is good and recovery is expected within a few days. This disease is caused by respiratory syncytial virus and typically seen in healthy infants. Such a disease in a child with congenital cardiac defect or immune deficiency may progress into respiratory failure.

Case 3

Four year old child presented with history of fever and cough for two days followed by breathlessness that worsened over next 12 hours. Child was apparently well prior to this illness. Fever was high with sick interfebrile period. Cough was mild. High fever with sick interfebrile period suggests bacterial infection and mild cough points to probable lung affection. Breathlessness starting two days after onset of fever denotes progression of infection likely to be a developing pneumonia.

Physical examination showed sick looking child, RR 40/min HR 105/min, intercostal chest retraction, chest movements reduced on right lower part anteriorly, TVF/VR increased, impaired note on percussion, bronchial breath sounds with few crepitations, other systems were normal. These signs are typical of pneumonia of right middle lobe. Investigations – Hb 11 Gm%, WBC 18000 P 78 L 22 E 0 Pl N Chest X-ray revealed haziness on right side suggesting diagnosis of **acute bacterial pneumonia**.

Child was treated with Amoxycillin-clavulanate and recovered well. Sequence and progression of symptoms are important to note as much as severity of each symptom. Breathlessness appearing two days after onset of fever and mild cough is typical of pneumonia. With proper treatment, breathlessness is first to improve followed by fever but cough increases in severity. This is because damaged part gets liquefied and nature tries to expel it through airways. It is not a worsening situation and parents must be counselled appropriately.

Case 4

Eight year old healthy child presented with high fever for a day followed by breathlessness that increased over next few hours requiring urgent hospitalization. Breathlessness in this child has come up within a day of onset of fever and increased in severity quickly. It suggests immune response and not just the extension of infection that would have taken longer time to manifest more so in older child. This suggests development of severe pleural effusion. As there has been no history of any preceding infection, it is likely to be occult infection like tuberculosis to which this child has reacted immunologically.

Physical examination showed highly febrile child, uncomfortable, RR 45/min HR 120/min, chest movements absent on left side, trachea and apex beat shifted to right, dull note on percussion up to second intercostal space, absent breath sounds, no foreign sounds.

These findings are classical of large pleural effusion. Etiology is a guess – most likely tuberculosis. Investigations – Hb 12 Gm% WBC 18000 P 80 L 15 E 2 M 3 Pl N. Chest X-ray marked haziness all over the left side with mediastinal shift to right, pleural fluid WBC 5000 P 75 Proteins 2.6 Gm suggestive of acute inflammation. Pleural fluid was negative for GeneXpert and also bacterial culture. Thus, diagnosis in this child is based on local epidemiology and ruling out other infections. So final diagnosis was **pleural effusion due to tuberculosis.**

It is worth noting that neutrophilic leukocytosis in blood and pleural fluid denotes acute inflammation – either infective or non-infective immune-inflammatory in origin. Progress of symptoms in a short time suggests non-infective immune inflammation. It is not unusual to confirm the diagnosis of tuberculosis in such a patient because the focus of tuberculosis in such a child is expected to be very small situated in the subpleural region that sets up a large immune reaction in the form of pleural effusion. Though every effort must be made to prove the diagnosis including contact tracing.

Case 5

Six year old child presented with acute onset of cough and breathlessness over the last 12 hours. The cough was severe and dry. There was no fever. The child had a similar episode a few months ago and was treated with some medicines – details not known. There was a family history of asthma in the father. This history clearly suggests bronchial asthma.

Even in absence of past and family history, one would have considered the same diagnosis because the acute onset of severe cough suggests airway disease and absence of fever denotes a non-infective cause.

Physical examination showed an uncomfortable child but not sick, RR 35/min HR 105/min, subcostal chest retraction, audible wheeze, chest movements bilaterally symmetrical, rhonchi + on auscultation. Other systems were normal.

The diagnosisis is clear – **bronchial asthma.** There is no need for any tests in this child. Eosinophilia is not diagnostic of asthma. Chest X-ray may reveal prominent bronchovascular markings and at times patchy haziness due to small areas of atelectasis due to bronchial obstruction. Serum IgE is also non-specific and does not add value to diagnosis. Pulmonary function tests are not reliable at this age as child may not be able to perform the test optimally. Allergy tests are reserved only in resistant cases as majority patients are allergic to house dust mites, pollens and not commonly to food items. Other irritants such as smoke, perfumes and at times stress worsen the disease.

Acute attack is best treated with nebulised salbutamol and steroids. Adrenaline is used only in case of inadequate response. Maintenance therapy may be required in a child with persistent asthma.

Case 6

Eight year old child presented with history of breathlessness over last 2 weeks, gradually increasing and cough off and on. She was apparently well two weeks ago when she felt out of breath while coming back from school. However, on rest, she felt better. Gradually she found it difficult to move about for which she sought medical attention. There was no significant past or family history. Gradually progressive breathlessness with cough may be due to respiratory or cardiac disease. Significant cough indicates airway affection and considering breathlessness along with it, could it be asthma? But asthma is typically episodic and not gradually worsening. Interstitial lung disease may present with breathlessness gradually increasing, though such increase is over long time and cough is not a feature. Lung parenchymal disease often is infective and so presents with fever. So, this child may be suffering from cardiac disease. In absence of significant past history, congenital heart defect is less likely. So, it is likely to be an acquired heart disease. Most common cause of acquired heart disease in children is due to complications of rheumatic fever. Though there is no past history suggestive of rheumatic fever in terms of arthritis, such an episode may be incomplete and not even diagnosed as rheumatic fever. Gradually worsening breathlessness suggests increased pulmonary venous congestion as in case of mitral valve affection – either stenosis or regurgitation or both.

Physical examination revealed uncomfortable child, RR 34/min HR 120/min BP 100/50 mmHg, peripheral pulses well felt, precordial pulsations, apex beat in 6th intercostal space just outside mid-clavicular line, hyperdynamic, cardiomegaly+, pansystolic murmur best heard at apex and conducted to axilla, P2 loud, liver 2F+, firm, mild tenderness, hepatojugular reflex +ve, spleen not palpable, chest occasional crepitations, other systems normal. It was diagnosed as **Rheumatic mitral regurgitation**. There was no evidence of active carditis. This was confirmed by chest X-ray, ECG and echocardiogram. Child was treated with oxygen and anti-failure line of therapy followed by long term penicillin prophylaxis.

It is important to differentiate cardiac diseases from respiratory disorders. Breathlessness in respiratory disease is either acute or very slowly progressive while in cardiac disease it evolves over a few days to weeks. Such a difference makes a child with a respiratory disease more hypoxic as compared to cardiac disease. However, there are always few exceptions.

Case 7

Two year old child presented with history of cough and breathlessness off and on and occasional episodes of fever since last one year. History of not gaining weight. Absence of fever each time rules out primary infective disorder. As cough and breathlessness in this child suggests progressive disease as evident by faltering in weight and hence asthma is ruled out. Chronic interstitial lung disease would not present with significant cough and hence not likely. So respiratory causes are ruled out and so it must be a cardiac problem. Recurrent cough and breathlessness suggest pulmonary congestion and so probably left to right shunt defect such as VSD – it being the common defect.

Physical examination revealed wt 8 kg, length 82 cm RR 40/min HR 120/min BP 90/50 mmHg, no cyanosis, peripheral pulses well felt, precordial pulsations, apex in 5th intercostal space outside midclavicular line, hyperdynamic, systolic murmur best heard in parasternal area on right side 3rd intercostal space, P2 loud, liver 3F+, firm, mild tenderness +, spleen not palpable, chest few creps+, other systems normal. These findings are in favor of ventricular septal defect with congestive cardiac failure – **VSD with CCF.**

Investigations include echocardiogram that confirmed moderate size VSD with pulmonary hypertension. Chest X-ray and ECG add value to final diagnosis as lung markings and other chest defects and rhythm disturbances are not detected on echocardiogram. Child was treated with anti-failure line of therapy and would need surgical correction at optimal time.

Congenital heart defect may present at variable time depending on severity of defect. Left to right shunt defects present only after few weeks after birth when pulmonary pressures are reduced and so blood can flow across the defect from high pressure on left side to lower pressure on right. Smaller the defect, later is the presentation. Atrial septal defect may remain undiagnosed even in adult life. Most of the cardiac defects are successfully repaired.

Case 8

Four year old child presented with breathlessness for last 12 hours that worsened over time and child became drowsy. He was suffering from asthma and was on regular compliant treatment and well controlled. On the face of it, it may appear to be an attack of asthma but there was no cough at all, besides, the fact that he was well controlled. This should raise suspicion about the diagnosis.

Physical examination showed RR 45/min, deep and rapid breathing, chest clear no foreign sounds, HR 110/min, drowsy child responding to being called. Other systems N. Deep and rapid breathing with clear chest denotes metabolic acidosis and one common cause that is often hidden to begin with is diabetic ketoacidosis. On direct questioning, this child did have polyuria, polydipsia and polyphagia for last one week prior to onset of this illness. Investigations confirmed the diagnosis of **diabetes mellitus.**

Child was treated accordingly. Metabolic acidosis presents with deep and rapid respiration and may simulate breathlessness, though there is no increased effort of breathing, hypoxia or any chest signs. Metabolic acidosis results commonly in case of severe diarrhea and also renal tubular disease. Both these conditions present with other symptoms and signs but diabetes mellitus presents with hidden symptoms that are often not reported or observed.

Take Home Message

Onset of breathlessness offers a clue to the diagnosis. Sudden development of breathlessness in minutes is often due to mechanical causes such as inhaled foreign body or pneumothorax or rarely pulmonary embolism in adults. Breathlessness occurring in few hours is usually immunological as in asthma or immune mediated pleural effusion, that presenting in few days may be due to infections like pneumonia, bronchiolitis or myocarditis. Cardiac breathlessness due to heart defects may present in short period but in the background of symptoms of heart disease.

MCQs

1. **Which statement related to breathless child is WRONG?**

A) Cough is always present in respiratory disease
B) Cough is present in left to right shunt
C) Cough may not be present in respiratory disease
D) Cough may not be present in cardiac disease

2. Cough is a predominant symptom in this disease

A) Bacterial pneumonia
B) Acute bronchiolitis
C) Left to right shunt defect
D) Chronic interstitial lung disease

3. This is the only physical sign in acute bronchiolitis

A) Bronchial breath sounds
B) Hyper-resonant note on percussion
C) Mediastinal shift
D) Fine crepitations

4. Which of the following statement related to chest retraction in breathless child is WRONG?

A) Not seen in acute bronchiolitis
B) Not seen in chronic interstitial lung disease
C) Not seen in pleural effusion
D) None of the above

5. Which of the following statement is RIGHT?

A) Wheeze is heard in asthma
B) Wheeze is heard in cardiac failure
C) Wheeze may be present in case of inhaled foreign body
D) All of the above

Answers to MCQs

Correct answers as follows:

Q1 A	Q2 C	Q3 B	Q4 D	Q5 D

58 General Weakness – A Vague Symptom

Introduction

General weakness is not only a subjective feeling of the patient but vague enough that demands seeking clarification by the physician before embarking on its analysis. It may connote different meaning to different people. When a mother complains about general weakness in her child, it depends on her subjective understanding of what child has. It may be far from what the real problem may be. Often a mother equates thin stature of a child to weakness.

Basic Concepts

Generalized weakness is a complaint that mostly does not refer to neurological disorder. However, one must make sure that weakness does not relate to paresis. Rarely though, severe hypokalemia in a malnourished child or in a sick elderly individual may present with generalized paresis and so also in case of progressive ascending polyneuritis. So, one must confirm that there is no paucity of movements in a child presenting with generalized weakness. Generalized weakness refers to tired muscles. Muscles are short of desired energy required for movement and so such a patient wants to move and also can move but finds it very tiring and so reluctant to move.

What do Muscles Need for Adequate Functioning?

Muscles need oxygen that is provided by the lungs, pumped by the heart and transported through hemoglobin to the required sites. Thus, a child with slowly developing lung or heart disease or anemia may fail to deliver adequate oxygen to muscles and so present with generalized weakness. If lung or heart disease or anemia develops rapidly, the child presents with acute breathlessness rather than generalized weakness. Thus, generalized weakness develops over time and rarely in a short time. Besides oxygen, muscles need glucose for energy. It is not hypoglycemia but hyperglycemia that fails to deliver enough glucose to muscles. If a child is hypoglycemic, presentation is acute with seizure or change in behavior. But in the case of hyperglycemia as in diabetes, muscle cells cannot utilize glucose in spite of its availability and hence remain deprived of necessary glucose. Thus, diabetes may present with generalized weakness. However, if a child with diabetes often presents acutely with diabetic ketoacidosis and preceding phase of weakness may be short and missed. Energy comes from calories – though carbohydrates are the major source of calories and thus child with severe protein-energy malnutrition (PEM) also has generalized weakness. He is reluctant to play and prefers to be inactive.

Muscles in such a child are wasted that causing generalized weakness, besides the fact that nutrients are also not available. Muscles also need intracellular ions such as potassium and magnesium for adequate function. However, hypokalemia or hypomagnesemia are mostly acute and when severe, they manifest paresis – neurological weakness. Though rarely renal disease may present with chronic hypokalemia presenting with generalized weakness.

Causes of Generalized Weakness

As mentioned in the discussion above, severe PEM is a common cause of generalized weakness though major symptoms pertain to acute infection that brings the child to a health facility. In addition, loss of weight and appetite predominate. In older children, PEM is secondary to chronic progressive disease as in the case of end-stage renal disease.

However generalized weakness may be the only presenting symptom in chronic lung diseases such as interstitial lung diseases (chronic bronchitis with emphysema is rare in children), chronic heart conditions (congenital heart defects, rheumatic heart disease and myocardial disorders) and chronic anemia of various etiologies (iron or Vitamin B12 deficiency, congenital hemolytic anemia and marrow aplasia). Diabetes as a cause of generalized weakness should be kept in mind and will be evident only if one asks for polyuria, polydipsia and polyphagia. As generalized weakness is a prominent symptom, other symptoms are often not complained of, unless asked for. Chronic hypokalemia is rare to present as generalized weakness.

Clinical Approach

History – it is important to confirm that the child can move limbs in all directions, thus ruling out paresis.

Onset and duration – acute onset within a few days is typical of diabetes that is evident by asking about thirst, increased urine output and increased appetite. Most other conditions present subtly over days or weeks.

Progress – fast deterioration is a risk if one misses diabetes while other conditions worsen slowly.

Localizing symptoms – chronic lung disorders are easily missed as patients get adapted to hypoxia and do not complain about breathlessness though they do have tachypnea that is not noticed and complained by the patient.

Palpitation may be a symptom in chronic cardiac conditions in older children while mother may notice **precordial hyperactivity** in younger child.

Cough may be a symptom in both cardiac disease but often absent in chronic interstitial lung disease.

Significant **pallor** is rarely missed by parents and often is a main compliant along with generalized weakness. So, it is easy to make out in history itself.

Physical Examination

General appearance – Tired and chronically sick look is common to all except child with diabetes who may look acutely sick especially if initial stage is missed. Child with PEM may be irritable or lethargic depending on severity of protein or calorie deficiency.

Growth parameters – growth faltering is the hallmark of PEM but also abnormal in other chronic conditions to a variable extent. Child with diabetes may have normal growth.

Pallor is striking in case of severe anemia while many other conditions may also be marginally pale.

Heart rate and respiratory rate – are important to pick up subtle cardiac and respiratory disorders. Mild tachypnea is easily missed unless one counts respiratory rate over a full minute and same is true with mild tachycardia in a cardiac disease. Such basic signs can pick-up chronic but otherwise silent cardiac or respiratory diseases that are otherwise missed.

Pulse-oximetry is now considered as bedside clinical maneuver as much as use of blood pressure in routine clinical practice. This is because it offers great help in early pick-up of respiratory and cyanotic heart defects. In fact, it is now being used routinely in every newborn for early diagnosis of congenital heart defect.

Systemic examination – murmur, cardiomegaly and signs of cardiac failure would suggest a cardiac disease. Mild increase in respiratory rate may be the only finding in chronic interstitial lung disease that is easily overlooked. Pulse-oximetry will show low oxygen saturation in such a case. One must make a habit of noting pulse and respiratory rate judiciously. In case of severe pallor, presence of hepatosplenomegaly suggests hemolytic anemia while absence indicates either deficiency anemia or marrow aplasia. Child with marrow aplasia looks sick while one with deficiency or hemolytic anemia are not sick looking.

Investigations

Specific investigations are planned according to the system involved. At times, there is no clue on history or physical examination. In such a case, chest X-ray and echocardiogram/

ECG may offer clue. However, if both these tests are normal and one is sure about the problem being pathological, further tests may be necessary to rule out cardiac disease (stress test) and interstitial lung disease (CT scan). Detailed hematological tests can define specific cause of anemia (serum iron or B12, hemoglobin electrophoresis).

Management

It would depend on specific diagnosis. What is important to note is a fact that generalized weakness is a vague symptom and cannot be passed on by prescription of a "tonic". There is a risk of missing life-threatening diseases. A child with PEM needs not only nutritional supplements but counselling for rehabilitation and ruling out comorbid conditions. Specific treatment depends on final diagnosis.

Take Home Message

Generalized weakness as a presenting complaint needs cautious approach because some of the conditions present with subtle clues on history as well as physical examination that are easily overlooked. Diabetes mellitus is easy to miss unless thought of and so also chronic renal tubular disease. Polyuria is common to both and personal history mostly focuses on oliguria and not polyuria. Thorough physical examination should start with actual count of respiratory and heart rate so as not to miss mild abnormality.

MCQs

1. Weakness to lay people may mean

A) Thin stature
B) Loss of weight
C) Paresis
D) Any of the above

2. Choose the RIGHT statement. General weakness to a doctor should mean

A) Wants to move but cannot
B) Reluctant to move due to severe pain
C) Reluctant to move in spite of no pain
D) Feels tired easily

3. Pseudoparalysis is characterized by

A) Severe pain
B) Normal power
C) Normal deep tendon reflexes
D) All of the above

4. Choose WRONG statement. General weakness in PEM is due to

A) Poor muscle mass

B) Hypoglycemia

C) Hypokalemia

D) None of the above

5. Choose the WRONG statement. Hypoglycemia may present as

A) Generalized weakness

B) Seizure

C) Unconsciousness

D) All of the above

Answers to MCQs

Correct answers as follows:

Q1 D	Q2 D	Q3 D	Q4 D	Q5 A

59 General Weakness – Needs a Cautious Approach

Clinical Application of Basic Concepts

Thin stature is often considered equivalent to weakness. Weakness is a vague symptom and refers to lack of energy. Energy is provided through nutrition and oxygen. Naturally, many organs are involved in providing energy and undue expenditure of energy also would lead to weakness. However, when generalized weakness is the only complaint, one needs to go into the details of history to find out presence of subtle symptoms that may have been overlooked. Weakness is also a term used for paresis and one must make sure to rule out neurological disease.

Case-Based Discussion

Case 1

Ten year old child presented with generalized weakness for last two weeks. There were no other symptoms. On direct questioning, this child had stopped going out to play for last few months though for no apparent reason. He would prefer to be sedentary. There is no history of palpitation or breathlessness or polyuria, polydipsia and polyphagia. Parents had not noticed any significant pallor.

It is obvious that this problem has existed for several months though may have been aggravated over last two weeks and hence presented now. This history suggests that this child has been getting progressively tired over months. Absence or palpitation, breathlessness and symptoms of diabetes rules out chronic lung, heart conditions and chronic anemia. So, we have no clue to diagnosis on history.

Physical examination showed no abnormality on casual cursory examination but on detailed observation, his respiratory rate was 30 per minute at rest and it was certainly abnormal. Oxygen saturation at rest was 92% that meant he was hypoxic. Though he was apparently comfortable. This finding is in favor of chronic interstitial lung disease. Investigations showed Hb 15 gm%, CBC otherwise normal, chest X-ray normal, HRCT showed evidence of interstitial lung disease. Thus, diagnosis of **chronic interstitial lung disease** was confirmed. Etiology is often not evident but may be related to environmental factors triggering immune response. Steroids are considered on such a probability.

History should start with confirmation of period of onset of the symptoms as subtle symptoms are often not reported. This case emphasises need for thorough physical examination including counting respiratory and heart rate for a minute. Chronic hypoxia may often be tolerated by patients as they get adapted to it as polycythemia often compensates mild chronic hypoxia and hence delay in the diagnosis.

Case 2

15 year old child presented with generalized weakness and on direct questioning he reported tiredness that was gradually increasing. Apparently, he had no other symptoms except mild cough. At the age of 6 years, he had suffered from rheumatic fever with arthritis, from which he had recovered completely.

Gradually increasing tiredness suggests slowly progressive disorder. In the background of rheumatic fever in the past, one may consider heart condition such as valvular damage. Tiredness in this child indicates deficient oxygen supply to muscles as a result of cardiac disease. It denotes pulmonary venous congestion due to back pressure from left side of heart. It may favor diagnosis of mitral stenosis. Mitral regurgitation may have been more symptomatic with breathlessness.

Physical examination revealed heart rate 92/min at rest, respiratory rate 27/min (both mildly increased), no obvious cardiomegaly but loud first heart sound and mid-diastolic murmur at mitral area. This suggests diagnosis of **rheumatic mitral stenosis.** Echocardiogram confirmed the diagnosis of mitral stenosis. This child needs surgical intervention.

Slowly worsening left sided heart function may present with exertional dyspnea that patients perceive as tiredness and hence complain of general weakness. This case illustrates how this vague symptom needs to be analyzed.

Case 3

Four year old child presented with generalized weakness for last four months that made him not to participate in play activities. Apparently, there were no other symptoms except mild cough. On detailed questioning, he would feel tired after playing for few minutes and would rest in between such activities. It suggested slowly worsening tiredness over several months. It could be either lung or heart disease. If it is a heart disease, it is unlikely to be congenital heart defect because he was normal during first three years of life. Rheumatic heart disease also can be ruled out as he has been too young to have suffered from damage to heart as a result of rheumatic fever. However other types of heart diseases such as primary myocardial or pericardial conditions cannot be ruled out. Chronic interstitial lung disease is a possibility as interstitial lung diseases have different etiologies including damage due to previous viral infections and also due to environmental exposure to toxic or pollutants.

Physical examination showed heart rate 104/min and respiratory rate 28/min (both on higher side), precordial pulsations, mild cardiomegaly, soft systolic murmur at mitral area not conducted with normal heart sounds. Chest examination revealed few crepitations at the base of lungs. This suggests probable primary myocardial disease. Echocardiogram confirmed diagnosis of **cardiomyopathy**. Etiology of such a disease is not easy to correlate as it may result from events that have occurred in the past with such a viral infection. Further investigations are necessary to rule out metabolic or storage disorders.

Case 4

Eight year old child presented with generalized weakness and tiredness over last two months that was gradually increasing. On direct questioning, he reported mild fever off and on during this period. But it did not disturb him and so was ignored. There were no other symptoms.

Mild fever off and on suggests probable infection that has affected either lung or heart. Absence of cough almost rules out infective lung disease. Valvular or myocardial diseases do not present with low grade long duration fever but pericardial affection is likely. It may be in the form of mild pericardial effusion or constrictive pericarditis. Mild pericardial effusion may not be symptomatic and if fluid accumulation increases, it may lead to breathlessness. However constrictive pericarditis may deteriorate slowly as fibrosis develops slowly in chronic infection such as tuberculosis. So, one must look for evidence of constrictive pericarditis in this child.

Physical examination showed mild tachycardia and tachypnea but no other cardiac findings. However, liver was enlarged and firm but not tender and neck veins were engorged without hepatojugular reflux. This suggests superior and inferior vena caval obstruction and so diagnosis of **constrictive pericarditis due to tuberculosis** was considered. Echocardiogram confirmed the diagnosis. Constrictive pericarditis hampers free heart movements during cardiac cycle. As the process evolves slowly, heart function does not deteriorate over short time as may happen in progressive pericardial effusion with cardiac tamponade. Hence patient feels increasingly tired over time and presents with weakness.

Case 5

Four year old child presented with generalized weakness and reluctant to participate in play activities over last six months. It was gradually increasing to an extent that he would refuse to go out to play. Earlier he used to be very active child. There were no other symptoms.

Gradually increasing tiredness indicates slowly worsening oxygenation either due to chronic lung or heart disease. Absence of cough rules out lung disease as well heart disease with pulmonary congestion. So, it may be due to heart condition with pulmonary oligemia – less of blood flowing through lungs resulting in lack of oxygen. However, such a child should develop cyanosis but if pulmonary obstruction is mild, cyanosis may not be noticed by parents. Though on direct questioning, parents may reveal probable cyanosis seen on crying. However, it can be easily overlooked.

Physical examination showed mild clubbing of nails that is suggestive of chronic hypoxia, systolic murmur at pulmonary area without cardiomegaly or cardiac failure. This is in favor of **pink Fallot's tetralogy.** An echocardiogram confirmed the diagnosis. He would need surgical correction. This case illustrates the fact that mild cyanosis is difficult to be noticed by the patient and also by the doctor. A pulse oximeter is now a part of physical examination that would pick up mild hypoxia that can be further evaluated.

Case 6

Six year old child presented with slowly progressive tired feeling over the last 6 months. He was normal prior to onset of present symptom and was very active. Initially he would run about but would need to rest – it was unusual for him though was ignored. When this problem increased over time to an extent that he would refuse to go out to play, parents sought medical advice. On direct questioning, he had developed cough over last two months that was also slowly worsening. Hence, there was slowly worsening tiredness and cough. It suggests probable space occupying lesion in the chest now compressing over airways leading to increasing cough.

Physical examination showed impaired note on percussion on right anterior side of the chest but it did not correlate with either lobes of lungs or pleura. It denotes probability of mediastinal mass in the chest. Chest X-ray confirmed **large mass in anterior mediastinum** and was proved to be benign. It was surgically removed.

Physical findings in the lung lesion are restricted to surface area of lobes of lungs – it means right upper lobe lesion has findings only in upper half of the chest anteriorly and right middle lobe only in lower half of chest anteriorly. Lower lobe is represented only posteriorly. Physical findings in pleural disease are seen below a particular intercostal space but all over the chest anteriorly, laterally and posteriorly. This is referred to as lobar or pleural distribution of signs respectively. When physical signs do not correlate with either of these two patterns, one considers space occupying lesion.

Case 7

Ten year old child presented with generalized weakness and tiredness for last one week. He was very active prior to onset of this symptom and in fact used to attend coaching for tennis. One week ago, he felt tired while playing though coach insisted on his continuing to play and next day he refused to go to play. Initially parents thought he was just being stubborn. But when his problem persisted, they visited a doctor. It was only on direct questioning that polyuria, polydipsia and polyphagia was apparent and so diagnosis of **diabetes mellitus** was confirmed. He would have come in diabetic ketoacidosis with unconsciousness within next few days had he been further ignored. This case illustrates importance of detailed personal history. As oliguria is more common than polyuria, such a symptom is often missed while eliciting history. Polyuria may be caused by diabetes mellitus, diabetes insipidus, renal tubular disorders or it may also be psychogenic.

Case 8

Two year old child brought by mother complaining of generalized weakness since the age of one year. According to mother, this child was doing well till the age of one year. He had grown well and weighed 10.5 kg at one year, his food intake was good. But thereafter he started making fuss about eating and in spite of trying various methods and tonics, there was no improvement. He had gained just 1.5 kg through entire second year. So, she was worried about his generalized weakness. On direct questioning, mother reported that he maintained his activity level and there were no physical complaints. Active child almost rules out any significant pathology.

Physical examination showed happy and active child, weight 11.5 kg, length 87 cms and there was no abnormality detected. So, this child was completely **normal**. This mother was interpreting "poor" intake of food and "poor" weight gain during second year as weakness. She required to be counselled rather than child needing any investigations or treatment. So, mother had to be managed. Health status is better judged by activity level and growth by length/height and not by weight. Weight gain is variable in a normal healthy children and all that we need to ensure is no weight loss and some weight gain over months. Weight gain in a normal child during second year is one third of that gaind in first year while length gain is half of what is gained in first year. Thus, every normal child looks thin during second year as compared to first year due to differential gain in length and weight. This is often reported by mothers as weakness.

Take Home Message

This case emphasises the need to understand terms used by the patient that may not correlate with real problem. There are several terms used by patients while describing their symptoms, meaning of which may be misinterpreted by the doctor. Weakness is one such term that may connote paresis or tiredness but also just a thin stature. Cold and cough are other such terms used to connote noisy breathing. Patients also use medical terms to describe their symptoms such as acidity, chest congestion or throat problem. Unless doctor tries to decipher correctly what patient wants to convey, further evaluation may proceed in wrong direction.

MCQs

1. Generalized weakness is the presenting complaint in this infectious disease

A) Acute UTI
B) Hepatitis A viral infection
C) Acute URTI
D) Acute meningitis

2. Which statement is RIGHT? The reason for generalized weakness in hepatitis A infection is

A) Sudden destruction of large number of hepatocytes
B) Development of jaundice
C) Liver failure
D) All of the above

3. Generalized weakness may be the presenting complaint in this chronic disease

A) Chronic sinusitis
B) Chronic UTI
C) Tuberculosis
D) All of the above

4. Which statement is RIGHT? The reason for generalized weakness in above diseases is

A) Low grade fever
B) Prolonged fever
C) Increased catabolism
D) All of the above

5. Generalized weakness in interstitial lung disease is easily missed because

A) Absence of cough or breathlessness
B) No chest signs
C) Respiratory rate not counted
D) All of the above

Answers to MCQs

Correct answers as follows:

Q1 B	Q2 A	Q3 D	Q4 C	Q5 D

60 My Child is not Gaining Weight!

Introduction

Children during their growing period must show age-appropriate weight gain, though undue weight gain at other age groups may be pathological. The rate of weight gain varies in different phases of life. Weight gain is maximum during adolescence when a child gains about 15–20 kilograms of weight over four years till puberty is achieved and continues to gain about 8-10 kilograms over the next four years. Average weight gain in the first year is about 5-6 kilograms and thereafter it slows down to about 2 to 2.5 kilograms per year till the adolescent spurt starts. Around 7-9 years of age, there may be a small increase in weight over the average, amounting to about 3-4 kilogram per year during those two years. While adults are expected to maintain weight but small gain in weight may continue even in adult life. However, the rate of weight gain not only depends on different periods of growth but also varies in individuals depending on the genetic endowment, environmental influences and lifestyle. Thus, if one child grows 3 kilograms a year after the first year and the other 2 kilograms a year, at the end of another 10 years, they end up with a difference of 10 kilograms in their comparative weight but both may be equally healthy. It is the trend noted by periodic weight records that is more relevant. This is important to note that weight is not the only criterion of health.

Make Sure What Parents Mean

Most parents don't know what the average weight should be at a particular age. It is often their perception that the child is not putting on adequate weight. This is a common complaint, especially in the toddler age group. It is because an infant gains about 6-kilogram weight and 25-centimeter length in the first year that drops to 2 to 2.5 kilogram weight and 12-centimeter length in the second year. Hence there is a disparity between weight and length gain in the second year as compared to the first year. Weight gain is 40% and length 50% of the respective gain in the first year. Thus, a child in the second year is perceived to be thinner in relation to length as compared to stature during the first year. Such a change is physiological. In addition, forced feeding that inevitably results in the second year compounds the problem. During subsequent years, a child's weight gain follows an individual pattern that may be different from the average. Parents often compare a child's weight with that of other children around the same age but they forget that two children of the same parents also differ in their stature and at times even twins differ. So, the doctor must make sure whether there is a real problem of poor weight gain or just an imaginary one.

Confirm "Not Gaining Weight?"

Healthy child is always active, playful and happy without any symptoms. This is much more so in younger children. As age advances, behavioral issues may come in the way of happiness in particular and also may affect activity level. However, most complaints about weight gain exist in case of toddlers and younger children and this is in spite of children remaining active and happy. With too much focus on weight instead of health, poor weight gain is often a universal complaint especially in middle and upper socioeconomic groups. Objective way to monitor weight is to maintain growth chart. As every child has different birth weight and weight velocity. Growth chart in a normal child is expected to maintain around same centiles through growing period. In simple words, growth of the child follows the line on growth chart which he/she has always been before. It indicates normal growth pattern irrespective of actual weight. Growth chart is also useful to monitor length/height till puberty is reached and head circumference in first two years of life as brain growth is nearly over by end of second year. Each child should have a growth chart and parents should maintain periodic charting, initially with the help of a doctor in infancy but later by themselves. Normal growth pattern as shown in linear records in a chart can assure parents about child's growth being normal. It also provides confidence to a doctor not to indulge in unnecessary laboratory tests.

Clinical Approach

First step is to confirm whether child is losing weight or weight is stationary for more than expected period or whether child gains weight but less than expected at that age. Loss of weight certainly is abnormal and needs explanation. In first six months of life, if an infant's weight remains the same even for a fortnight, it is considered abnormal because this is an age of fast growth. In subsequent months of infancy, if weight has remained the same over a period of one month, one needs to look into probable cause. Beyond infancy, absence of weight gain over three months period should be considered abnormal. Once it is confirmed that weight gain has faltered, **next step** is to find probable cause. In an otherwise asymptomatic infant, most common cause is inadequate nutrition, mainly due to faulty feeding such as over-diluted milk or delayed introduction of complementary feeds. In an otherwise asymptomatic toddler, feeding problems such as bottle or breast addiction and forced feeding by parents are common reasons for absence of weight gain. In such an infant or toddler, appropriate correction of faulty feeding settles the problem and there is no need for any medical help.

However, in an older child in spite of being asymptomatic, weight loss or absence of weight gain over three months may need proper assessment to exclude pathological causes. Of course, if child is symptomatic at any age with weight loss, it clearly calls for finding the cause. Such children are sick to a varying extent, have poor appetite and are cranky. So, they are easy to recognise.

Pathological Causes

In every acute short-lasting illness, there may be weight loss recorded but such a child would regain weight in a short time again. All that one needs to do is to confirm regaining of weight. It calls for no more intervention. However. if a child after a weight loss fails to regain original weight, one must observe for some more time and take appropriate action if weight does not pick-up. It may indicate incompletely cured disease or underlying silent disease. In a chronic illness, significant weight loss is expected and it would take longer time to regain lost weight but on recovery, child should stop further loss of weight and then start, at least, gaining little weight. Regaining weight to original level may not occur after severe loss of weight during prolonged illness though on all other counts, child should have improved especially in terms of energy level and appetite.

Weight Loss in Absence of Obvious Illness

It is a real challenge. One must get into details of history to find any clue to a hidden problem. Such problems could be low grade infection such as tuberculosis or slowly evolving organ dysfunction. Loss of appetite, behavior change such as irritability or lethargy, disinterest in play or activities that he/she loved earlier are some of the signals of hidden disorders. It may be ideal to monitor body temperature by thermometer to pick-up any low-grade fever that would necessitate investigations for infections. In absence of documented fever, hidden organ dysfunction must be scrutinized. Subtle symptoms often are not reported by patients or parents of children and doctor must inquire about them. Mild puffiness of eyelids in the morning may indicate renal disease. Vague abdominal pain or distension and change in bowel pattern may signify hidden intestinal disease such as lymphoma or inflammatory bowel disease. Unexplained pallor is due to hematological disorder and may present only with mild enlargement of spleen. Undue tiredness after accustomed exertion may suggest either a lung or heart defect or diabetes mellitus. Acquired or inborn metabolic disorders may present initially without any obvious signs on physical examination. Doctor must inquire about subtle symptoms or look for subtle signs on physical examination to pick up a hidden cause of poor weight gain or loss of weight.

Take Home Message

Parents often complain of children not gaining weight but it may be just a wrong perception. It could easily be evident when you see such a child being active, playful and happy. Further, growth chart helps in objective assessment. However, once the problem is confirmed to be genuine, there would be a need to pinpoint the cause. At times, cause is hidden and detailed inquiry and focused physical examination can offer a clue. It is irrational to prescribe a "tonic" without proper evaluation for a child who is not gaining weight. Anyway "tonic" mostly does not help.

MCQs

1. This symptom is seen in both healthy and diseased child

A) Active
B) Playful
C) Loss of appetite
D) Happy

2. This is most dependable in deciding whether problem is genuine or not

A) History
B) Physical signs
C) Investigations
D) Growth chart

3. Indicator of a genuine problem on growth chart is

A) Weight at first visit
B) Velocity of weight
C) Both
D) None

4. Which of the following statement related to infant's weight gain is RIGHT?

A) Must gain every month
B) Must gain every two months
C) Must gain every week
D) All of the above

5. Which of the following statement is WRONG? This may be the hidden cause of not gaining weight

A) Acute infection
B) Chronic organ dysfunction
C) Chronic infection
D) All of the above

Answers to MCQs

Correct answers as follows:

Q1 C	Q2 D	Q3 B	Q4 A	Q5 A

61 Poor Weight Gain – Needs a Proper Evaluation

Basic Concepts for Clinical Application

Healthy children of the same age vary a lot in their weight and hence a record of weight at one single point may fail to judge whether child is failing to gain weight. Growth chart shows a range of normal weight expected at a particular age, upper level being at 97th percentile and lower at 3rd percentile, 50th percentile being the mean. A child who starts at 3rd centile and maintains same level over years is considered normal. It is only downward trend that signifies weight loss. It is different than not gaining weight. Weight of children beyond infancy may remain the same even over three months' period and it is normal. This is because normal weight gain at this age may be as small as 500 grams over three months that is not even easy to assess. Hence when child presents with not gaining weight, doctor must make sure whether it is true or just perceived. Most of the times, it is a perception of parents without monitoring child's weight.

Case-Based Discussion

Case 1

Mother of 18 months old child complained of poor weight gain for last 8 months and poor appetite for last 6 months. There were no other symptoms. Child was gaining weight well in first six months and thereafter gained less weight over next 4 months. But last 8 months, there has been hardly any gain in weight. On direct questioning, child remained active, had normal bowel movements and urination and slept well. On this history, it is clear that this child is unlikely to have any significant disease as he has been active and playful. So, we need to look at his growth chart to decide whether he has been faltering in his weight centiles. It would help to decide the probable cause of faltering, if any.

Physical examination did not reveal any abnormality. The growth chart showed that he had maintained his weight centiles and so also his length and head O. Hence this is **a normal child**. Many mothers perceive poor weight gain around the second year of their child. This is physiological in the sense that weight gain slows after the first year. But add to the problem of misconception, most mothers start forcing to feed the child and it becomes a vicious cycle. The more the mother forces the child, the more he refuses and starts hating food. This pattern ends up in poor eating in the third year and the child may even start losing weight. Counseling is an important part of the management of such a problem and not the "tonics".

Case 2

Four year old child was brought by parents because of poor weight gain after the first year of life and poor appetite. There were no other symptoms. Previous growth records showed that his weight centiles had come down from 75th to 25th level though his height was maintained above 50th centiles through last four years. He remained active and playful and had normal development.

History suggests that this child has genuinely faltered in his weight centiles without any symptoms or change in his activity and energy level. It mostly rules out any active disease. As his height has maintained a centile level, it may suggest the recent poor intake of nutrition. However, parents complain about the poor intake of food from the age of one year. Had it been a poor intake of nutrition over the last three years, his height also would have started showing a decline in centiles. This kind of disparity suggests that his intake of food is sufficient for his energy and activity level though his parents perceive it to be poor. After all, metabolism decides how much you use out of what you eat. It is similar to a fact that the amount of study is not proportional to the success achieved but a lot depends on how much you use.

Physical examination did not reveal any abnormality. Thus, we can conclude that this child is deriving enough energy from his food irrespective of what his parents consider to be poor intake. So, it is likely to be constitutional thin stature. This child is "programmed" to be thin but healthy. It may be a familial tendency. On direct questioning, it was revealed that his father used to be thin during childhood though now he is obese. This is a **normal child** and in fact, should take adequate care not to become obese later in life. This child does not need any drugs or investigations but parents should be properly explained and counseled.

This case illustrates a fact that weight below the expected average may not be pathological but just a constitutional or genetic factor. A growth chart helps to allay the anxiety of parents.

Case 3

One year old infant presented with poor weight gain since birth. He was born at the end of full-term with a birth weight of 1.4 kg. His cry was poor at birth and required bag and mask ventilation with oxygen for half an hour. He was fed with a nasogastric tube for 2 days followed by spoon feeding and then on breastfeeding. He did not need any other intervention and was discharged after 10 days. His weight has always been below the 3rd centile, his length on the 5th centile and head O on the 10th centile. His motor milestones are delayed as he has started to sit but with support but his other milestones are near normal. His mother had suffered from prolonged febrile illness during the second trimester and had lost 6 kg weight in this illness.

This history suggests a lack of fetal nutrition and explains his poor birth weight as well as remaining below the expected centiles at one year of age. In view of the absence of any other symptoms, it is unlikely that this child has any other disease.

Physical examination at one year – weight 6.8 kg, length 71 cm, head O 44 cm, mild pallor +, no other abnormal findings. He has gained 5.4 kg in one year which is within normal limits. Birth length was not recorded. So, this child is **normal** and expect him to catch up over time to near-normal adult parameters.

In malnutrition, weight goes down first and if nutrition continues to be poor, length starts faltering after a few months. However, head O remains within normal limits. This is the way nature protects the brain even in malnutrition. The only exception is when malnutrition starts early in the first trimester of pregnancy.

Case 4

Two year old child presented with poor weight gain over last year. He was born after full-term delivery with a birth weight of 3 kg, was breast-fed exclusively for the first 6 months and thereafter was on complementary feeds along with breastfeeding. The mother continued to breastfeed this baby even now though milk yield had been very scanty. The child gradually started fussing to eat but would demand breast milk. Initially, forced feeding worked for a short time but he learnt to vomit food, if forced. Thus, his intake of food had gone down drastically over the last few months and was surviving only on a small quantity of breast milk. He had started going to playgroup and since then used to get frequent episodes of cold and cough with occasional fever. He was constipated and suppressed the urge of passing stool to avoid painful defecation. His sleep was disturbed and he was getting cranky.

This history clearly suggests a significant deficiency in nutritional intake. Recurrent episodes of cold, cough and occasional fever relate to contact with probable viral infections and are aggravated by malnutrition. It is unlikely to be malnutrition secondary to chronic disease and so is likely to be due to primary malnutrition because of breast addiction and refusal to eat solid food.

Physical examination showed significant pallor, and signs of rickets in terms of frontoparietal bossing and beading of costochondral junctions. There was generalized hypotonia of muscles. No other abnormal findings.

Laboratory tests confirmed severe iron deficiency anemia and an X-ray of the wrist showed signs of rickets. This child's poor weight gain is due to **breast addiction** that led to fussy eating resulting in the mother forcing the child to eat and it started a vicious cycle ending with poor nutrition and poor weight gain. This child needs to be de-addict from breastfeeding. The mother should be counseled about it though it is a challenge at this stage. After all, any addiction is difficult to get rid of without strong willpower.

This case illustrates the importance of ideal feeding practices. Breast addiction and bottle addiction are not uncommon but forced feeding during early life is a rule with many parents. Such habits come in the way of proper weight gain. The best time to prevent breast addiction is when it begins. While breastfeeding may be continued in the second year, one must consider the risk of addiction leading to malnutrition and such an addiction is difficult to change.

Case 5

Two year old infant presented with poor weight gain since the age of 3 months. He was born after full-term normal delivery with a birth weight of 2.5 kg. He was exclusively breastfed during the first four months but was supplemented with formula feed because of suboptimal weight gain during the fourth month. In spite of supplementation, the child did not gain weight as per the expected standard. He was also seen to lag behind milestones in all domains. He suffered from recurrent respiratory infections since the age of 9 months. This history suggests multiple problems in this child besides poor weight gain. So, it must be a disorder that has disturbed multiple systems but has not been worsening. Such a static disorder may be either congenital malformation or chromosomal disorder or one-time damage to the brain early in life. There is no history suggestive of perinatal or postnatal events and so is unlikely to be one-time damage to the brain. It may be a syndromic disorder.

Physical examination revealed a weight of 8.5 kg (birth wt 2.5 kg), length 84 cm, head O 45 cm, generalized hypotonia and dysmorphic features with developmental delay suggestive of chromosomal abnormality.

It suggests the diagnosis of Down's syndrome that is confirmed by the chromosomal study. Thus, poor weight gain in this child is due to **Down's syndrome** and needs no intervention as far as weight is considered. However, this child requires physiotherapy and occupational therapy. Syndrome refers to the conglomeration of several abnormalities. It is often a genetic disorder and may involve defects in multiple organs. Growth failure is common in many of them besides abnormal facies and congenital defects.

Case 6

15 year old child presented with fever followed by severe anorexia, vomiting and jaundice for the last 4 days; fever subsided over another few days but jaundice kept on worsening over the next one month. At the end of a month, the entire skin became yellow and there was severe itching. The child had lost appetite completely during this month and had lost 4 kg weight. Jaundice subsided thereafter slowly and so also itching disappeared and appetite was slowly returning to normal. However, child had not started gaining weight for which mother brought the child for opinion. On direct questioning, it was found out that mother had restricted many items from routine diet as advised by many friends.

Physical examination showed no abnormality. Laboratory investigations showed no active liver disease though serum proteins were lower than normal and IgG HAV was positive confirming diagnosis of hepatitis A recovered infection. So this child's poor weight gain was due to **undue restriction i**mposed by the family.

Mother needs to be counselled about importance of good nutrition during the stage of recovery from hepatitis A disease and harm caused by undue restriction of diet. It is a myth to restrict items of routine diet in a child suffering from acute hepatitis due to hepatitis A virus.

This case illustrates that prolonged illness would result in significant loss of weight as expected but on recovery, a normal child should start gaining weight. At such a time, patient should be encouraged to eat a balanced food to an extent possible without undue restriction. Myths prevail about restriction of food during and after illnesses affecting intestines and liver in particular. It is often harmful.

Case 7

8 year old child presented with fever off and-on-and loss of appetite for last one month. There were no other symptoms. He was treated with two antibiotics over last one month but without any response. Several laboratory tests and chest X-ray were normal except mild anemia and ESR 75 mm.

History suggests subacute infection or non-infective disorder that has not shown any localization even at the end of one month. It is probable that this is infective disease with hidden localization such as TB or hidden lymphoproliferative disorder such as lymphoma. Such a child needs review of focused physical examination and repeat relevant tests.

Physical examination at the end of one month revealed enlarged liver, firm, not tender without signs of liver dysfunction in the form of pedal edema or splenomegaly. Neck veins were engorged but hepatojugular reflux was absent. This suggested block in superior vena cava and enlarged liver a manifestation of block in inferior vena cava. This gave away a diagnosis of constrictive pericarditis most likely to be due to Tuberculosis. There was no easy way to confirm diagnosis of tuberculosis in this child as BAL was also negative. Based on circumstantial evidence, anti-TB therapy was started and child was afebrile within two weeks. Final diagnosis in this child was **tubercular constrictive pericarditis.**

Unlike in younger children, poor feeding/eating habits lead to poor weight gain in apparently normal and active children, weight loss or initially no weight gain of unknown origin is always a challenge in older children and adults that is likely to be due to a pathological cause. Hidden cause may be a chronic infection, organ dysfunction or malignancy. Often there are clues enough to suspect one of these conditions only if one is careful in history taking and physical examination.

Case 8

One year old child presented with poor weight gain and loss of appetite over last four months. This child was born after full term and normal delivery with birth weight of 3 kg. Was exclusively breastfed till the age of 6 months and then started on complementary feeds consisting of home-made gruel of cereals and pulses. Child was gaining weight well till the age of 8 months but had not gained any weight thereafter in last four months. Mother complaind of abdominal distension and occasional loose stools for which no medical help was sought. There were no other symptoms.

Only localizing symptoms in this child were abdominal distension and occasional loose stools. On direct questioning, mother informed that abdominal distension waxes and wanes at times and so abdominal distension is due to accumulation of gas and hence suggestive of intestinal disease. As there is no history of fever, infection is unlikely. However, as this child developed loss of appetite, it must be non-infective inflammatory disorder that has resulted in malabsorption. As onset of this problem nearly coincides with introduction of complementary feeds, it may be related to one of the food items, wheat being the common culprit. So, it may be celiac disease.

Physical examination revealed gaseous abdominal distension and moderate pallor. There were no other abnormal findings. This supports intestinal disorder but cause should be found out by further investigations.

It was confirmed to be **celiac disease** with presence of IgA tTG antibodies. Further confirmation can be achieved by duodenal biopsy though avoiding wheat may show improvement and is a rational way of proving the diagnosis in absence of duodenal biopsy.

Malabsorption is a hidden cause of poor weight gain or weight loss. If malabsorption is immune mediated, loss of appetite is a predominant symptom with or without fever. However appetite may be normal or even voracious in spite of loss of weight if malabsorption is due an enzyme defect,

Take Home Message

Constant weight in infancy should be taken as loss of weight. However, in subsequent years, constant weight for a few months is not abnormal though throughout childhood, weight must increase over time. Poor weight gain in infants and toddlers is often a misconception and in such a situation, child is always active and happy. Even hidden pathology leads to disturbed well-being and is noted in terms of poor appetite, lack of energy and change in behavior such as lethargy or irritability. Growth chart is the best objective measure that helps not only to differentiate normal from abnormal but also suggests a probable diagnosis by analyzing onset, duration and progress of weight loss.

MCQs

1. In assessing poor weight gain, this is the most important point in the history

A) Mother's perception
B) Appetite
C) Activity and energy level
D) Change in behavior

2. In assessing poor weight gain, this is the most important point in clinical examination

A) Present poor weight
B) Tracing weight centiles
C) Abnormal physical findings
D) All of the above

3. Weight gain may be poor at one year in this situation

A) Birth wt 1.8 kg in a neonate born after 32 weeks gestation
B) Birth wt 1.2 kg in a neonate born after 32 weeks gestation
C) Birth wt 2.4 kg in a neonate born after 38 weeks gestation
D) All of the above

4. Which of the following statement is WRONG? Weight gain may be poor in a normal child because

A) Breast addiction
B) Myths and beliefs about feeding
C) Constitutional
D) None of the above

5. Which of the following statement is WRONG? This cause of poor weight gain may be hidden

A) Tuberculosis
B) Insufficient breast milk
C) Celiac disease
D) Syndromic child

Answers to MCQs

Correct answers as follows:

Q1 C	Q2 B	Q3 B	Q4 D	Q5 B

62 My Child is Short!

Introduction

Height (of) achievement is always a dream and hence short stature in a child is a concern for parents. Length/height depends upon nutrition in infancy, thyroid and growth hormone beyond infancy in childhood and sex hormone during adolescence besides genetic factors. Once puberty is achieved, growth nearly stops but the timing of puberty varies in individuals. If puberty is delayed, it ends in tall stature while if puberty is achieved early, it results in comparatively a short stature. Girls active in sports tend to achieve puberty a bit later than those who tend to be sedentary. In an adequately nourished infant with a normal status of thyroid function, growth hormone and sex hormone, height will be decided by genetic factors alone and it cannot be changed. Thus, a child of short parents is most likely to be short. It is a myth that height increases with pull-ups or any other exercises or supplements.

Is there any Difference Between Length and Height? How are they Measured?

For practical purposes, both are nearly equal though the length is slightly more than the height by 0.5-0.7 cm. This is because, on standing, there is a small reduction in intervertebral spaces. Measuring length or height accurately is not as simple as one thinks. For accurate measurement of height, the person must stand erect with occiput, buttocks and heels touching against stadiometer (ruler on a stand) and horizontal headpiece resting on head. Length is measured with infant lying supine on an infantometer (horizontal ruler with a movable foot-end piece) with head placed at one end and foot-end moved to touch heels with outstretched legs. Ideally measurement is considered accurate only if three consecutive readings are same. However, in routine practice, single reading suffices as interpretation does not vary significantly. Though for research purposes, utmost accuracy.

Average Length/Height Gain in Childhood

Infant gains 25 cm in length in first year of which 15 cm are gained in first 6 months and 10 cm in later half of first year. In second year, length is increased by 12 cm and thereafter 5-6 cm per year till adolescence. During adolescence, height increases by 10-12 cm per year. Though there are many variables and so, even normal children grow at different velocity.

Can Adult Height be Predicted in Childhood?

In normal healthy child, Tanner formula can roughly predict adult height taking into account mid-parental height with a range of 8.5 cm on either side. Target height = (father's height

+ mother's height) divided by 2 + 6.5 cm for boys and minus 6.5 cm for girls with a range of 8.5 cm upwards or downwards. Indian Academy of Pediatrics has published simplified growth chart for calculation of mid-parental height.

Confirm Short Stature

Height below 3rd centile on growth chart or 2nd standard deviation below the mean for that age is considered short stature meaning child is short in height. The best way to judge is to monitor height velocity over time period or to follow the trend of height gain. It is only when short stature is confirmed that one must try to find out probable cause.

Common Causes of Short Stature

Early onset of chronic malnutrition is the most common cause seen especially in underprivileged community. In such a situation, child will never attain normal adult height. Other pathological causes include endocrine disorders such as Cushing's, hypothyroidism and growth hormone deficiency, syndromic abnormalities (Down, Noonan, Russell-silver, Prader-Willi and Turner syndrome in girls),chronic systemic diseases, chondrodystrophy such as achondroplasia and rickets. In absence of any such pathology, short stature may be genetic or constitutional. A child with constitutional short stature does attain normal adult height with spurt in height gain during adolescence while a child with genetic short stature does remain short in adult life.

Clinical Approach to Short Stature

First step is to confirm short stature. Parents often compare growth of their children with those of the peers or other children in extended families. Even two children of the same parents vary in their growth pattern.

Once short stature is confirmed, it is important to find out **time period of origin** of the problem. If it has started very early in life, it is mostly primary nutritional or at times secondary nutritional due to severe systemic diseases.

Child with systemic disease resulting in short stature is **sick looking** with many other symptoms and signs besides short height. Most of other conditions presenting with short stature do not manifest sickness. Growth hormone deficiency typically presents after the age of 3-4 years of age.

Delayed cognition is typical of hypothyroidism along with abnormal facies and are also in mucopolysaccharidosis with hepatosplenomegaly and bony defects.

Bony defects are typical features of chondrodystrophy and rickets. Abnormal facies, delayed development and structural malformations in different organs are features of syndromic problems. Proportionate or disproportionate trunk and limbs may help in assessing bony abnormalities. In absence of any of the above-mentioned abnormalities, short stature may be genetic or constitutional. Assessment of mid-parental height and periodic growth monitoring including height velocity would help differentiate one from the other.

Investigations in a Child with Short Stature

Bone age is estimated radiologically by the Tanner-Whitehouse method which can report bone age in weeks. Routinely, an X-ray of one hand is used to estimate bone age because it includes 20 bones in one single plate. Routine X-ray of bones fails to assess bone age correctly as it can at best offer a range in years that is not useful. Bone age denotes bone development or maturity.

Height age is the age at which a normal child achieves the said height. It denotes bone growth. For example, if six year old child has a height of 100 cm then his height age is 4 years because a normal child attains 100 cm at 4 years of age.

Chronological age is an actual age in years and months. Comparing chronological age with bone and height age and assessing height velocity gives a clue to the probable diagnosis. Bone age is delayed in hypothyroidism and growth hormone deficiency and may be mildly delayed in malnutrition. If chronological age is more than height age which is more than bone age, it suggests hormonal deficiency that can be further proved by specific tests. In fact, hypothyroidism should be suspected at birth by cord blood tested for TSH and further confirmed by free T4. Early detection of hypothyroidism is important to avoid delayed brain development as thyroid supplements can be started before brain function is affected. If chronological age is equal to height age but more than bone age, it is likely to be genetic or due to small birth weight for gestational age (both the conditions have normal height velocity) or chromosomal disorder (abnormal height velocity). If bone age and height age are equal but less than chronological age, it is likely to be constitutional (normal height velocity) or chronic diseases (abnormal velocity). Once a probable diagnosis is made, specific tests can be planned to confirm the diagnosis.

Management of Short Stature

There are no supplements or physical exercise that increase height. So, management depends on the cause. Growth hormone replacement therapy is now freely available and would help a child with GH deficiency. It is also approved for idiopathic short stature and in children with some of the syndromic problems such as Turner syndrome in girls. It may also be useful in severe systemic diseases with growth failure. Thyroid replacement should start at the earliest as mentioned above. Vitamin D deficiency rickets can be treated with Vitamin D supplements. Systemic diseases may have specific treatment, if available.

Take Home Message

Short stature, once confirmed, is best assessed by periodic monitoring of growth and plotted on a standard chart. It helps to pick up early deviation in growth parameters and would lead to rational management, if possible. Treatable conditions should not be missed and in particular, hypothyroidism is best diagnosed at birth with cord blood screening. Growth hormone replacement is now possible and economically affordable. After all, height (of) achievement is everyone's aim in life.

MCQs

1. Which of the following statement is WRONG? Short stature is considered if

A) Single height measurement falls below 3rd centile on growth chart

B) Single height measurement falls below 2nd standard deviation from the mean at that age

C) Only if height velocity is abnormal

D) All of the above

2. Which of the following statement is RIGHT? Growth is proportionate in

A) Hypothyroidism

B) Growth hormone deficiency

C) Rickets

D) Mucopolysaccharidosis

3. Delayed development is a feature of

A) Hypothyroidism

B) Syndromic problems

C) Mucopolysaccharidosis

D) All of the above

4. Which of the following statement is WRONG? Bony defects are seen in

A) Rickets

B) Achondroplasia

C) Mucopolysaccharidosis

D) None of the above

5. There are no abnormal physical findings in

A) Genetic short stature

B) Constitutional short stature

C) Idiopathic short stature

D) All of the above

Answers to MCQs

Correct answers as follows:

Q1 C	Q2 B	Q3 D	Q4 D	Q5 B

63 Everyone Wants to Reach "Height"

Basic Concepts for Clinical Application

Short stature is defined as a height 2 standard deviation below the mean for the age and must be confirmed before embarking on finding the cause. The cause of short stature can be guessed clinically. A detailed history should include sick or not sick, proportionate or disproportionate, bony defect or not, mental development normal or abnormal, abdominal distension or not and family history of short stature and physical examination for malnutrition, abnormal facies and other congenital malformations. Linear growth measurements including the velocity of growth and mid-parental height offer clues to the probable cause of short stature. Further, a comparison between chronological age, height age and bone age (as measured radiologically) along with height velocity can almost confirm the cause of short stature. Hormonal estimation or other specific tests for storage disorders may be necessary to stamp the diagnosis.

Case Based Discussion

Case 1

Two year old child was referred for not gaining weight and height as compared to the previous child. He was irritable and not very active for the last year. There were no other specific complaints. He was growing well till about 8 months of age but thereafter his weight and height gain was very poor. On direct questioning, this child was exclusively breastfed till one year of age and thereafter mother tried to introduce family food but the child would refuse but insist on breastfeeding. His intake of semisolid food was very little. His elder brother and parents were of average height.

History of the gradual faltering of weight and height after the age of 8 months and irritability with poor nutritional intake suggests **primary malnutrition** as the cause of growth failure.

Physical examination confirmed poor weight and height and there were no other significant abnormal findings. There is no need for any investigations in this child and all that is required is to de-addict him from breastfeeding and ensuring adequate intake of family food together with supplements of vitamins and minerals. Parents often complain of poor weight and subnormal length is noted by the doctor. On direct questioning, parents may have observed poor length. It is clear that when both weight and length are faltering but weight is more affected than length, the problem is related to poor nutrition – either primary or secondary. Primary malnutrition is considered in children below the age of two years. Generally, no investigations are necessary for primary malnutrition but It is important to note that bone age is minimally delayed in malnutrition but it is easy to rule out endocrine disorders.

Case 2

Two year old child was referred for recurrent fever, cough and loose stools since the age of 3 months and also not gaining weight and length. He was born after full-term normal delivery with a birth weight of 3 kg and was exclusively breast-fed in the early months. However, while on exclusive breastfeeds, he developed the first episode of fever and cough and thereafter continued to suffer infections at periodic intervals. Over time, parents noticed poor weight and height gain. This infant on exclusive breastfeeding started suffering from recurrent febrile illnesses and so it suggests abnormal host status. In view of the two systems involved – respiratory and intestines – it may be either immune deficiency disorder or cystic fibrosis. It is likely to be a progressive disorder as evident by poor growth. So **secondary malnutrition** due to host abnormality is the cause of poor growth.

Physical examination revealed sick-looking child, irritable with evidence of respiratory tract infection besides poor weight and length, weight affected more than length. It is typical of severe malnutrition. This child needs investigations to diagnose the exact cause of recurrent illnesses. This child was proved to be suffering from cystic fibrosis resulting in secondary malnutrition.

Malnutrition starting in early infancy in an infant born with normal birth weight and during exclusive breastfeeds is always due to abnormality in the host, either immunological, structural (congenital malformation especially in urinary tract or lungs) or functional (as in cystic fibrosis). There may be few clues on history and physical examination but investigations are necessary to make a final diagnosis.

Case 3

Eight year old female child presented with not gaining height noticed over last few years. Parents realized it when a younger sibling outgrew this child's height. There were no other complaints. This child was healthy, active and doing well in his studies. Parents were of average height and there was no family history of short stature. History rules out genetic causes, chronic malnutrition and hypothyroidism. Growth hormone deficiency, constitutional delay, turner syndrome and skeletal disorders are possibilities that can be differentiated on physical examination.

Physical examination showed a weight 22 kg, height 110 cms, and proportionate limb-trunk growth. The child looked happy and active and there were no abnormal findings. This rules out Turner syndrome (short neck, increased cubital angle, wide-spaced nipples, high arch palate) and also skeletal disorders. So now we are left with growth hormone deficiency and constitutional delay. This can be differentiated by height velocity on the growth chart. He was diagnosed with **constitutional delay** based on maintaining the same height velocity each year.

Growth hormone deficiency results in decreasing height velocity (height velocity. Normal height gain each year beyond 2 years of age till adolescence is around 5-6 cm per year and in GH deficiency, it goes on decreasing every year, generally starting from 2 years of age. It is not uncommon to find that one of the parents was short in height in childhood but picked up to normal height during an adolescent growth spurt. This is typical of constitutional short stature.

Case 4

Eight year old child was referred for short stature. Parents had noticed it since the age of 3-4 years but thought he might catch up with improving nourishment and exercise. He has no other symptoms; he was active and good in his studies. His both parents were short. History suggests genetic short stature though we must make sure that there is no other cause because genetic or familial short stature is a diagnosis of exclusion.

Physical examination showed a weight of 20 kg, height of 110 cm and no other abnormality. We need to look at the growth chart. It showed a height velocity of 4.5 cm each year and it was maintained the same over years. Mid-parental height revealed that this child's target height (height expected in adulthood) fell within mid-parental height. This confirms the diagnosis of **genetic or familial short stature**. There is no need for any investigations, however, in case of doubt, one may estimate bone age and compare it with chronological and height age.

A child born to parents with short stature may not necessarily be short in adulthood. Hence it is always necessary to confirm the absence of any other cause for short stature in such a child.

Case 5

Six year old child presented with developmental delay noticed since the age of 9 months and short stature noticed since the age of 3 years. Parents were more worried about the developmental delay and so did not seek advice about height. Unfortunately, the doctor had not measured height either and so it went unattended. On direct questioning, he was constipated and passed hard stools once in 2-3 days.

A combination of developmental delay and constipation along with short stature suggests multisystem affection starting early in infancy. It favors the possibility of hypothyroidism or storage disorder such as mucopolysaccharidosis.

Physical examination showed a weight of 21 kg, a height of 96 cm, dysmorphic features, coarse dry skin, hoarse voice, puffiness of eyelids, umbilical hernia, abdominal distension loaded with feces and developmental delay mainly in cognition. These findings are typical of **congenital hypothyroidism**. His chronological age is six years, height age is nearly 4 years. It was confirmed with low T3, low T4 and high TSH. Bone age in this child was 3 years – lower than height age which in turn was lower than chronological age. He needs thyroxin supplements for life. However, his mental condition would not improve, height may pick up a little but he would always remain short though his constipation would improve on treatment.

Congenital hypothyroidism ideally is diagnosed at birth by cord blood screening as it offers a chance for normal mental development as well as target adult height. Such screening is now done routinely in most of the general hospitals in India. It is cost-effective. In absence of such screening, one must look for clues for early diagnosis such as delay in passing meconium at birth and subnormal length at birth with wide posterior fontannel suggestive of delayed bone growth. If not picked up at that age, permanent damage is most likely.

Case 6

Six year old child presented with short stature noticed two year back when a younger sibling had surpassed the elder brother's height. There were no other complaints. Initially, the parents were not much worried as they both were also short but now the child himself was concerned about it. So, parents sought medical advice. On direct questioning, parents were sure that this child looked normal in height in the first few years. History suggests height faltering after the first few years and progressively going down but the child maintained good health. This history may suggest familial or genetic stature but if height velocity is progressively going down, it may be due to growth hormone deficiency. A growth chart would offer clues.

Physical examination showed a weight 21 kg and a height 102 cm without any other abnormality. His height age is four and a half years. However, height velocity was going down every year from the age of 3 years – initially, it was 6 cm in the fourth year, 5 cm in the fifth year and now 4 cm in the last year. It strongly suggests **GH deficiency**. However, one should confirm it with appropriate tests as familial short stature is a possibility. Investigations ordered for him included serum IGF 1 – insulin-like growth factor that correlates well with the level of growth hormone. Growth hormone can be estimated with a stimulation test in which basal level is assessed followed by a level after a challenge with a drug like clonidine. The absence of an increase in GH after a challenge is diagnostic of GH deficiency. Growth hormone is now freely available, and very safe though the cost is a factor though it is getting more affordable. Ideally, therapy should be continued till the target height is achieved.

Case 7

Two year old child presented with poor height and weight since early infancy. This child was born after full-term with a birth weight of 1.6 kg. There was no major problem at birth through direct breastfeeding was not possible for the first few days and had to be fed with a spoon. Over the next few months, the mother noticed poor growth and after the age of six months, he suffered recurrent respiratory or intestinal infections. History suggests growth failure that started in utero and is further contributed by recurrent infections. It was not an isolated short stature but chronic severe malnutrition.

Physical examination showed a weight of 5.5 kg, length of 70 cm, head O 44 cm, moderate pallor, poor subcutaneous fat, and poor muscle mass. There were no other localizing signs. He had gained 4 kg weight (normal neonate gains 4 kg in the first 6 months) so his weight age is just 6 months. We did not know his length at birth, however considering it to be around 45 cm he had gained 25 cm (normal neonate gains 25 cm length in 12 months), so his height age is around 12 months. His head O at birth is not known but considering it to be near normal or slightly lower than normal, it may have been 32 cm, so he has gained 12 cm (it corresponds to one year of age). Thus. he is lagging behind in all three growth parameters. He is also developmentally subnormal. It is typical of intrauterine growth restriction. However, his weight is much lower as compared to his height and head O, it is because of his recurrent illnesses with poor nutritional intake. So his growth failure is due to **IUGR** further worsened by **poor nutrition.** Ideally, he does not need any specific investigations though one must make sure that there is no other cause for recurrent infections such as immune deficiency.

Fetal malnutrition starting in the first trimester of pregnancy affects brain growth as evident by subnormal head O. This would result in learning disability in such a child besides remaining short in adulthood.

Case 8

Six year old female child presented with short stature noticed over the last four years and also mild developmental delay. There was no history of constipation or any frequent illnesses. Short stature with developmental delay suggests abnormal growth and brain development. One may consider hypothyroidism but the absence of constipation is against it. However, not every child with hypothyroidism would have all the typical symptoms.

Another possibility is any syndromic abnormality that shares both growth and brain dysfunction.

Physical examination showed a weight of 18 kg, height of 98 cm, wide webbed neck, low set ears, wide cubital angle, presence of heart murmur and mild developmental delay. Dysmorphic features with a heart murmur in a female child is typical of **Turner syndrome**.

This was confirmed by a chromosomal study showing a 45 X pattern. Such children are often detected late in childhood or later because of delayed sexual maturity. There are many other syndromes with short stature along with other abnormalities. As a rule, short stature in a female child demands to rule out Turner syndrome.

Take Home Message

Growth monitoring with periodic measurements of weight, length/height (till puberty) and head O (during the first two years of life) is important in all children. Of course, weight should be monitored periodically throughout life. A growth chart with periodical plotting of measurements helps not only in the diagnosis of short stature but also in evaluating the cause of many other diseases as the origin, duration and progress of diseases is objectively evident.

MCQs

1. Which of the following statements is WRONG? This child with short stature also has a developmental delay

A) Hypothyroidism
B) Turner Syndrome
C) Constitutional delay
D) Mucopolysaccharide defect

2. This child of short stature has proportionate limb-trunk growth

A) GH deficiency
B) Hypothyroidism
C) Chondrodystrophy
D) Mucopolysaccharide defect

3. This child of short stature is likely to catch up to normal target height

A) Constitutional delay
B) Familial short stature
C) Hypothyroidism
D) Turner syndrome

4. Weight is more affected than height in this child of short stature

A) Chronic malnutrition

B) GH deficiency

C) Hypothyroidism

D) Constitutional delay

5. This child of short stature does not need any investigations and/or therapy

A) Turner syndrome

B) Constitutional delay

C) GH deficiency

D) Rickets

Answers to MCQs

Correct answers as follows:

Q1 C	Q2 A	Q3 A	Q4 A	Q5 B

64 Ensure the Child is Developing Well

Introduction

Childhood is the period of not only just growth but also development. Growth refers to an increase in physical size while development denotes the maturity of function. As much as growth is mainly measured by an increase in weight, height and head circumference reflecting an increase in brain size, development is assessed in four major domains – gross motor, fine motor, cognition (social-adaptive) and language. At times, only one of the domains is delayed, it is referred to as differential developmental delay. If two or more domains are affected, it is referred to as global developmental delay. Global developmental delay is a result of brain dysfunction but may not be equal in all domains. However, isolated developmental delay in one domain may result in spite of normal brain function as in the case of gross motor delay due to musculo-skeletal disorder and language delay due to hearing impairment. Maturity of brain functions mostly occurs in first two years of life and to a small extent may continue till five years of age, thus it is most vital to assess development in first two years of age though mild dysfunction may manifest later in childhood.

Developmental Milestones

There occurs sequential achievement of milestones in each domain.

Gross motor domain

Head control, rolling over from prone to supine and thereafter in both the directions, sitting with support and thereafter without support, crawling (some children may skip crawling), stand with support and thereafter without support, walking, going up the staircase and thereafter down the staircase, running, hopping and jumping.

Fine motor domain

Puts hands to mouth, holds object given in the hand, reaches for objects when shown, transfer object from one hand to other, releases object when asked for, pincer grasp (picking up small size object with two fingers), drinks from a cup, turns pages thereafter even a single page at a time, can thread a bead, use scissors to cut a paper.

Cognitive domain

Keeps quiet when picked up, focuses on eyes, follows moving object, recognizes mother, social smile (smile on response), recognizes other family members, responds when called, pick-a-boo, understands 'no', says bye bye, follows simple orders, points to body parts, scribbles and sequentially achieve ability for strokes, circle, cross, square, triangle etc., puts on one block over the other thereafter tower of several blocks, imitation play, turns pages of a book thereafter able to turn each page separately, recognizes shapes and colors, identifies objects in pictures

Language domain

Receptive language develops before expressive language. Receptive language refers to understanding the language while receptive language refers to response either in the form of gestures (non-verbal) or spoken words (verbal) that is speech. Expressive non-verbal language (gesture or sign language) develops before verbal language (speech). Even a newborn responds to human words especially high-pitched sounds of the mother and stops crying when talked to. This represents early receptive language. Cooing, babbling follow thereafter. When called by name, infant of 4-5 months of age looks towards the direction of the caller. It represents expressive language. This is followed by monosyllables, bisyllables and then on to words, meaningful words, sentences. Many of these milestones involve more than one domain such as cognition, language and fine motor together.

Developmental Assessment in office Practice – A Screening Test

Detailed developmental assessment is necessary only when a developmental delay is suspected on the screening test. The screening test can evaluate developmental status at **3 months of age** (head control, recognizing mother, social smile, cooling/babbling, hand to mouth), at **12 months of age** (sitting definitely and also may be standing, pincer grasp, response when called by his name, pick-a-boo) and finally at **18 months of age** (walking, few words a must).

Assessment at 3 months of age picks up developmental delay if any arising from antenatal or perinatal events (usually head size is smaller than expected), that at 12 months helps to pick up minor defects and autism spectrum disorder (a disorder of social communication presents as language delay, absence of eye to eye contact, purposeless hyperactivity and repetitive behavior) and that at 12 months of age to confirm autistic spectrum disorder and other minor delays.

Developmental Delay – Static or Progressive?

Static developmental delay results from one-time damage to the brain that may have occurred before, during or after birth, especially during the first two years of life. Early recognition and prompt management can improve developmental status at least to some extent. Progressive developmental delay is due to active disease and would worsen over time, if not recognized early enough and managed in time. Ideally, such defects need to be picked up on routine screening at birth or early in life. However not all such progressive disorders are amenable to diagnosis, control or correction and hence outcomes are usually poor.

Common Causes

Prenatal

Congenital malformations of the brain, chromosomal disorders, congenital infections (maternal infection transferred to the fetus through the placenta) and adverse effects of drugs or radiation exposure to the mother during pregnancy.

Perinatal

Hypoxic-ischemic brain injury, bilirubin encephalopathy (result of severe unconjugated bilirubinemia) problems in preterm neonates such as periventricular hemorrhage, periventricular leukomalacia, hypoglycemia, polycythemia), hypoglycemia in a neonate born to diabetic mother.

Postnatal

Intracranial infections, severe head injury, hemorrhage due to coagulation defects, inborn errors of metabolism, hypothyroidism, Autism spectrum disorder

Investigations

MRI of brain helps to detect site of damage that may offer a clue to probable etiology. Genetic tests including chromosomal study and metabolic tests are necessary in suspected conditions. The classical presentation of cerebral palsy and autism spectrum disorder may not need any specific tests. Assessment of vision and hearing may demand tests such as VER – visual evoked response and BERA – brainstem evoked response audiometry.

Prevention

Low birth weight and preterm delivery may be preventable with proper antenatal care at least in some situations. Blood group Rh incompatibility is preventable by administration of antibody to Rh –ve mother immediately after the birth of Rh +ve neonate. Ideal intranasal care may prevent damage such as due to hypoxic-ischemic encephalopathy. Prevention of brain damage due to inborn errors of metabolism can be prevented by neonatal screening for specific disorders and is now available for about 6 common conditions including hypothyroidism in many centers in India. However western countries routinely test for 20 conditions.

Management

Physiotherapy to prevent contractures, occupational therapy to make a child independent as much as possible, speech therapy and sensory integration (coordinated use of sensory inputs) are the mainstay of management that should be started as early as possible for a better outcome. Behavioral modification may be necessary. Other areas that deserve attention are constipation, gastro-esophageal reflux, nutritional deficiencies – especially vitamin D deficiency, general hygiene, immunization, visual and hearing aids if necessary and special education. Thyroid hormone replacement therapy should be started at birth or as early as possible. Drugs are necessary only in case of epilepsy or rarely to control excessive hyperactivity in a child with an autism spectrum disorder.

Take Home Message

Developmental screening is important for the early detection of delays, if any. Earlier in life a developmental delay is picked-up, and more is the chance of a better outcome. Cause of developmental delay can be guessed on clinical parameters and may need confirmation by specific tests. Management mainly consists of non-pharmacological therapies and drugs are rarely needed. The outcome of progressive disorders is generally poor. Ideal antenatal and perinatal care may prevent some of the causes of static developmental delay. Prevention of damage due to metabolic defects is possible only when there is an index case in the family or by universal neonatal screening.

MCQs

1. This gross motor milestone may be skipped in a normal child

A) Rolling over
B) Sitting without support
C) Climbing staircase
D) Crawling

2. This is the earliest age at which a child may accidentally inhale a foreign body

A) One year
B) 8 months
C) 5 months
D) 3 months

3. Global developmental delay is considered when

A) Any of the two domains are affected
B) Any of the three domains are affected
C) All domains are affected
D) All of the above

4. Which of the following statement is WRONG? This condition may manifest with language delay in spite of normal hearing

A) Tongue-tie
B) Global developmental delay
C) Autism Spectrum disorder
D) All of the above

5. This disorder can be diagnosed and prevented at birth

A) Down's syndrome
B) Congenital malformation of the brain
C) Congenital hypothyroidism
D) Birth injury

Answers to MCQs

Correct answers as follows:

Q1 D	Q2 B	Q3 D	Q4 A	Q5 C

65 Early Pickup of Developmental Aberration for Timely Action

Clinical Application of Basic Concepts

Development refers to functional maturation and is assessed in terms of four domains – gross motor, fine motor, cognitive or social adaptive and language. The brain is the major organ responsible for development in all domains. However, in spite of normal brain function, the developmental delay could be due to the affection of other systems. Gross motor delay could be due to musculoskeletal problems and language delay from hearing impairment. Visual defects can lead to pseudo-developmental delay. The first two years of life are crucial for brain development and also to a small extent up to five years. Thus, major defects in development manifest early in life though minor defects such as learning disability may be detected later. It is important to monitor development in the early years of life. Beyond five years of age, school performance can detect aberrations, if any. Grossly, developmental assessment at the age of three months can detect major abnormality arising out of antenatal or perinatal events, at one year of age, autism spectrum disorder and hearing impairment can be made out and further confirmed at eighteen months of age. Developmental delay in two or more domains is referred to as global developmental delay. It is important to decide whether the delay is static (milestones are achieved at the same slow speed) suggests one-time damage or progressive (development speed is slowing down and so worsening) indicates ongoing damage.

Case-Based Discussion

Case 1

The mother of one year old infant complained about her child not able to sit without support, did not speak any words and was not gaining weight well. On further inquiry, the mother was 35 years old when this child was born after full-term with normal delivery but his birth weight was only 2 kg. He did not cry at birth but had spontaneous breathing on stimulation and was normal thereafter. The mother on direct questioning said that he appeared to be a bit slow in his activity but it did not bother her much. He had been constipated. He held his head at 6 months and rolled over at 10 months. He recognized her at 3 months of age, could reach for the object by 6 months of age, he is very social and goes to anyone who picks him up and is a loving happy child.

History suggests that he has a developmental delay in all four domains that are static and so it must be due to one-time damage. There has been no significant problem at birth and so the cause of this delay must be due to antenatal factors. This mother was delivered at the age of 35 years that carries a high risk of chromosomal disorder.

Physical examination revealed weight 7 kg, length 70 cm, head O 40 cm, dysmorphic features suggestive of Down syndrome, microcephaly, generalized hypotonia, developmental quotient around 50%, no other neurological abnormality, grade 3 systolic murmur, no other abnormality in heart or any other systems.

This child has a static global developmental delay with a congenital heart defect and dysmorphic features suggest the diagnosis of **Down syndrome**. It can be confirmed with chromosomal analysis and parents must be counseled about avoiding future pregnancies. In fact, they should have been counseled before or during early pregnancy about prenatal tests to diagnose such defects.

There is no specific treatment but the child can do better with physiotherapy and occupational therapy. At present, heart defect does not need any intervention except periodic monitoring for timely action. He may need diet advice and relief for constipation. Such children have borderline developmental quotient and can be educated to an extent. But ultimately, they should be trained in areas that need more physical than intellectual inputs.

Case 2

The mother of one year old infant complained about the developmental delay in her child. He had started rolling over at 11 months of age, barely reached for the object, could recognise his mother and other family members but had no vocalization. He was generally irritable and constipated. This child was born after full-term with normal delivery in a primipara at the age of 22 years and had no problem at birth but his weight was 1.5 kg. Mother suffered from severe vomiting during first three months and later developed eclampsia for which she had to be hospitalized.

History suggests severe intrauterine growth restriction as a result of maternal illness during pregnancy. As there was no significant birth problem, cause of developmental delay must be due to antenatal factors and one of such factors could be poor nutrition right from early fetal life. Any other cause needs to be considered based on physical examination.

Physical examination showed weight 6 kg, length 68 cm, head O 39 cm, signs of calorie malnutrition and anemia, irritable child, generalized hypotonia with poor muscle mass, no localizing signs in any other systems.

This child is severely malnourished – wasted (very poor weight) and stunted (poor length) with microcephaly suggesting severe malnutrition that must have started very early in fetal life as also evident by history. So, this child's developmental delay is due severe fetal malnutrition **IUGR.**

There is no need for any investigations. Treatment is to improve nutrition, though this child will remain short and small in stature and also will have some brain dysfunction. However, with improved nutrition and adequate stimulation, this child's disability can be minimized to an extent possible. It is important to realize that it is only when malnutrition sets in so early in fetal life that results in developmental delay. Otherwise, any severe malnutrition resulting during the latter part of pregnancy or after birth is not likely to affect brain function severely though mild defects such as learning disabilities may manifest especially if malnutrition started early during infancy.

Case 3

One year old adopted child presented with developmental delay. Parents had taken custody of this child two months ago and were concerned about this child not standing without support and not speaking any words. Though he seemed to understand spoken words. He did not show stranger anxiety. Otherwise, he appeared to be happy, feeding well and had gained one kg weight in the last two months. Apparently, they were not informed about earlier milestones but were told that the child was normal. History suggests that this child is lagging behind in milestones and his present development is like a 9-month-old child. However, there are no clues to probable cause.

Physical examination showed a weight of 8 kg, length of 72 cm, head O 42 cm, and no other significant abnormality. This child's weight and length are appropriate for 9 months and his head O is on the lower limit of normal.. His milestones are not much behind the expected level and considering that this child was reared for the first 10 months in a shelter home, there may have been a lack of stimulation and it could explain the mild delay, especially in speaking. Language development occurs first in the receptive domain and then follows by expressive ability. This child did respond to spoken words which means that he had developed receptive language. Thus, our impression would favor a normal child with a **lack of stimulation** in early infancy. It is expected that this child would pick up lagging milestones within a short time with interaction with parents.

This case illustrates the importance of early stimulation in terms of communicating with the neonate and infant. It is the best way to achieve maximum developmental potential. This is equally important in normal and abnormal neonates and infants. In fact, communication with the fetus during pregnancy has shown benefits, though not easy to evaluate.

Case 4

One and half year old child presented with complaints of not able to walk without support.

He was born after full-term with normal delivery, birth weight of 3 kg and had been normal without any significant problems. He was exclusively breastfed for the first 6 months and then was started on complementary feeds while continuing to breastfeed that he takes even now. He gained weight well in the first year but had not gained only 800 gm in the last 6 months. He had achieved all milestones in time during the first 6 months but had started sitting without support only at one year and then standing at 14 months. The doctor had said that it was within normal limits. But now that he was not able to walk without support, his parents were worried. His other milestones were all normal as he could speak words with meaning and respond appropriately to his age.

History suggests a well-nourished child without any disease and is lagging behind only in gross motor milestones sometime after the first 6 months and his other domains are all normal. So, he has an isolated delay in gross motor milestones starting sometime after the age of 6 months in spite of normal brain function. Obviously, the fault lies in the musculoskeletal system and not in the peripheral neurological system as he can stand and so does not have any paresis. Acquired motor delay in a well-nourished child is often due to vitamin D deficiency rickets contributed by a predominantly milk diet.

Physical examination showed a weight 11.5 kg, length of 78 cm, head O 48 cm, signs of rickets, no other abnormality. Diagnosis of **vitamin D deficiency rickets** was confirmed by biochemical (low or normal serum Ca, low serum P and high serum alkaline phosphatase) and radiological tests (cupping and fraying at the epiphyseal end of bones with demineralization) He needs a therapeutic dose of vitamin D– 6 lakhs unit to heal rickets and repeated twice more to replenish the store. Ideally vitamin D supplements should be given every day for the next three months but often lacks compliance and so a massive dose is often prescribed. His parents should be counseled about diet. He may have been breast-addicted and so consumes mainly milk without much solid food.

Case 5

Two year old child presented with inability to speak and not responding age-appropriately. Though his motor milestones were normal. He was born after a full-term with normal delivery and had achieved all the milestones in time except speech development. When consulted about this delay, the doctor had said that such a delay was familial in this child as his uncle also was a late talker. They were advised to check their hearing ability and was found to be normal. But now a year had passed without any improvement and so parents were worried. On direct questioning, it was realized that he was hyperactive, often kept on moving without purpose, engrossed in activities with repeated maneuvers, had no eye-to-eye contact, would not respond when called by his name and would not follow any orders. However, he would sit for a long time in front of the television. Unfortunately, this aspect remained ignored. So, this child has a communication disorder with attention deficit.

Physical examination confirmed his abnormal behavior but had no abnormality in any other system. Diagnosis of **Autism spectrum disorder** was confirmed by standard tests done by psychologists – DSM 5 – developmental manual test.

He would need long-term therapy under the guidance of a developmental pediatrician. Surely, he would improve at least to some extent but only with strong commitment from his parents. Ideally, he should have picked up at about one year. A simple screening test for autism spectrum disorder is to see whether the child responds to his name being called at least by one year. If there is no response, one should check hearing ability and brain function in other domains and if found to be normal, such a child should be referred to a developmental pediatrician. If diagnosed early and treated properly, there would be a much better outcome. There are no drugs for such a problem though occasionally hyperactivity may need some medications. Such disorders are on the rise, maybe due to awareness but also may be due to nuclear families with limited social interaction with inappropriate use of TV, mobile phones, and computers.

Case 6

The mother of one year old child complained of inability to hold head, not recognizing her, and no smile or cooing. This child was born after full-term cesarean section delivery done for fetal distress. He did not cry at birth, required oxygenation and ventilation for the next 4 days, had few seizures on D2, was on IV fluids and subsequently fed through a nasogastric tube. He also developed sepsis which was treated with antibiotics. He was discharged on D 20. He was prescribed anticonvulsant drugs. He had three more episodes of seizures and had poor weight gain. He was on physiotherapy without much benefit. History clearly suggests severe **hypoxic-ischemic birth injury** resulting in severe developmental delay and seizure disorder.

Physical examination showed a malnourished infant with global developmental delay, microcephaly and severe spasticity with signs of bilateral upper motor neuron lesion. It confirms the diagnosis of spastic cerebral palsy with remote symptomatic epilepsy (due to one-time damage) and severe malnutrition.

In such a typical presentation, there is no need for neuro-imaging as it does not add to any more relevant information. Neuro-imaging is reserved in a child suspected to have cerebral palsy only in case of absence of microcephaly, presence of abnormal birth history or family history of a similar problem. Treatment is palliative in the form of physiotherapy to prevent contractures, occupational therapy and anti-epileptic medications, nutritional rehabilitation and care of non-neurological problems such as constipation, gastresophageal reflux, skin and bladder care and vitamin D supplements. Prognosis in such a child is guarded. Hypoxic-ischemic birth injury is preventable to an extent with adequate prenatal and intranatal care.

Case 7

Two year old child presented with delayed standing and inability to walk without support. He was born after 30 weeks of gestation with normal delivery. He did not cry at birth and required resuscitation with a bag and mask ventilation and oxygenation. He also required tube feeding for one week but thereafter was discharged. He was under regular follow-up and had gained initial milestones a bit more delayed than normal. He held his head at 5 months, rolled over at 7 months, and sat at 10 months. Cognitive and language milestones were also developed a bit late but he was talking now at two years of age and also had a normal understanding. He had no other complaints. This history suggests mild global delay that has improved to near normal except the inability to walk without support at 2 years of age which is disproportionately delayed. We may have to find an answer on physical examination.

Physical examination showed normal nutritional status with cognition and language development within normal limits, bilateral upper motor neuron signs in lower limbs but not in upper limbs. There were no other abnormalities. Bilateral pure motor UMN lesion without sensory loss rules out spinal disease. As pyramidal fibers innervating both lower limbs are affected, the lesion in the brain is periventricular. The lesion is static and so the diagnosis is **spastic diplegic cerebral palsy.** This must have resulted from the probable milder grade of periventricular hemorrhage. This type of cerebral palsy has near-normal brain function. There is no need for neuro-imaging as it is unlikely to give any more relevant information. Physiotherapy would improve this child and the prognosis is good.

Cerebral palsy is a static brain disorder of tone and posture in a developing brain with or without affection of domains other than the gross motor. Thus, in cerebral palsy, the motor delay is always a predominant finding.

Case 8

The mother of one year old child complained of developmental delay. This child was born after a full-term and normal delivery. The child had cried immediately and there was no problem at birth. He was discharged on D 3 with exclusive breastfeeding. However, on D 5, he developed an acute episode of vomiting followed by seizures and unconsciousness for which he was hospitalized. There was no fever. He was put on IV fluids and anti-convulsant drugs and some investigations were sent. Over the next 2 days, he improved and looked normal. Pending reports, he was discharged without any medicines. However, he returned with similar events within the next two days.

This history rules out any birth injury as his problems started only after four days with normal birth events. Sudden onset of severe neurological symptoms in an apparently normal neonate and then quick recovery within two days on IV fluids, suggest **inborn error of metabolism.**

In such a disorder, an abnormal metabolite is formed from one of the constituents of ingested feed due to a lack of a specific enzyme and this abnormal metabolite is toxic to the brain. Specific abnormality can be diagnosed only on detailed metabolic investigations. If not recognized in time, it results in ongoing brain damage that is fatal. Even if an abnormality is diagnosed and an offending agent from the ingested feed is withdrawn, irreversible damage may have occurred and one can hope to prevent further damage.

Ideally, such diseases are best diagnosed by neonatal screening to prevent damage but can be considered mostly if an index case exists in the family. However neonatal screening is carried out routinely in western countries for more than 20 such diseases, selected on the basis of their incidence in the community. In India, many centers have started neonatal screening programs for 5-6 common diseases and are cost-effective considering the common prevalence of these diseases in the community.

Take Home Message

Developmental screening must be done by every doctor at 3, 12 and 18 months and if found to be delayed, detailed testing is necessary. This is the only way one can pick up early deviation in development and take appropriate measures to achieve maximum developmental potential. This is an important part of monitoring a young child in the initial years. Subsequently, school performance can be a guide to any such delay.

MCQs

1. Malnutrition during this period is likely to result in severe developmental delay

A) Early in fetal life
B) Late in fetal life
C) Early in infancy
D) Late in infancy

2. Global developmental delay refers to delay in

A) Two domains
B) Three domains
C) All domains
D) Any of the above

3. Which of the following statement regarding cerebral palsy is RIGHT?

A) Head O is normal
B) Head O is small
C) Head O is big
D) Any of the above

4. Delayed speech development may be seen in

A) Hearing impairment
B) Autism spectrum disorder
C) Normal child
D) Any of the above

5. Autism spectrum disorder is suspected by

A) Poor social communication skills
B) Purposeless hyperactivity
C) Delayed speech
D) Any of the above

Answers to MCQs

Correct answers as follows:

Q1 A	Q2 D	Q3 B	Q4 D	Q5 D

Section 3

Analysis of Other Symptoms Seen at Times in Office Practice

Analysis of Other Symptoms Seen at Times, in Office Practice

There are a few other symptoms that may not be as common as those discussed in the previous section but may present as an only complaint or at times, be a part of multiple symptoms. Thus, they also need to be addressed. Some of these problems are ignored by patients and doctors alike and at times not even be recognized as an important contributor to the diagnosis or general ill-health.

66 Skin Rash – A Challenge

Basics

Skin rash may appear red, swollen, itchy or irritated and also may present change in texture (rough – sandpaper rash in scarlet fever). Rash is not pathognomonic of any disease as similar rash is seen in many diseases. We need to look at morphology (macular, popular, vesicular, nodular, pustular, purpuric, confluent), progression (spread, peeling – dying skin, pigmentation), areas involved (hands and feet, trunk and back, face - rashes that spare hands and feet are scarlet fever and impetigo), blanching (becoming white or pale after pressure as in inflammatory rash), time of appearance of rash (usually appear in first few days (often an infection), but if after a week, mostly inflammatory diseases), accompanying symptoms and signs, history of allergy and drugs, family history of similar disease.

Common Causes Related to Morphology

Centrally distributed maculopapular rash (viral infections, rickettsia, inflammatory diseases, drugs), confluent blanching erythema (Kawasaki, scarlet fever, toxin induced rash), vesicular rash (varicella, herpes simplex, enteroviral infection, skin-scalded syndrome, Steven-Johnson syndrome), urticarial rash (coxsackie virus, HBV,HCV, vasculitis, malignancy, drug, allergy), purpuric rash (HUS, DIC, ITP, leukemia, meningococcemia, vasculitis, hemorrhagic viral fever),nodular (TB, fungal, rickettsia, erythema nodosum), circular scaly rash with raised border, skin in the middle of the lesion appears normal (ringworm), red, itchy with prominent borders, scaly, blisters that may ooze and form crusts (contact dermatitis, allergic eczema), red blisters, itchy (hand, foot and mouth disease), red, wet and irritating (diaper rash), silvery scaly with sharp defined borders, may be itchy, often on scalp, elbows, knees and back (psoriasis), butterfly rash on face sparing nasolabial fold (Systemic lupus erythematosus), painful swollen red rash with fever (cellulitis), pimples or blisters, extremely itchy, scaly, raised white lines (scabies), white or yellow scaly patches that flake off, areas are red, greasy or oily (seborrhea), red skin all over sparing hands and feet, sandpaper rash (scarlet fever).

Clinical Approach to Skin Rash

Does it represent underlying serious disease?

In every disease, physician must rule out serious disease even before embarking on finding the cause. In such cases, patient appears sick with change in behavior and often febrile accompanied with other symptoms besides skin rash.

Purpuric rash suggests severe and often life-threatening diseases such as meningococcemia, disseminated intravascular coagulation abnormality as in sepsis or hemolytic uremic syndrome with renal involvement, vasculitis of different etiologies including malignancy, leukemia and bone marrow aplasia. Gangrenous rash is typical of rickettsial infection. Vesicular-bullous rash in a sick looking child denotes probable drug reaction as in Steven-Johnson syndrome. These conditions merit hospitalization and prompt management.

Does it represent a potential evolving serious disease?

Skin rash with inflammation of mucous membranes, fever and/or multisystem involvement indicate diseases that may worsen over time as in case of Kawasaki disease (may develop coronary artery dilation leading to myocardial infarction) and toxic reactions to staphylococcal or streptococcal infections (prolonged fever with risk of fatality). Such suspected diseases ideally need referral for expert opinion for investigations and management.

Once seriousness is ruled out, is it primay skin disease or systemic disorder?

Such diseases are usually benign though they need correct diagnosis to prevent chronicity (scabies, eczema, contact dermatitis- need proper treatment or referral to a dermatologist) and close monitoring to rule out complications, if any (infectious disease such as measles, varicella, mumps).

Rash itches or itch rashes?

It is important to assess what started first – was it a rash or an itch? Unless asked for, such a history does not come forth and even then, most patients or parents of children might not have noticed the sequence of appearing itch and rash as both may follow in quick succession. Itch at the onset without a rash may suggest autonomic nervous system abnormality (worsened by anxiety or stress), diabetes or increase in bile salts as in obstructive jaundice. Such primary conditions causing itching are often missed. Rarely Hodgkin's lymphoma or other immune disorders may present with itching before other symptoms and signs manifest.

Management

Life threatening and potential serious conditions are managed by experts. Infections may be self-limiting or may need antibiotic as in case of scarlet fever or skin infection such as scabies, cellulitis or impetigo. Many other conditions are managed with palliative measures more than curative treatment. It is ideal that dermatologists manage primary chronic skin diseases. Oral antihistamines are necessary for severe allergic or itching disorders. Local application of steroids, antibiotics, antiseptics, moisturisers and soothing agents may be required.

Ointment contains 80% oil and 20% water whereas **cream** contains 50% of each oil and water. So, ointments are preferred for dry skin as they provide moisture and also possess antiseptic properties. **Lotion** is dilute form of cream.

Home remedies – cold compress help temporarily to offer relief from severe itching. Oatmeal bath is recommended as it works as anti-inflammatory and antioxidant. Aloe vera has medicinal properties and is present in many skin creams. Coconut oil is a moisturizer and also has antibacterial activity.

Take Home Message

Physician must rule out life threatening and potentially serious conditions that may present with skin rash and then try to be rational in approach to probable etiology. It is important to differentiate primary skin disease from a systemic disease (fever and other symptoms) presenting with skin rash. Timely referral for hospitalization in serious disease is important to save life. Potentially serious conditions must be suspected in time with necessary investigations. Referral to a dermatologist is important especially in chronic primary skin conditions.

MCQs

1. This helps the most in the diagnosis of skin rash

A) Morphology

B) Progression

C) Distribution

D) Accompanying symptoms and signs

2. Skin rash in relation to fever may appear on

A) First day

B) Within 2 -3 days

C) After a week

D) All of the above

3. Which of the following statement is WRONG? Peeling of skin is seen in

A) Varicella

B) Kawasaki disease

C) Severe inflammation

D) Severe infection

4. Which of the following statement is WRONG? This type of skin rash suggests potential seriousness

A) Purpuric
B) Gangrenous
C) Vasculitic
D) None of the above

5. This type of application is ideal for dry skin

A) Cream
B) Lotion
C) Ointment
D) All of the above

Answers to MCQs

Correct answers as follows:

Q1 D	Q2 D	Q3 A	Q4 D	Q5 C

67 Fainting Episode – A Diagnostic Challenge

Basics

Sudden fainting referred to as syncope presents with sudden brief loss of postural tone and consciousness due to transient cessation of cerebral blood flow as a result of either hypotension or bradycardia. Typically attack occurs while standing due to blood pooling in lower limbs due to gravity resulting in fall in blood pressure resulting in transient hypo perfusion of brain. It is frequently preceded by feeling of warmth or nausea. If attack is prolonged, seizure may occur. Skin is pale and sweating, eyes are closed and there is no bladder or bowel incontinence. Symptoms other than fainting may also be present such as drowsiness, headache, unsteadiness or feeling weak. Several mechanisms are involved in causation of such an episode and include autonomic nervous system dysfunction, auto-dysregulation of cerebral blood flow, endogenous vasodilator and low serum ferritin. Autonomic nervous system exercises control over many functions such as heart rate, blood pressure, bowel and bladder and such control is involuntary.

Causes

It may occur in healthy individual as a vasovagal attack triggered by anxiety, fear, stress, pain or hunger and is typically experienced by an older school-going child while standing at morning assembly. But sudden fainting attack may also be caused by variety of disorders such as heart defects (rhythm disturbances, arrhythmias including tachycardia, WPW syndrome or long QT syndrome, myocardial dysfunction, hypertrophic cardiomyopathy, outflow tract obstruction), nervous system disorder (seizure, stroke, transient ischemic attack, migraine, normal pressure hydrocephalus. autonomic nervous system dysfunction), severe anemia, hypoglycemia, dyselectrolytemia, sepsis, toxins and drugs. Other situational syncope includes dehydration, hyperventilation, cough and micturition syncope. Postural hypotension is seen in elder people due to sudden change in body stance.

Differential Diagnosis

Syncope has to be differentiated from primary seizure disorder or vertigo. Besides, underlying cause of syncope has to be established. History is most important to be obtained from a witness with second-to-second details of the event. Such detailed history is often unavailable but attempts must be made to obtain as much information as one can get. This assumes far more importance because often physical examination does not reveal any abnormality. Subsequent investigations and management depend on provisional diagnosis.

Clinical Approach

First step is to confirm a fainting episode as syncope. A single episode of a standard pattern in a healthy child occurring in a typical situation does not pose a problem. Prolonged attack or recurrent episodes need careful assessment.

Seizure may occur in any position, eyes are open and attack is followed by post-ictal drowsiness, at times with bladder incontinence of tongue biting as against eyes are closed, there is no bladder incontinence, tongue biting or drowsiness following syncope. In fact, a child with a syncope stands up immediately after a momentary period of unconsciousness.

Vertigo presents with feeling of spinning, unsteadiness, dizziness without loss of consciousness or feeling surrounding objects rotating. It is worsened with change in position and is often accompanied with nausea or vomiting.

Next step is to find the cause, once syncope is confirmed. A single typical episode with a quick and complete recovery in an otherwise healthy child without any physical examination abnormalities or obvious disorder does not need any investigations and patient or parents must be assured of its benign nature. However, in case of **first attack occurring during physical exercise** such as playing indicates probable heart defect. Besides, **prolonged attack or recurrent episodes** justify further assessment.

Physical examination may reveal evidence of heart or neurological disease, severe anemia or other acute conditions and further relevant tests can be ordered or patient referred for specialty opinion. Repeated physical examination and also in different positions may detect autonomic nervous system abnormality. Real challenge is to plan investigations in absence of any clue on physical examination. It is important to rule out cardiac rhythm disturbance especially long QT syndrome or any other silent heart defect, for which ECG or Holter monitoring and echocardiogram would be necessary. EEG may be abnormal in a seizure disorder, however normal EEG does not rule it out. Video-EEG may be considered if seizure is highly suspected that could record tracings for longer hours. Neuro-imaging is rarely necessary. Tilt-table test can detect changes in heart rate and blood pressure on sudden changing position from lying down to sitting and standing. Fasting blood sugar is considered to rule out hypoglycemia.

Management

Appropriate therapy depends on specific cause of syncope and is best left to a specialist. In an apparently benign and situational syncope, preventive measures may be considered. They include diet modification such as small frequent feeds, adequate amount of salt and water, sleep with elevated head, slow change of body position and avoiding caffeine or alcohol. Biofeedback may be tried. It consists of mind-body technique that involves using auditory or visual feedback to gain control over involuntary body functions such as blood flow, heart rate and blood pressure. Essentially it is a form of relaxation technique and meditation and it is useful in cases of chronic stress, anxiety or pain.

Take Home Message

Diagnosis of syncope is based on history obtained from a witness and cause is commonly benign. However, if syncope occurs during physical exercise or if it is prolonged or recurrent, it needs further investigations and specific management. In benign syncope, relaxation technique and meditation is useful.

MCQs

1. Which of the following statement is WRONG? These are other symptoms of poor cerebral blood flow

A) Drowsiness
B) Headache
C) Nausea
D) Feeling weak

2. Which of the following statement related to syncope is WRONG?

A) Eyes are open
B) It occurs in standing position
C) It lasts for very short time
D) It takes time to revive consciousness

3. Physical examination in a child with syncope may be normal in

A) Presence of heart defect
B) Presence of neurological defect
C) Both of the above
D) None of the above

4. Which of the following statement is WRONG?

A) Every child with syncope must be investigated
B) Syncope occurring during physical exercise must be investigated
C) Recurrent syncope must be investigated
D) All of the above

5. Syncope due to autonomic nervous system abnormality can be suspected by

A) Changes in heart rate

B) Changes in blood pressure

C) Changes in body temperature

D) All of the above

Answers to MCQs

Correct answers as follows:

Q1 C	Q2 D	Q3 C	Q4 A	Q5 D

68 Squint - A Straight View

Introduction

It is a condition in which both eyes do not look in the same direction. This happens when eye muscles of both eyes do not work together. When one eye is focusing at an object, other eye is off direction. Affected eye does not look at the direction of gaze. Affected eye is turned inwards, outwards, upwards or downwards though most commonly eye turns inwards or outwards and rarely up and down. It is also termed as strabismus. It may be mild and not easily noticeable. Such a child may turn head or neck to one side to suppress the vision from the affected eye to avoid double vision. It may be intermittent or present all the time. Intermittent squint is normal in first two months of life and It disappears by the age of 4 months. It may develop transiently in a normal person when tired.

Types of Squint

It is referred to as esotropia when affected eye is turned inwards, exotropia when eye is turned outwards, hypertropia when turned upwards and hypotropia when turned downwards. It may be constant or intermittent squint. It may manifest when eye is open or when eye is covered referred to as latent squint. In concomitant squint, degree of squint is same in all the directions which means all eye muscles are working but not synchronously as their movements are not aligned. Non-concomitant squint manifests only in one direction but not in the other direction.

Causes of Squint

Some babies are born with a squint, if it persists beyond the age of four months,it is permanent. Exact cause of such a congenital squint is not known. Often it is familial. However, squint may develop anytime later in life as a result of refractive errors (myopia, hypermetropia), diseases of eye muscles (including paralysis of muscles), retinoblastoma, brain defects (midbrain lesions involving 3rd, 4th and 6th cranial nerve nuclei, cerebral palsy, abnormalities such as Down's or Noonan syndrome) and also affection of nerves.

Is Squint Harmful?

A child with a squint may stop focusing with the affected eye called as amblyopia or lazy eye resulting in disuse of neural functioning and is at the risk of permanent loss of vision if not corrected in time. Binocular vision is due to vision focused from both the eyes together and it results in three-dimensional view of the object as perceived by brain. Thus, a child with a squint may not develop binocular vision. However, in case of children with squint, both eyes focus on different spots but brain learns to ignore out of focus image and so there is usually no double vision unlike in adults. Squint in a child also is a cosmetic problem that affects the child psychologically causing diffidence.

Clinical Approach

Generally, it is the parents who report a squint in their child but a physician also should look for it, especially if it is mild and ignored by parents to seek advice or when it is latent. Squint persistent beyond the age of four months or worsening squint at any age needs proper evaluation. First step is rule out neurological disorder. Signs of raised intracranial pressure, paresis including that of eye muscles and cerebellar signs must be looked for and so also developmental delay in a child with abnormal physiognomy. Once neurological disease or defect is ruled out, it is ideal to refer the child to an ophthalmologist. It is not easy to check refraction or fundus examination in a young child. Routine testing of vision at birth and again at 6-8 weeks of age, thereafter at preschool and school age is ideal. Squint and amblyopia should be diagnosed as early as possible for better outcome.

Management

Glasses may be required for refractive errors. Amblyopia is treated with a patch on a normal eye so as to force the brain to use the affected eye. Vision therapy is to improve visual skills and abilities, it is a training with the help of lenses, prisms, filters, patches, electronic gadgets and balance boards. It is used for improving lazy eye and improve binocular vision problems. At times, corrective surgery may be necessary though under-correction or over-correction is a possibility.

Take Home Message

Persistent squint beyond four months of age in an infant should not be ignored. Sudden occurrence of a squint may be due to neurological disorders and need appropriate investigations and management. Non-neurological squint should be referred to an ophthalmologist as early as possible for proper evaluation and treatment to avoid long term vision problems.

MCQs

1. Which of the following statement is WRONG? Squint

A) Is normal in first two months

B) It may be evident when tired

C) May disappear by itself

D) Is always fully correctable

2. Which of the following statement is WRONG?

A) Squint may be present since birth
B) Squint may develop anytime in life
C) Squint may not be evident
D) None of the above

3. Which of the following statement regarding squint is WRONG?

A) It may result from myopia
B) It may result from hypermetropia
C) It may result from Amblyopia
D) No cause may be found

4. Clinical examination in a child with squint should include

A) Refractive error
B) Movements of eyes in all directions
C) Fundus examination
D) All of the above

5. Early diagnosis of squint is important to prevent

A) Loss of vision
B) Loss of binocular vision
C) Psychological disturbance
D) All of the above

Answers to MCQs

Correct answers as follows:

Q1 D	Q2 D	Q3 C	Q4 D	Q5 D

69 Mouth Ulcers

Introduction

Mouth ulcers are common in the community seen at all age groups, while most of them are benign and self-limiting, one must be cautious to rule out any systemic disease.in the background. Mucous membrane of the mouth is very delicate and is easily damaged even by trivial factors. These lesions are seen in all the parts of mouth including base of gums. They are painful and cause difficulty in eating, drinking and speaking.

Causes

Two most common causes include **local trauma** and **aphthous ulcers**. Local mechanical injury may be induced by accidental biting of cheeks or lips while chewing hard food items, sharp tooth, poorly fitting dentures or braces, chemical injury by spicy food or thermal injury due to hot drink. Ulcers caused by local injury heal within 1-2 weeks. Aphthous ulcers are also localized to mouth but they recur every few months and may take longer time to heal. While exact cause is not known, it is likely to be triggered by genetic predisposition, stress, Vitamin or iron deficiency and hypersensitivity to tooth pastes or smoking. Both these causes are restricted to mouth only without much systemic symptoms.

Next common causes include **infections** and **vitamin/iron deficiency**. Viral infections such as coxasachie A (hand, foot, mouth disease), herpes, varicella, EB virus, HIV, bacterial infections such as scarlet fever, fungal infections, syphilis etc. Deficiency disorders include vitamin B12, folate and other B complex vitamins and iron deficiency.

Rare but serious causes include **autoimmune disorders** such as SLE, juvenile idiopathic arthritis, dermatomyositis, vasculitis syndromes, inflammatory bowel disease, **drug reactions** such as Steven-Johnson syndrome and occasionally **leukemia**. Some of these disorders may start with mouth ulcers before other manifestations appear and, in such situations, correct diagnosis is difficult in initial stages. However, such patients are often disproportionately sick. Mouth represents transition between skin and GI tract and hence mouth ulcers are often associated with skin lesions or GI disturbances.

Clinical Approach

First step is to differentiate between localized benign lesions and mouth ulcers representing a probable systemic disorder. Systemic disorders generally present with sickness besides other symptoms such as fever, skin rash, joint involvement etc. Sickness is different than discomfort caused by painful lesions and though it is a subjective impression, experienced physician can make out a difference between discomfort and sickness. However, at times it could be tricky and one has to be cautious in pronouncing a benign lesion.

Once a benign disorder is considered, detailed history may suggest local injury and if not, one may look at family history to consider aphthous ulcers and also assess probable vitamin B12 or folate deficiency (knuckle pigmentation) and iron deficiency (koilonychia). Past history of similar disease favors diagnosis of aphthous ulcers as they are recurrent. History of drug therapy may be a clue to cause of mouth ulcers.

However one must be cautious to keep in mind that isolated mouth ulcers may be the only initial presentation of systemic disorders and so must look for evidence of systemic disease on physical examination such as evidence of viral infection, skin rash, nail abnormalities, joint swelling, restriction of joint movements or pain, pallor, lymphadenopathy, hepatosplenomegaly and signs of other organ involvement.

Investigations

Isolated mouth ulcers without evidence of any other physical findings in an otherwise normal child does not call for any investigations. In case of accompanying pallor, peripheral blood smear along with CBC can suggest deficiency anemia. Aphthous ulcers is a clinical diagnosis based on circumstantial evidence and do not justify any tests.

If mouth ulcers don't heal within two weeks or in case of doubt about probability of systemic disorder, CBC, ESR/CRP are initial tests that may support a systemic disease – either infective, autoimmune or malignant diseases. Further investigations depend on initial test results. In case of suspected fungal infection, work up for immune deficiency including HIV is necessary as fungal mouth ulcers are seen in immune-compromised individuals with an exception of a neonate or an individual on long term antibiotic therapy.

Treatment

Benign lesions are self-limiting and don't need any specific drug therapy. It is best to avoid spicy and hot food, drink plenty of fluids, keep mouth clean and rinse mouth with warm water with pinch of salt by keeping water in mouth for few minutes. Local application may be tried such as ghee or butter or local anesthetic agents. Local steroids are not helpful but analgesics may be tried. Withdrawal of probable offending drug is necessary if suspected to be drug induced mouth ulcers. Replacement therapy is necessary for vitamin and iron deficiency disorder.

Viral infections are also self-limiting and don't need any specific treatment. However, disseminated herpes infection needs to be treated with acyclovir or ganciclovir. Streptococcal infection is treated with first generation cephalosporin or amoxicillin. Fungal infection is treated with local anti-fungal drug unless it is disseminated that needs systemic therapy. Treatment of other serious disorders must be left to a specialist.

Take Home Message

Mouth ulcers are usually benign and self-limiting but we must look for any systemic disorder in the background that may not be initially evident, unless specially looked for. However, if lesions persist beyond two weeks, we must investigate to rule out a systemic disorder. Local lesions heal on their own and while local application may be tried, healing takes a natural course.

MCQs

1. Which if the following statement is WRONG? Mouth ulcers may be

A) Progressive
B) Migratory
C) Both likely
D) One of them likely

2. Which of the following statement is WRONG?

A) Single ulcer is due to local cause
B) Single ulcer is due to systemic cause
C) Multiple ulcers are due to systemic cause
D) Multiple ulcers are due to local cause

3. Which of the following statement is WRONG? Self-limiting mouth ulcers may be

A) Due to local cause
B) Due to systemic cause
C) Never associated with fever
D) Always associated with pain

4. Which of the following statement is WRONG? Fungal infection in mouth may be seen in

A) Immunocompetent individual
B) Immunocompromised individual
C) Normal neonate
D) None of the above

5. This helps the most in healing of mouth ulcers

A) Local anesthetic agent
B) Local steroid
C) Nature
D) Analgesic

Answers to MCQs

Correct answers as follows:

Q1 C	Q2 B	Q3 B	Q4 D	Q5 C

70 Epistaxis

Introduction

It is a common condition, often due to benign causes but at times may represent more serious diseases. Epistaxis refers to bleeding from nostrils, nasal cavity or nasopharynx, mostly from anterior part of nasal cavity. Blood dripping from posterior nasopharynx may be due to epistaxis, but occasionally, massive epistaxis may be confused with hemoptysis or hematemesis.

Causes

Fragile capillaries in the anterior part of nose are vulnerable to rupture due to extreme environmental temperatures and is one of the most common benign cause of epistaxis. Nose pricking may also lead to epistaxis and so also accidental injuries to nose or head injuries with basal skull fracture. Foreign body in the nostril may also present with epistaxis but it is unilateral. Epistaxis may be the manifestation of underlying hematological or vascular disorder. Common hematological diseases include platelet disorders (destruction or lack of production of platelets or platelet dysfunction in spite of normal number of platelets) and coagulation disorders (congenital or acquired deficiency of coagulation factors), vascular disorders such as vasculitis and different types of vascular malformations. Hypertension is not the cause of epistaxis in children as hypertension is mostly acute unlike in adults in whom chronic progressive hypertension may present with epistaxis.

Clinical Approach

First step is to make sure that it is blood. Many times, blood-stained kerchief is shown to the doctor as evidence of blood. Rarely, a child can intentionally cheat the parents and doctors both. Next step is to locate exact site in the nasal cavity.

History

It should find out whether epistaxis was unilateral or bilateral, time taken to stop bleeding, recurrence of bleed within short time, relation to environment or injury, any accompanying symptoms such as fever, bleeding from other sites, past history of similar episodes and family history of bleeding disorder.

Physical examination

It should first ensure that child is hemodynamically stable and then start with inspection of nasal cavity, ideally with a nasal speculum. During active episode, local examination may not be possible unless bleeding stops but throat examination may reveal dripping of blood from nasopharynx. In such case, firm pressure should be applied over the nostril for two minutes to stop bleeding. If it fails or takes time to control bleeding, further evaluation or referral is mandatory. Bleeding is easily controlled by pressure in common benign causes and physical examination should rule out presence of foreign body. Physical examination should focus on abnormal findings such as sick look, purpura, and ecchymosis, bleeding from other sites, hepatosplenomegaly or lymphadenopathy.

Investigations

Tests are necessary only when one suspects hematological or pathological vascular causes of bleeding. Sick child, bleeding from other sites, difficulty to control bleeding and presence of abnormal physical findings are pointers to justify further evaluation with relevant tests. Hemoglobin level can estimate degree of blood loss. Besides CBC, platelet count and PT/PTT are basic screening tests to give a clue to type of bleeding disorder. Further tests can define subtypes such as bone marrow in case of low platelet count and coagulation factor assessment and liver function tests in case of coagulation defects. In case of suspicion of vasculitis, special tests may be required.

Management

Usually firm pressure over nostrils controls bleeding. However, if it fails, topical epinephrine 1:10000 and 4% lidocaine may help to control bleeding. Nasal packing with gauze has been a traditional method that is now replaced with balloons, tampons or compressed sponge. Specific treatment is necessary in case of hematological or vascular causes.

Take Home Message

Occasional self-limiting epistaxis in a healthy child is often a benign problem and does not call for any specific intervention. However, it could be the first and only a single manifestation of hematological or vascular disorder that would need proper evaluation. Usually, detailed history and thorough physical examination does point to a probable systemic disorder.

MCQs

1. Epistaxis could be

A) Unilateral
B) Bilateral
C) Variable
D) All of the above

2. Which of the following statement is RIGHT? Degree of blood loss can be assessed with

A) Detailed history
B) Area of kerchief/towel soaked with blood
C) Pulse rate
D) All of the above

3. Which of the following statement is WRONG? Epistaxis in a healthy child may be due to

A) Local cause
B) Platelet disorder
C) Coagulation disorder
D) Vasculitis

4. Which of the following statement is WRONG?

A) Recurrent epistaxis should be investigated
B) Recurrent epistaxis may not need investigations
C) Isolated first episode should not be investigated
D) None of the above

5. Epistaxis in such a child must always be investigated

A) Recurrent nose bleeds
B) Family history of nose bleeds
C) Difficult to control bleed
D) All of the above

Answers to MCQs

Correct answers as follows:

Q1 D	Q2 C	Q3 D	Q4 D	Q5 D

71 Sleep Problems

Introduction

Sleep is not a luxury but a necessity. Adequate sleep is necessary to boost health and work performance. Neonate sleeps for 18-20 hours a day including day time naps, infant about 12-13 hours, toddler around 10-12 hours and adult should sleep for 7-8 hours a day. Day nap should not be more than 20-30 minutes if at all taken by adults. However, majority adults and many children are sleep-deprived because of changes in life styles, especially in cities. Sleep pattern is often ignored as an important part of health and so rarely discussed unless it poses a significant problem.

Inculcating Ideal Sleep Habits

Most of the neonates sleep very well during the day and remain comparatively awake during night hours. This pattern settles down to natural rhythm by next few weeks. Thereafter, babies sleep for 3-4 hours at a time and get up for a feed to sleep again. However, as infant grows and develops ability to interact with the surroundings, sleep is easily disturbed and infant remains awake for more time. Many times, infant fights sleep in order to be with parents and other family members. It is at this time around 6 months of age that parents should try to set healthy sleep pattern. Parents should set a fixed sleep schedule that should be followed each day to an extent possible.

It is important to put the baby on the bed when sleepy but awake so that infant learns to fall asleep. Mother should maintain physical contact with the baby while putting the baby to sleep and even sing a song to sooth the baby but not form habit of breast feeding or rocking to get to sleep. Warm water bath often helps to induce the baby to sleep. Sleep hygiene consists of providing comfortable quiet environment avoiding light or sound. Once this routine is repeated every night, infant gets habituated to sleep at that particular time. Initially baby shares parent's bed and subsequently a toddler could share parent's room but separate bed. Such healthy habits need to be sustained in subsequent years. Older children and adults must plan a dinner time at least two hours prior to sleep time and also avoid ingestion of stimulant like coffee and exposure to electronic gadgets to facilitate good sleep.

It is known that bright light including TV screen disturb initiation of sleep because melatonin - hormone from hypothalamus – is secreted in poor light inducing sleep process. Meditation and other relaxation techniques such as concentrating on breath or body scan, light music or reading a book help to calm the mind and relieve stress.

Common Sleep Problems in Children

Normal infant in initial months does get up for a feed but goes back to sleep immediately at the end of the feed. Most infants towards latter half learn to sleep through the night without need for a feed. Occasional sleep disturbance is common in children and is due to minor illness or environmental disturbance. However, when it happens frequently, one must attend to it as a problem such as difficulty in initiation of sleep, interrupted sleep and day time sleepiness.

Initiation of Sleep

Parents may find it difficult to put the baby to sleep. This is usually due to failure of timely instilling sleep habit. Even older child may also face same problem. Most households are busy till late in the night with many activities and this is deterrent for young child to go to sleep. Older children may be stressed with studies or fights that make them not get to sleep quickly. They waste time in bed trying to sleep and then find it difficult to get up in time.

Interrupted Sleep – Arousal Disorders

Infant may wake up several times due to hunger but often due to habit formed by mother to feed on breast or by bottle to put him back to sleep. Once this habit is formed, infant wakes up for sucking pleasure rather than for hunger. Older children may get up due to obstructed airway presenting as snoring or sleep apnea – transient cessation of breathing in sleep that may go unnoticed but results in day time sleepiness. Nightmares are other reasons for waking up in sleep, they occur after a dream and children are able to remember the event when fully awake. At times, older child wakes up half-asleep, is confused and agitated and performs simple activities such as sitting up or mumbling, complex activities such as screaming and becoming aggressive – night terrors or even more complex activities such as sleep walking. Children have no recall of such activities as against in nightmares where the child remembers entire event. Restless leg syndrome is another problem where a child gets severe urge to move legs and hands due to perception of aching, itching, tingling or creeping sensations. This is a result of stress, anxiety or depression.

Day Time Sleepiness

Inadequate sleep due to difficulty in initiation of sleep and need to get up in time for school or work and interrupted sleep due to variety of reasons lead to day time sleepiness. School going children burn late night oil to study specially during examination time and it is a common cause of day time sleepiness. Some of them are habituated to go to bed at late hours at all times.

Common Sleep Problems in Adults

Most of the problems faced by older children are also prevalent in adults and mainly arise from stress and tension at work place and at home. Chronic respiratory disorders such as chronic bronchitis and emphysema, asthma, sinusitis, chronic cardiac diseases, diabetes, chronic GI problems, other degenerative disorders of joints and physiological old age issues such as aches and pains as well as enlarged prostate in males are other reasons for sleep problems.

Consequences of Sleep Problems

Sleep disorders can take a toll on mental and physical health besides on mood, energy, memory issues, weight gain, ability to handle stress and poor performance at study and work. It is a silent problem but has serious negative impact on life.

Management of Sleep Problems

Prevention is better than cure and it is important for parents to inculcate healthy sleep habits that are as vital as other habits related to diet and exercise. It is also necessary to develop emotional and psychological health that helps to cope up stresses in life effectively. Sleep problems must be recognized early to manage well. Parents should try to change wrong habits in children with cooperation and firmness. Pathological conditions are tackled appropriately such as adenoidectomy and tonsillectomy for obstructed sleep apnea. Stress, tensions, depression need proper counselling and at times expert referral. Rarely investigations may be necessary to diagnose correctly the cause of sleep problems. Sleep laboratories are now available in major centers for sleep study that involves continuous monitoring of several physiological parameters during sleep. Such a study can reveal apnea episodes and other breathing disorders and may need special intervention.

Take Home Message

Sleep problems are common in children and adults but remain unrecognized or ignored. Inculcating healthy sleep habits and providing sleep hygiene for infants and children are important steps for parents. While transient disturbance in sleep is common, frequent disturbances in sleep need early recognition, proper evaluation and management.

MCQs

1. Ideal amount of sleep every day for adults is

A) 5-6 hours
B) 7-8 hours
C) 9-10 hours
D) Amount that keeps an individual happy

2. Day time sleep

A) Is not recommended

B) Is a must

C) Is ideal for 20 minutes

D) Is fine as per the need

3. This organ in the body is responsible for sleep initiation

A) Cerebral cortex

B) Hypothalamus

C) Thalamus

D) All of the above

4. This system dysfunction is common cause of disturbed sleep

A) Respiratory

B) Cardiac

C) Neurological

D) GI

5. A child with nightmare wakes up with

A) Inconsolable crying

B) Aggressive behavior

C) Confusion and disorientation

D) Normal behavior

Answers to MCQs

Correct answers as follows:

Q1 B	Q2 C	Q3 B	Q4 A	Q5 D

72 Flatulence – "Gas" Problem

Introduction

Flatulence refers to accumulation of gas in gastrointestinal tract. Normally, gas is formed in the large intestine as a result of bacterial (helpful bacteria exist in intestine) action on digested food (bacterial fermentation) that produces gases like methane, nitrogen and carbon dioxide which exit out. Gas also may be swallowed while eating or drinking rapidly, eating gas-producing food items, soft aerated drinks and chewing gums. Flatulence may also result from indigestion caused by food intolerance, food allergy or gastrointestinal diseases. Whenever excessive gas is produced or normally produced gas does not exit, it results in retention of gas in alimentary canal. Flatulence leads to bloating of abdomen as well as frequent farting and burping. It produces discomfort and embarrassment.

Gas-Producing Food Items

It is mainly the carbohydrates in food that produce gas as a result of their digestion while proteins and fats contribute to a little gas. Among sugars, lactose (dairy products) and fructose (some fruits like mangoes, grapes, oranges, sweet lime, figs) cause excessive gas though other sugars also may do so especially if ingested in excess. Complex sugars such as starch are difficult to break down and so produce excessive gas as happens in consumption of potatoes, corn, noodles and wheat. Rice produces very little gas. Beans, cabbage, broccoli, sprouts, green leafy vegetables produce excessive gas. However, it is important that many of such gas-producing food items are also beneficial in many other ways and hence food intake should be balanced with proteins, fats, carbohydrates, vegetables, fruits and dairy products based on what suits individual's digesting system the most.

Common Causes of Flatulence

Flatulence is often a result of wrong eating habits including imbalanced food consumption and constipation that upset digestive processes causing flatulence. This does not represent any disease process. However gastrointestinal diseases also lead to flatulence and at times may be the only symptom of developing disease.

Food intolerance is an individual person's inability to handle food effectively and while it is not a disease but an isolated defect that demands avoiding food items to which a person is intolerant.

Food allergy results from abnormal response to ingested food that worsens over repeated exposure to an offending agent unlike in case of food intolerance in which there is no worsening symptoms.

Gluten induced allergy – **Celiac disease** is due to allergic reaction to wheat, barley, oats is a classic example of food allergy that is often seen.

GERD – gastresophageal reflux disease – may present with burping in addition to retrosternal discomfort (heart burn), vomiting and aspiration into airways leading to cough.

Lactose intolerance is due to lack of lactase – an enzyme that is necessary to break down lactose – that presents with flatulence, abdominal bloating and pain often with watery stools. This is seen often secondary to acute intestinal infection in children, is transient and self-limiting. It is also more prevalent in old age, especially in those individuals who are not used to consume dairy products.

Inflammatory bowel disease may present with flatulence in addition to abdominal pain, abnormal stools often with blood and deteriorating health. In such cases, other systems may also be involved such as joints, eyes, kidneys etc.

Irritable bowel syndrome presents in similar way but with normal health status and is mainly due to stress rather than any intestinal pathology.

Chronic intestinal infections including parasitic disease such as amebiasis and giardiasis also present with flatulence. In fact, chronic intestinal disorders of any cause including GI **malignancy** may result in flatulence.

Clinical Approach

First step is to note whether symptoms pertain to frequent passage of gas (farting or burping) or just abdominal bloating with discomfort without passing gas. Acute onset bloating of short duration with severe abdominal pain is the hallmark of surgical abdomen such as acute intestinal obstruction and presents with vomiting.

Those who present with excessive farting also have bloating and abdominal discomfort. If such a person is otherwise healthy and not sick, it may be due to imbalanced diet or irritable bowel syndrome. However, if such a person is sick, one needs to evaluate more sinister causes that include inflammatory bowel disease (IBD), chronic intestinal infections including TB, parasitic diseases and even malignancy. Physical examination often fails to diagnose such conditions and would need further relevant investigations. If burping is a main presenting symptom, one may consider upper GI disorders such as GERD, esophagitis or malignancy in old age with other accompanying symptoms or simply an imbalanced diet in an otherwise healthy person.

Investigations

Healthy individual with chronic problem does not justify any investigations as problem lies often in eating habits. Similarly, no tests are necessary in case of strong clinical suspicion of irritable bowel syndrome.

Stool microscopy may reveal evidence of chronic parasitic infection. Occult blood in microscopic stool examination or **fecal calprotectin** may indicate presence of intestinal inflammation.

Reducing substance in stool (lactose) is seen in every loose stool and does not suggest per se lactose intolerance and hence not routinely asked for.

CBC may show neutrophilic leukocytosis with thrombocytosis in IBD along with low serum albumin.

ESR may be useful in monitoring course of the disease rather than diagnosis of a specific condition. Serum IgA **anti-tTG** antibody is a screening test for celiac disease.

Imaging may be necessary in selective conditions such as GERD, IBD, intestinal TB, malignancy but with limited use.

Colonoscopy and intestinal biopsy help in diagnosing IBD, celiac disease. Upper GI endoscopy with biopsy is necessary to diagnose GERD along with 24 hour esophageal pH monitoring. However, tests for celiac disease or GERD must be further supplemented with **therapeutic trial** as all such tests have limitations and at best are highly suggestive but nor confirmative by themselves.

Management

It depends on the cause. Life style and diet modification is the key to many benign conditions. Home remedies include eating low carbohydrate containing fruits such as berries (blue, black, straw), apricots, grapefruit, peach, watermelon and low carb vegetables such as carrots, tomatoes, green beans. Rice and fermented items like Idli produce less gas. Knee-chest position, hot water, ginger help to relieve gas.

In pathological disorders, diet modification to avoid offending agent is the standard management in allergic disorders as in celiac disease in which wheat, barley and oats should be avoided. Diet change (elemental diet) is also necessary in other intestinal disorders such as IBD besides immune-suppressive drugs. Prokinetic drugs, H2 blockers and PPI –proton pump inhibitors may help in case of GERD. Chronic intestinal infections are treated with specific antibiotics. Surgical treatment may rarely be necessary in GERD as fundal plication or rarely in IBD – especially ulcerative colitis with fistula formation as seen more commonly in adults.

Take Home Message

Flatulence is a common problem in the community presenting as abdominal bloating or discomfort, excessive farting or burping. Diet and life style related issues predominate in apparently healthy persons. However, flatulence of sudden onset or as a persistent symptom in a sick individual demands further evaluation to rule out significant gastrointestinal disorder.

MCQs

1. Which of the following statement related to symptoms caused by flatulence is WRONG?
A) Abdominal bloating
B) Abdominal pain
C) Excessive burping
D) None of the above

2. Which of the following statement is WRONG?
A) Farting may be normal
B) Burping may be abnormal
C) Farting is always abnormal
D) None of the above

3. This type of carbohydrate is responsible for excessive gas production
A) Lactose
B) Fructose
C) Starch
D) All of the above

4. This produces least gas
A) Rice
B) Wheat
C) Sprouts
D) Dairy products

5. This condition needs drug treatment
A) Inflammatory bowel disease
B) Irritable bowel syndrome
C) Chronic intestinal infections
D) Gastresophageal reflux disease

Answers to MCQs

Correct answers as follows:

Q1 D	Q2 C	Q3 D	Q4 A	Q5 B

73 Dental Health – Mostly Neglected!

Introduction

In general, teeth are the most neglected part of the body in Indian population with few exceptions. Parents of infants are concerned about timely eruption of teeth and thereafter blame every disease either to erupting teeth or even during pre-erupting stage. Younger generation is concerned with cosmetic aspects of teeth with emphasis on well aligned sparkling white teeth. But almost no one is concerned about dental health.

Basic Information

First tooth may appear anytime from 6 months to as late as 18 months of age. Rarely neonate is born with a tooth that may have to be extracted because of fear of slipping into throat and downwards but almost there is no human without teeth. (Though such a condition is reported). Primary teeth have shorter and thinner roots and thin enamel that looks white. They are 20 in number. They primarily act as "space-maker" for permanent teeth to be placed. Around 6 years of age, deciduous teeth start falling to create a space for permanent teeth and this process continues till all 20 teeth are replaced by 32 teeth. Wisdom teeth may appear as late as 18-25 years and often at least one of them is impacted in many individuals. Though appearance of primary as well as permanent teeth may vary a great deal in normal individuals but number remains universally the same. Though, extra teeth or appearance of permanent teeth before falling of primary teeth are also known but rare.

Dental Care

Care in early childhood

It should start right from the time first primary tooth erupts. It is ideal to use a finger or finger-brush with rice-grain size smear of fluorinated toothpaste and by the time all primary teeth erupt, one may need to use a pea size dollop of toothpaste. In place of toothpaste, tooth powders of various types can be used as per the prevalent cultural practices. Bottle feeding, prolonged breast feeding or night feeding should be avoided to prevent tooth decay.

Care at other age groups

Soft bristled brush is ideal and must be used with gentle pressure. Vigorous pressure damages the enamel. One must follow correct technique of brushing. Brush must be held at 45-degree angle to the gum line and use rotational movement. Molars – the teeth at the back must be properly brushed as most food particles are stuck there. Foods and drinks with acidic pH tend to damage enamel if you brush immediately after consumption of such items, so brushing must be delayed by 30-60 minutes. Brushing should be only two times a day and not after each meal. Cleaning gums with finger and mouth wash are important to maintain hygiene. It is important to clean the teeth, gums and mouth with water each time immediately after eating anything. Sugary drinks should not be consumed in a lingering way. Eat raw fibrous fruits such as apple, pear, carrot, and cucumber that help to keep teeth white. They help to remove plaque over the teeth that are responsible for yellow staining of teeth. Such fibrous foods also need extra chewing and so generated saliva neutralises acid that may erode teeth.

Water fluoridation helps to prevent tooth decay by 20-40%. It is ideal to use fluorinated toothpaste. Permanent teeth start getting yellowish over time and one may use a whitening toothpaste that has an abrasive ingredient such as silica that scrubs the surface of teeth and make it white. Periodic floss or interdental cleaning helps maintain oral hygiene.

Dental Diseases

90% of adults in India have some tooth decay after the age of 20 years. It is seen also in younger children with temporary teeth but usually starts during adolescence due to lack of proper maintenance.

Tooth pain

It is a common problem that may result from infection of tooth or its structures but also may indicate other conditions such as cracked tooth (fractured tooth), chipped tooth, impacted tooth and exposure of nerve endings in a cavity.

Dental caries or cavities

Commonly known as tooth decay, it is caused by breakdown of the tooth enamel as a result of bacteria on teeth that acts on foods and produce acid that destroys enamel and results in tooth decay. With worsening destruction, nerve endings are exposed resulting in sensitivity to cold items that leads to sudden and severe pain. Cracked tooth is a fracture that may cause pain on biting or on release of biting pressure and at times may result in cold sensitivity with inflammation of pulp. Pain may also be due to infection in a decaying tooth.

Gingivitis

It is the infection of gums that is caused by a plaque formed of sticky bacteria. It may localize to form an abscess. Such infections may spread to nearby areas and may even be the cause of brain abscess in a child with congenital cyanotic heart defect. They also may cause halitosis – bad smell to breath and mouth. If left untreated, it causes bone loss and tooth may become loose and shift.

Impacted wisdom tooth

50% of adults may have at least one impacted wisdom tooth. It may damage the adjacent tooth, may result in gum disease, a cavity or misalignment.

Stained teeth

Teeth are often stained due to pigments in food or drugs. Iron deficiency anemia being so common in India, oral iron is the cause of staining of teeth. Tobacco chewing is also common in India and is a cause of staining.

Crooked teeth

Teeth may be crooked and poorly aligned or there may be a gap between teeth that may come in the way of good hygiene.

Bruxism

It refers to grinding of teeth. It may occur in sleep or even at day time. It may result from stress, sleep problems, malaligned teeth or respiratory allergy and may result in headache, cracked tooth and jaw pain.

Monitoring Dental Health

Periodic dental check is ideal right from the time first tooth erupts. Infants and toddlers commonly visit pediatricians or health facility for immunization and hence there are opportunities to not only monitor growth but also dental health. Subsequently parents need to be sensitized to continue maintaining good oral hygiene. Visit to dentist happens only when routine measures fail. Early detection of dental problems is the only way to preserve good teeth. Unfortunately, this aspect is universally ignored in India.

Management of Dental Problems

Dental care has advanced a great deal applicable even for young children and it is out of scope of this article. Aim is to prevent dental diseases and correct naturally present defects at the right time. Treatment of neglected diseases always would leave behind permanent damage though at least would prevent further worsening.

Take Home Message

Dental health is a neglected area and community including doctors need to be sensitized to attend to it. Prevention of dental diseases is easy and cost-effective. Early detection is ideal but needs a periodic visit to a dentist even in absence of any symptoms.

MCQs

1. **Which of the following statement is WRONG?**
A) Permanent teeth are always 32 in number
B) Timing of appearance of teeth is variable
C) Primary teeth are whiter than permanent teeth
D) Impacted third molar is rare

2. **Which of the following statement is RIGHT? Eruption of primary teeth may cause**
A) Loose stools
B) Fever
C) Mild discomfort
D) Convulsion

3. **Brushing of teeth should start when**
A) First permanent tooth erupts
B) First primary tooth erupts
C) Set of primary incisors erupt
D) Child can spit out

4. **Which of the following statement is WRONG? Tooth pain may be caused by**
A) Infection
B) Injury
C) Impacted tooth
D) Crooked teeth

5. **Which of the following statement about bruxism is WRONG?**
A) It may be due to stress
B) It may cause headache
C) It may cause tooth pain
D) It occurs only in sleep

Answers to MCQs

Correct answers as follows:

Q1 D	Q2 C	Q3 B	Q4 D	Q5 D

74 Urine Output – A Marker of Renal Health

Introduction

Urine output is an important parameter that is easy to judge on direct inquiry and offers useful bedside information (It is difficult to judge in young infants but measurement of 24 hour urine output is rarely necessary). Patients can also keep a note of it and therefore it forms a part of personal history that every doctor must inquire. Reduced amount of urine – oliguria – is the common occurrence in disease states but excessive amount of urine – polyuria may also be a manifestation of a disease process.

Urine output less than 400-500 ml per 24 hours in adults is considered as oliguria. In infants, it is less than 1 ml/kg body weight/hour and in children less than 0.5 ml/kg/hour. (Urine output more than 2.5 litres per day in adults is considered polyuria and it is more than 5 ml/kg/hour in infants and 4 ml/kg/hour in children).

Basics Revisited

Glomerular filtration is the first step to make urine through which excess of water and waste products from the blood are excreted out of the body. Kidneys are supplied with 20% of cardiac output that amounts to more than one liter per minute in an adult.

Afferent arterioles deliver blood to a glomerulus for filtration while efferent arterioles carry the filtrate into excretory system and venules carry the blood back into the circulation.

Renal autoregulation can dilate or constrict afferent arterioles which counteracts changes in blood pressure within limits. Rate at which kidneys filter blood is called glomerular filtration rate (GFR). Serum creatinine increases only after GFR is reduced considerably to less than 30 ml/min from normal 100-120 ml/min and hence is a late indicator of impaired renal function.

Common Causes of Oliguria

Reduction in blood supply to kidneys, impairment of glomerular function and obstruction to urine outflow are main groups of mechanisms that produce oliguria. Poor perfusion of kidneys may result from dehydration due to various causes (poor intake of water specially in hot weather, severe diarrhea or vomiting, severe burns, shock), capillary leak (dengue shock syndrome), poor cardiac output, systemic hypertension or renal artery disease (stenosis or arteritis).

Glomerular dysfunction may be caused by glomerulonephritis (endothelial and interstitial diseases) and renal failure of different etiology.

Obstruction to urine outflow presents with oliguria in spite of normal renal function as in case of bilateral pelvic-ureteric junction defect or posterior urethral valve. Neurological disorders may also lead to retained urine.

Clinical Approach to Oliguria

First step is to confirm reduced urine output. It may be obvious or rarely may need to measure urine quantity especially in ICU setting. Poor intake of fluids in a sick individual may also have oliguria but it is not severe and also not a presenting feature.

Enlarged bladder denotes either mechanical obstruction or neurological disorder, in spite of normal urine formation. Once obstruction is ruled out, one must look for signs of dehydration (tachycardia, dry mucosa, loss of skin turgor) or shock (cold extremities, hypotension, increased capillary refill time and encephalopathy) or cardiac failure (pedal edema, engorged neck veins, cardiomegaly).

Hematuria (high colored urine), facial puffiness, systemic hypertension suggests endothelial glomerular disease such as acute glomerulonephritis due to different causes or signs of renal failure (encephalopathy with deep rapid breaths suggestive of metabolic acidosis) of various etiology.

Investigations

Routine urinalysis is a simple test that may reveal primary renal glomerular disorder. Urinary specific gravity and electrolytes are important in specific conditions. GFR can be estimated roughly – referred to as eGFR by following simple equation. (There are other complicated methods of calculation).

eGFR = 0.5 X (height in cms divided by serum creatinine mg%) Serum creatinine and blood urea are other renal function tests. Relation of blood urea and serum creatinine may vary between 10:1 to 20:1. Increased ratio suggests pre-renal conditions due to poor perfusion as in case of dehydration or cardiac failure.

Other relevant tests would depend on probable diagnosis and include estimation of electrolyte and acid-base imbalance, imaging (abdominal USG, upper GI study, echocardiogram) and diagnostic tests for infections.

Management

It would depend on final diagnosis. Not every patient with oliguria would need intravenous fluids. It would be necessary only in case of dehydration or intravascular constriction. It may be harmful in case of cardiac failure and useless in case of obstructed urinary system. Similarly diuretic drugs are not required for every oliguric patient. Other details are out of scope of this article.

Clinical Approach to Polyuria

It is important to ask for polyuria because physicians generally focus on oliguria, it being much more common. Polyuria is at times confused with frequency without increased volume of urine. Thus, it is not merely the number of times urine passed but quantity of urine passed at each time. Young infants tend to pass urine more often and it is dilute, hence polyuria is not easy to assess. Common causes include diabetes (polyphagia and polydipsia along with polyuria), renal tubular disorders (child is sick with acidosis and other metabolic abnormalities) and rarely psychological disorders (compulsive water-drinking).

Take Home Message

Oliguria – reduced urine output may be due to insufficient formation of urine or due to obstruction to outlet of urine in spite of adequate production. If it is due to reduced formation, one needs to differentiate between prerenal condition from renal pathology. It can be assessed easily on the basis of history and physical examination before embarking on investigations. Polyuria should be differentiated from frequency due to local irritation and is easy to miss in young children unless specially asked for.

MCQs

1. For routine office practice, oliguria must be
A) Estimated by periodic physical collection over 24 hours
B) Measured by 24 hours collection by catheterization
C) Assessed by frequency and amount passed each time
D) Any of the above

2. Which of the following statement about oliguria is WRONG?
A) It may result due to renal glomerular disease
B) It may be due to renal tubular disease
C) It may occur in spite of normal kidneys
D) None of the above

3. Pre-renal oliguria may be due to
A) Cardiac disease
B) Intestinal disease
C) Capillary leak syndrome
D) All of the above

4. Edema in case of oliguria is seen in

A) Dehydration

B) Capillary leak syndrome

C) Obstruction to urine outflow

D) None of the above

5. Hypertension in case of oliguria is seen in

A) Glomerulonephritis

B) Cardiac failure

C) Renal failure

D) All of the above

Answers to MCQs

Correct answers as follows:

Q1 C	Q2 B	Q3 D	Q4 B	Q5 D

75 Voiding Dysfunction

Introduction

Voluntary control on passing urine develops over first few years with child remaining dry initially during the day and thereafter also by night. Depending on toilet training, most children achieve control during day by 3-4 years and night by 5-6 years. Though few children continue to wet the bed at night for longer duration. Ideal time for toilet training in children should start only after child demonstrates urge to pass urine by gestures or maneuvers and should proceed slowly as per the child's response. Urination appears to be a natural and simple process but a complex mechanism is involved for bladder to do what brain orders. However, the problems may arise at any age. Voiding dysfunction is a broad term used to describe conditions in which there is inconsistent coordination between urinary bladder and urethra. Normally urinary bladder allows filling of urine coming from the kidneys, stores it and releases it at appropriate time under voluntary control within limits. Voiding dysfunction occurs when there is a problem with either filling, storage or emptying.

Back to Basics

Once bladder starts filling to its normal capacity, it sends a message to the brain requesting an order to release. If facility does not exist, brain orders to wait for some more time and orders release as soon as possible. But there is a limit to which bladder can distend and hold on. If order to release does not come in time, bladder decides to release urine by itself without the brain order, even without proper facility and incontinence results. In normal health, such a neurological network works well and maintains dry state.

This network includes sympathetic and parasympathetic nerve, their connections in spinal cord, center of micturition in pons that relays information to brain cortex to get final order and pass on to spinal centers. Several muscles are involved such as bladder detrusor, external sphincter muscle and pelvic floor muscles. When detrusor contracts, sphincter must open and pelvic floor muscles must relax to allow urine exit. Any abnormality in this circuit results in voiding disturbances.

Symptoms

Voiding problems manifest in various ways such as frequency (passing urine number of times more than usual), urgency (strong urge to pass urine), hesitancy (difficulty in initiating act of urination), straining, slow, weak or interrupted stream of urine, retention (not emptying completely), overflow incontinence, dribbling and bed wetting (enuresis beyond the expected age of control). Such symptoms may be transient as in case of UTI or may also be intermittent or persistent. If left untreated, may cause renal damage.

Causes

Broadly causes can be divided into neurogenic and non-neurogenic. Neurogenic problems arise from cerebral cortex, pons, spinal cord or nerves due to various causes that result in detrusor-sphincter dyssynergia (incoordination between detrusor and sphincter – when detrusor contracts, sphincter also contracts resulting in functional obstruction to passage of urine). Non-neurogenic problems present as overactive, underactive or dysfunctional bladder and may arise from weak pelvic muscles, use of alcohol, caffeine or drugs like antihistamines or atropine, urinary tract infection, overweight and life style issues. Anatomical obstructive malformation in lower urinary tract and constipation are other important causes of voiding problems and recurrent UTI.

Chronic constipation results in distension of rectosigmoid that presses on urethra and also may be due to common sharing of neural pathways. Enlarge prostate is a common cause in old age. Young children tend to hold urine for long by ignoring urge to pass urine while busy with playing or at times avoiding unclean wash rooms in schools. It may lead to daytime wetting. Giggle incontinence results while laughing in children who are susceptible to detrusor instability and generally it disappears as child grows. Urethral irritation due to local fungal infection may cause frequent urination and at times urgency or incontinence.

Clinical Approach

Detailed history of voiding helps to define the type of a problem. Urgency is the hallmark of overactive bladder, child often has daytime urinary incontinence and tries to hold urine by standing on tiptoes, crossing of legs or squatting with heels pressed into perineum. Infrequent urination is the hallmark of underactive bladder and such children strain while voiding. History of constipation is often overlooked as a contributory factor to voiding problems. Neurological examination may pick-up lower motor neuron lesion in lower limbs with distended bladder with overflow incontinence or continuous dribbling without bladder distension. Examination of lower spine may reveal subtle signs such as tuft of hair indicating lower spinal cord defect. Upper motor neuron diseases may also result in voiding problems but major presentation is other than just voiding issues such as change in sensorium or seizures. It is important to observe flow of urine and patient's maneuvers while passing urine that gives clues to type of voiding problems.

Investigations

Routine urinalysis may reveal evidence of UTI that should further be confirmed with urine culture. Imaging studies include USG to assess post-void residual urine volume and rarely

CT scan or micturating cystourethrogram may be necessary. EMG of pelvic muscles may help to define status of these muscles. Urodynamic studies are required in selected cases of suspected detrusor-sphincter dyssynergia. In case of neurological disorders, relevant investigations are necessary.

Management

Non-neurological voiding problems are treated with behavior modification, bladder retraining, biofeedback and Kegel exercises to strengthen pelvic floor muscles. Drugs are rarely necessary but may be required in selected cases such as prophylactic antibiotics for patients with high infection risk or anticholinergics for temporary use. Neurological causes need relevant surgical correction or medical palliative management such as repeated bladder catheterization to avoid residual urine retention.

Take Home Message

Voiding problems are often not reported in time by patients, especially in case of non-neurological issues. These problems need timely intervention to prevent permanent renal damage besides disrupting normal life. Toilet training is important in early childhood and delayed or too early enthusiastic attempts may both lead to problems.

MCQs

1. Toilet training in children

A) Should start as early as possible
B) Urination is a natural process, training is not necessary
C) Should start only when child shows urge to pass urine
D) Should start when child can follow oral instructions

2. Which of the following statement about voiding problems is RIGHT?

A) It may be physiological
B) It may be pathological
C) It may be functional
D) All of the above

3. Which of the following statement about symptoms of voiding problem is WRONG?

A) Incontinence
B) Oliguria
C) Urgency
D) Hesitancy

4. Nocturnal enuresis may be a symptom

A) In a normal child
B) In a child with neurological disorder
C) In a child with anatomical urinary tract malformation
D) All of the above

5. Voiding problem may need

A) Surgical procedure
B) Antibiotics
C) Behavior modification
D) Any of the above

Answers to MCQs

Correct answers as follows:

Q1 C	Q2 D	Q3 B	Q4 D	Q5 D

76 Abnormal Movements – Movement Disorder

Introduction

Movements are under voluntary control that help us perform different tasks efficiently including maintaining body balance and working with hands. Such control is exercised mainly by basal ganglia and other related structures. Movement disorders result from loss of voluntary control – referred to as involuntary movements. However, at times, abnormal movements may also occur in spite of normal neurological system and then are considered to be physiological. Movement disorders often present as isolated or major symptom but may also be accompanied with affection of many other brain areas.

Types of Movement Disorders

They may often be involuntary but occasionally voluntary and may be either hyperkinetic (increased movements) or hypokinetic (decreased movements as in Parkinsonism). Hyperkinetic abnormal movements may include ataxia, dystonia, tremors, chorea, athetosis, myoclonus, hemiballismus, tics or Tourette syndrome.

Characteristics of Movement Disorders

Hyperkinetic Ataxia

Loss of truncal balance resulting in instability and swaying and/or intentional tremors (tremors on intentional movement of limbs – when made to move the limbs) and incoordination (as demonstrated by finger to nose test and many other clinical maneuverers) with hypotonia.

Dystonia

Increased muscle tone with twisting seen at rest or brought out on stimulation, sustained for variable time.

Tremors

Distal, fast, rhythmic, small amplitude movements, may be seen at rest or on stimulation or stretching hands out. May be physiological due to anxiety, stress or fear and are also seen in hyperthyroidism and liver cell failure.

Chorea

Proximal, chaotic, fast, non-rhythmic, large amplitude with emotional instability and hypotonia Athetosis –writhing movements, distal, slow, rhythmic, large amplitude, often together with chorea – choreoathetosis.

Myoclonus

Shock-like jerky movements of group of muscles, fast, arrhythmic. At times, such movement may be benign as in sleep myoclonus with normal neurological system.

Hemiballismus

Wide flinging movements of half side of the body (fly removal movement – movement while removing a fly coming on to your face), large amplitude.

Tics

Suppressible, paroxysmal stereotype muscle contractions

Tourette syndrome

Frequent, repetitive, jerky localized movements often involving face and neck with vocal tics in the form of grunting, throat clearing, shouting or barking, usually getting better by the age of 20 years

Hypokinetic

Slow movements as shuffling gait in Parkinsonism with other features such as tremors, stiffness of limbs and trunk, incoordination and impaired balance.

Causes

Can be etiologically classified as follows: Immune mediated (rheumatic chorea), Infection (TB meningitis with choreoathetosis and hemiballismus), Genetic (degenerative disorders), Metabolic disorders (Wilson disease), Vascular (strokes), Tumor (cerebellar tumor), Toxins (chronic hepatic disease or inborn error of metabolism), Drugs (anti-emetic, anti-convulsant).

Clinical Approach

First step is to characterize abnormal movement based on following criteria (as depicted above). Proximal or distal, fast or slow, rhythmic or arrhythmic, small or large amplitude. This may be confirmed by observation or supporting clinical maneuverers. Typical characteristic may help guess probable etiology based on common presentation. Second step is to confirm that abnormal movement is definitely pathological as tremors or myoclonus may be physiological. Next step is to ascertain whether abnormal movement is the only abnormality or whether there is evidence of affection of other areas of brain.

Presence of other symptoms and signs such as change in sensorium, pyramidal tract signs, cerebellar signs, meningeal signs, cranial nerve affection and evidence of involvement of other systems such as liver or thyroid disease. Thus, anatomy of disease can be found out. Pathology and etiology are guessed on history of presentation (acute, subacute or chronic, static or progressive) as well as past history (rheumatic fever), family history (consanguinity as in Wilson disease) and drug history.

Investigations

Provisional diagnosis is a prerequisite to ordering tests. Obviously specific test may vary in each case. CT or MRI scan may show basal ganglia lesion and affection of other areas if any. But may not be necessary in each case. For example, diagnosis of rheumatic chorea is often clinical with typical presentation and neuro-imaging will not help in defining the cause. Stroke may be confirmed with neuro-scan and if performed in early stage, damage can be reversed. CNS infection can be diagnosed with CSF examination, Wilson disease is confirmed with biochemical tests. Tics do not justify any tests.

Treatment

Symptomatic therapy

Abnormal movements may be controlled by drugs such as Haloperidol for rheumatic chorea, levodopa or beta-blocker for Parkinson tremors and other drugs like antidepressants and anticholinergics. Duration of symptomatic treatment depends on natural progress of the condition. Abnormal movements in Rheumatic chorea are usually controlled in few weeks but at times they may recur. Prolonged treatment is necessary in degenerative conditions.

Specific therapy

It depends on the cause. For example, Penicillamine for Wilson disease, anticoagulant and aspirin for strokes, anti-infective for infections and penicillin prophylaxis for rheumatic chorea as per the standard guidelines.

Take Home Message

Abnormal movements may be physiological or pathological. Characteristics of abnormal movement help in classifying movement disorder and guessing probable etiology. Brain imaging is necessary in selective conditions depending on availability of specific therapy. Symptomatic therapy is necessary for variable period.

MCQs

1. Which of the following statemen is WRONG? Abnormal movements may be

A) Voluntary
B) Involuntary
C) Physiological
D) None of the above

2. This abnormal movement can be suppressed

A) Dystonia
B) Tremors
C) Tics
D) None of the above

3. This abnormal movement can occur in sleep

A) Tremors
B) Myoclonus
C) Tics
D) All of the above

4. Which of the following statement is RIGHT?

A) Tremors are distal and slow movements
B) Chorea is proximal and repetitive movement
C) Dystonia is increased tone with twisting
D) None of the above

5. This abnormal movement disappears over years by itself

A) Tourette syndrome
B) Tics
C) Tremors
D) Ataxia

Answers to MCQs

Correct answers as follows:

Q1 D	Q2 C	Q3 B	Q4 C	Q5 A

77 Excessive Weight Gain – Obesity

Introduction

Malnutrition exists in the form of undernutrition as well as overnutrition. Unfortunately, India faces a dual burden of malnutrition. Prevalence of obesity has increased over last decade, more so in urban areas, but also in rural parts of the country and in all socioeconomic groups. Obesity in children is likely to persist in adulthood with its dire consequences that manifest in early adult life with significant morbidity and shorten productive life. Childhood obesity is mostly preventable with timely intervention to inculcate ideal life style.

Difference Between Overweight and Obesity

Overweight is defined as weight between 85th and 95th percentile for same age and sex while obesity refers to weight above 95th percentile for same age and sex. Both the conditions usually have abnormal or excessive fat accumulation in the body that carries risk to health. Overweight if not controlled progresses into obesity. Severe degree of obesity is referred to as morbid obesity.

Methods of Measurement

Periodic charting of weight and length/height right from birth up to puberty (completion of growing period) and thereafter weight is most essential to pick up early deviation in these parameters. This is the simplest way to track growth pattern though weight within normal range does not exclude excess accumulation of fat.

Body Mass Index (BMI) is calculated by dividing weight in kilograms by height square in meters. Body composition of growing children vary with age and sex but also is different in Indian children as compared to children in western countries. Hence, we must use Indian growth charts for assessing growth parameters including BMI. Indian Academy of Pediatrics has developed these charts, latest version is published and can be easily downloaded from IAP website as well as one can search them on internet.

However, BMI is also a rough guide but most practical way of measurement and so is widely used. IAP charts are user-friendly to an extent that one need not calculate BMI by the equation mentioned above but charting weight and height of a child on BMI chart can give an answer. There are three lines on BMI friendly chart – upper line – OB - represents obesity, middle line – OW - overweight and lower line – UW - underweight. Weight and height are charted and the point where they meet decides BMI.

If this point falls at or below UW, person is underweight, between UW and OW, person is normal. If this point lies between OW and OB, he is overweight and if point lies at or above OB, he is obese. It suffices for appropriate action. Waist-hip ratio is another practical and simple way to judge not only fat accumulation but also fat distribution. Waist circumference is divided by hip circumference is below 0.9 in males and below 0.8 in females DEXA scan is the best way to assess fat content of the body. Many Indians have excess of fat, even in an apparently thin body stature and are referred to as "thin fat Indians". Such individuals are also at high risk of complications.

Causes of Overweight/Obesity

Balance between consumption of energy (calories from food) and expenditure of energy (metabolic state and physical exercise) decides the outcome. Excess intake of calories and/or lack of physical exercise are the most common causes of overweight/obesity in the population. This is referred to as exogenous obesity. Onset of such an imbalance may start even in infancy, especially in infants fed on formula feeds or may start at later age due to wrong life style.

Endocrine disorders also present with obesity and they include primary hypothyroidism and Cushing's syndrome or secondary to pituitary disorders.

Children with developmental delay tend to be obese due to either lack of physical exercise or as in syndromic disorders such as Prader-Willi or hypothalamic disorders. Leptin deficiency may present in early infancy with obesity (Leptin hormone controls intake of food).

Clinical Approach to Obesity

First step is to confirm overweight/obesity by charting weight, height, BMI and waist/hip ratio. Once it is confirmed, next step is to find out probable cause. As a general rule, tall and obese is due to exogenous factors (excess intake of energy and/or lack of physical exercise) while short and obese are due to endocrine causes. Developmental delay or mental retardation points to hypothyroidism (lethargy, constipation are other features) or syndromic abnormalities (dysmorphic features and other associated malformations).

Rapid weight gain over short time indicates primary adrenal disorder such as tumor or hyperplasia (hypertension is a feature) and it may also be secondary to pituitary disorders (evidence of other hormonal disorders and increased intracranial tension in case of pituitary tumor).

Investigations

Exogenous obesity does not justify any tests to confirm the diagnosis. However due to inherent risk of consequences of obesity, periodic check on blood pressure, blood sugar, lipid profile and relevant tests for assessment of function of other organs is ideal.

Endocrine disorders should be confirmed by relevant tests. Imaging studies may be necessary in case of suspected pituitary or adrenal tumor as well as for determination of bone age as in case of hypothyroidism. Genetic tests may help to confirm syndromic abnormalities.

Complications

Obesity is a multisystem disease and severity of which depends on duration and degree of obesity. Many organs are affected though the functional disturbances are not evident clinically, they need to be monitored by relevant tests. Diabetes, hypertension, myocardial dysfunction, hypoventilation, fatty liver, osteoporosis, constipation, indigestion, immune dysfunction and mental health disturbances are common and need periodic monitoring.

Prevention

Exogenous obesity can be prevented to a large extent by healthy life style that should be inculcated from infancy. Periodic growth charting (both weight and height) right from birth onwards up to puberty and thereafter monitoring weight every month is a simple way to keep a track of weight and therefore health status. With it, one can take necessary action if weight increases to higher centiles. Weight for height is a better index to monitor and ideally, both weight and height should maintain similar centiles. Change in weight to higher centile needs explanation and appropriate action such as diet control and increase in physical exercise. Ideal life style is far more important in case of genetic propensity to exogenous obesity. It is sad to see the child being attended by the doctor since early infancy without growth monitoring and then come to attention, only when obesity has already been established. At that stage, outcome is usually poor in spite of good efforts.

Management

Exogenous obesity is managed by controlling excessive or imbalanced intake of energy and increasing energy expenditure by appropriate physical activities. Ideally, entire family should follow the same regime. Sustaining efforts is difficult for most patients and hence outcome is poor with its future consequences.

Endocrinal obesity would be treated according to the cause while syndromic obesity poses challenge in management due to multiple issues other than obesity.

Associated problems of obesity require proper management as in case of diabetes, hypertension and other organ dysfunctions.

Bariatric surgery is a debatable method of management and should be reserved for morbid obesity.

Take Home Message

Prevalence of obesity in all socioeconomic groups is fast increasing. Exogenous obesity must be prevented by ideal life style and by monitoring growth parameters regularly. Management of established obesity has poor outcome as sustained compliance is near impossible. Endogenous obesity develops more rapidly and is accompanied with many other symptoms and physical signs. Early diagnosis and prompt management is the way to expect better outcome.

MCQs

1. Which of the following statement is WRONG?

A) Obesity and overweight always go together
B) Overweight person may not be obese
C) Thin person may have excess of fat
D) All of the above

2. Which of the following parameters is the best indicator of obesity?

A) Weight
B) Height
C) Weight for height
D) All of the above

3. Which is the most reliable parameter of excessive body fat?

A) Weight for height
B) Body mass index (BMI)
C) Waist-hip ratio
D) Dexa scan

4. Rapid onset of excessive weight gain is likely to be

A) Exogenous obesity
B) Hypothyroidism
C) Cushing's syndrome
D) Syndromic obesity

5. Which of the following statement is WRONG? Obesity may affect

A) Kidney
B) Brain
C) Liver
D) None of the above

Answers to MCQs

Correct answers as follows:

Q1 A	Q2 C	Q3 D	Q4 C	Q5 D

78 Concept of Untold Symptoms

History taking is a process of "thought in action" in which, leading questions can unfold hidden physical symptoms to offer a clue to a diagnosis. However, there exist symptoms that are never expressed by patients and so, never taken into consideration by doctors in the management of diseases.

Patients do not voice them as they feel these symptoms do not relate to the disease process in the body. But they don't know that these very symptoms have direct relevance to the outcome of a disease. Such symptoms arise from the mind and they include anxiety, fear, uncertainty, depression, frustration, self-pity and even self-blame. The disease affects both the body and mind.

It is natural both need to be addressed in the management of diseases. While science (drugs) helps to treat the body, doctors must take care of the mind through ethical practice with empathy, proper communication and counseling, it is a measure of a doctor's concerns, commitment, accountability, responsibility, transparency and honesty.

It instils faith in the mind of a patient, calms his mind and improves compliance with treatment with a better outcome.

Every doctor must take note of such untold symptoms that are universally present in every patient, though to a varying extent and provide holistic care with the help of brain (science), heart (compassion), mind (commitment) and soul (inner conscience).

PREFACE TO PART 3

The power of observation is often undervalued and underutilized in the scheme of physical examination. Observation is beyond mere seeing. We are endowed by nature to observe. However, it is said, "what mind does not know, eyes cannot see". So, we need to train our mind to observe, the combination of critical thinking and vision. The power of observation can be extended to listening to sounds, not just hearing. (Listening is different than hearing, the same way as observation is different than seeing). One may be surprized to find what all can be assessed before touching the patient, that is the power of observation. Time spent for observation is worth and with repeated practice, it does not take time as it becomes a habit. The following chapters discuss the power of observation to help in the diagnosis of diseases of different systems and emphasize its importance in clinical practice.

Dr. Y. K. Amdekar

Part 3
Power of Observation

79 Power of Observation

You see but not observe

– Sherlock Holmes

Introduction

Observation refers to the ability to notice minute and significant details. Many a time, we see what is more obvious and what we expect to see but not what actually exists. Thus, we may miss some important clues. Observation helps us to see unexpected things. We must learn to focus outwards beyond what is striking to the eye. It is an important part of the physical examination, the medical diagnostic process, next only to the detailed history.

How to Develop Observational Skills?

Observation can be formal (planned) or informal (spontaneous). Physical examination starts with an inspection. Medical students are taught standard patterns of inspection as a part of general examination and examination of various systems. Beyond this formal approach, one must develop an eye for informal or spontaneous observation. Observational skills are developed by repeated mindful practice that makes us see beyond what two eyes can see, as if with the third eye – committed mind and critical thinking. Analysis of detailed history can prompt us to focus our observation on minute details. A role model teacher can sensitize a student to develop such skills. Of course, it is never too late, one can learn it through repeated practice.

Observation to Assess "Seriousness"

A mere look at the patient can alert us about something going wrong. A **change in behavior** of the patient often is the first clue to impending trouble. A patient suffering from high fever for the last 12 hours, looked confused with irrelevant talking. It was enough to suspect encephalopathy – the affection of the cerebral cortex. It could be either due to poor perfusion or oxygenation of the brain. Immediate intervention would need IV fluids and administration of oxygen. This patient was confirmed to be suffering from meningococcemia leading to circulatory collapse and could be saved because of astute observation. If the change in behavior in such a patient is missed, it could be fatal in the next 24 hours. So important is to note any change in behavior. No test can substitute such an observation.

A patient was operated for acute appendicitis and was noticed to be lethargic on postoperative day 3. There was no fever and the abdomen was soft without any guarding or tenderness. This patient was confirmed to be in early compensated septic shock due to infection. There are many such examples where observation saved the day.

ABC – airway, breathing, circulation – can be assessed by observation in a few seconds. One must confirm patent airway. The obstructed airway is evident by gurgling sounds in the throat suggesting the pooling of secretions Hissing nasal sound indicates obstructed nasal passage, inspiratory stridor and subcostal retraction evidence of upper airway inspiratory obstruction, wheeze with subcostal retraction suggests lower airway expiratory obstruction while grunting denotes probable pneumonia. Fast respiratory rate and depth of respiratory movements are easy to note. Mild tachypnea can warn impending respiratory failure, cyanosis being too late a sign. Deep and rapid breathing suggests acidosis. Circulatory status can be assessed by peripheral parts of the body being pale and cold. Such findings can be further confirmed by tachycardia, low blood pressure and increased capillary refill time.

Other facts such as hemorrhagic or gangrenous **skin rash,** greyish-white **membrane over a tonsil** (probable diphtheria) and **abdominal distension** are other observable findings that may need immediate further assessment.

Sudden excessive sweating may suggest autonomic disturbance due to sudden severe insults such as hypoglycemia or myocardial infarct.

Thus, irrespective of what the patient presents to us, it is necessary to assess "seriousness" if any, before embarking on history and physical examination. It does not take more than half a minute to do so.

Observation at the "First Look"

We must try to differentiate between acute sickness (short duration illness), chronic sickness (progressive long duration illness) or comfortable status (not affecting health in spite of symptoms). Nutritional status, growth (weight, height) and development (mental status), general body stature, posture and head-to-toe abnormalities and skin rash are other findings easily evident on observation. One can also note the way the patient walks into your chamber, sits, talks and behaves. We must make a habit of minute general observation; it helps a lot.

Eight-month-old infant presented with persistent high fever for 6 days without apparent localization. Cursory physical examination and laboratory tests failed to arrive at the diagnosis. Astute observation revealed a small nodule over the scalp that paved the diagnosis of secondary from primary neuroblastoma. Without such an observation, the diagnosis would have never been made.

Observation in Neurological Diseases

Neurological examination is mostly observation-based. One needs to touch a patient only to examine for deep tendon reflexes and sensations, all other parts of the examination are judged by observation.

Higher functions, motor system (power, tone, incoordination, nutrition and abnormal movements), most of the cranial nerves, vision, hearing, head (skull), and the spine can be assessed by observation.

Higher functions – It is enough to note whether the patient is alert and aware of time and space, if not does he respond to voice, if not, does he respond to pain and whether he is unresponsive. Even a mild change in behavior such as a confused state can be made out on observation. Memory can be tested by asking simple questions appropriate to age.

Motor system - **weakness** of limb movements can be obvious but mild weakness needs simple maneuvers for detection. For example, pronator drift (pronation of a weak side when hands are outstretched) suggests the mild weakness of the upper limb.

Gait (hemiplegic, waddling, wide-based, toe-walking, shuffling) should be observed closely which may bring out specific muscle weakness. Posture can reveal **muscle tone**. When pulled to sit or made to stand, one can observe a change in muscle tone if any (hypotonia or hypertonia). Dystonia (increased tone with twisting) may be evident on movements and so also a few types of **abnormal movements**, though, they may be observed even at rest. Incoordination, ataxia and nystagmus are easily noticeable. Wasting or hypertrophy of specific muscles needs close observation.

Speech (motor component of language) can also help in anatomical diagnosis.

Cranial nerves – Olfactory nerve is rarely affected but can be tested through the sensation of smell. The acuity of vision, field of vision and color vision can be assessed with simple techniques and so also fundus examination. Eye movements can detect affection of 3rd, 4th and 6th nerves. Ptosis is easy to note suggestive of 3rd nerve or cervical sympathetic nerve palsy. The corneal reflex can be tested (5th and 7th nerve affection) along with facial muscles. Inability to close the eye can differentiate between upper and lower motor neuron 7th nerve palsy. 8thnerve can be tested with the help of a tunic fork. Gag reflex and palatal movements are easily noticeable and so also shrugging of shoulders and tongue movements. Thus, all cranial nerves can be assessed by observation either directly or through simple maneuvers.

Vision and **hearing** can be assessed to some extent by observation though would need further relevant tests for confirmation.

Head size (microcephaly or macrocephaly) can be judged by observation and so also the abnormal **shape** of the skull as in craniostenosis, rickets or chondrodystrophy. Lordosis, kyphosis or scoliosis must be observed closely and so also any localized swelling or gibbus. Abnormal structure at the sacral **spine** such as a tuft of hair may suggest spinal cord anomalies. Neck stiffness or retraction may suggest a meningeal irritation besides any local pathology. Laxity of the anal sphincter and suprapubic fullness may suggest bowel and bladder involvement.

An old man with severe diarrhea and poor oral intake was found to be lying in a pithed frog-like posture suggesting severe hypotonia. The paucity of movements of limbs denoted quadriparesis. However, he was conscious and well-oriented. It was clear that he had developed lower motor neuron generalized disease. Considering the background of age, diarrhea and poor oral intake, severe hypokalemia was considered and confirmed. IV fluids with appropriate composition made a quick recovery. The only test ordered was serum potassium and no other neurological tests were done. Such an observation saves time and undue expenses.

Observation in Hematological Disorders

The probable cause of anemia (three major groups – deficiency, hemolytic or bone marrow disorders such as aplasia or infiltration) can be judged by observation. Comfortable patient with severe anemia without abdominal distension suggests chronic nutritional deficiency anemia either due to iron or vitamin B12. Further, koilonychia or knuckle hyperpigmentation would suggest iron or vitamin B12 deficiency respectively. On the other hand, a comfortable patient with severe anemia and abdominal distension indicates chronic hemolytic anemia. Such a patient may also have mild jaundice, abnormal facies and short stature. A similar presentation without abnormal facies and short stature may indicate acquired hemolytic anemia. Sick looking patient with severe anemia is likely to be either bone marrow aplasia (without abdominal distension) or infiltration (with abdominal distension) such as leukemia. Besides anemia, there may also be evidence of purpura due to thrombocytopenia or significant lymphadenopathy. Thus, comfortable or sick, abdominal distension or not and other supporting observational findings such as jaundice or short stature, abnormal facies can almost diagnose the cause of anemia. Further specific tests would be necessary to arrive at a final diagnosis.

Bleeding disorder can be another manifestation of the hematological disorder. Purpura indicates platelet dysfunction (comfortable patient in immune-mediated thrombocytopenia while sick in marrow disease) while bleeding at deeper sites is usually a coagulation defect. Generalized lymphadenopathy and/or hepatosplenomegaly as suggested by upper abdominal distension are other useful observational findings.

Observations in Pulmonary Disorders

Microanatomy of the pulmonary system consists of airways (upper and lower), lung parenchyma, pleural and interstitium. One can observe respiratory rate, depth of breathing movements, chest movements (symmetrical or asymmetrical), chest retractions (suprasternal, subcostal, intercostal or all of them). Respiratory sounds (stridor, wheeze, grunt, hissing sound and different types of cough sounds – dry or wet) beside sick or not sick. A severe cough can be evident in the observation that suggests primary airway disorder. Tachypnea with mild cough in a febrile patient may suggest pneumonia (grunting and intercostal retraction), pleural effusion or bronchiolitis (both of them without chest retraction, pleural effusion is localized with poor chest movements on the affected side while bronchiolitis is generalized with emphysema). Thus, microanatomical localization is possible and common pulmonary diseases can be suspected only on observation.

Observation in Liver Diseases

For clinicians, the liver has four parts – hepatocyte (liver cell), biliary tract, venous system and reticuloendothelial system (RE cells). One should observe the degree of sickness or well-being, severity of jaundice, pallor, abdominal distension (Generalized with fullness of flanks or localized to upper abdomen), edema and itching marks. Acute liver disease manifests with jaundice with or without encephalopathy and bleeding. Chronic liver disease presents with edema and upper abdominal distension. Biliary tract disease has intense jaundice , clay-colored stools and itching, disproportionate to general well-being until disease also involves hepatocytes (hepatobiliary disease). Venous system disorders (portal hypertension) manifests with hematemesis and splenomegaly without jaundice (presinusoidal portal hypertension), chronic disease with hepatosplenomegaly, ascites and jaundice in sinusoidal portal hypertension as in cirrhosis and hepatomegaly, ascites without jaundice in post-sinusoidal portal hypertension as in hepatic vein obstruction (Budd-Chiari syndrome). RE cell involvement presents as hepatomegaly without liver cell dysfunction and subsequently may affect other organs as in storage disorders or disseminated tuberculosis or localized tumors such as hydatid cyst or hepatoblastoma.

Observation in Renal Diseases

Microanatomy of the kidney has three main parts – glomerulus (endothelium, epithelium and interstitium), tubules (proximal and distal) and collecting system (upper and lower). Acute renal disorders present with mild edema and sick patient (acute glomerulonephritis), generalized massive edema and comfortable patient (nephrotic syndrome) or sick with high fever but without edema (acute pyelonephritis). Short stature, pallor, edema in a chronically sick patient may represent chronic renal glomerular disease while chronically sick, a malnourished patient without edema but with rickets and deep rapid breathing (metabolic acidosis) indicate a tubular disorder.

Localized fullness in the suprapubic region may suggest an enlarged bladder due to obstruction to the outflow of urine or localized fullness in the lumbar region may denote renal mass without other renal manifestations.

Observation in Cardiac Diseases

Microanatomy of cardiovascular system consists of heart (myocardium, endocardium and pericardium), major vascular system (aorta and pulmonary blood vessles) besides probable congenital defects. Tachypnea suggests left ventricular disease while edema of feet, engorged neck veins and upper abdominal distension indicates right ventricular disorder (CCF). Precordial pulsations on the chest wall indicate volume overload while precordial bulge suggests cardiomegaly with pressure overload. The "Suck-rest-suck" cycle in an infant suggests exertional dyspnea indicating cardiac failure. Severe cough and intercostal chest retractions indicate increased pulmonary blood flow as in the case of left to right shunt across VSD or PDA. Excessive sweating may be an indication of cardiac failure.

Observation in Endocrinal Disorders

Common endocrine disorders in clinical practice relate to thyroid, adrenal and pituitary diseases.

Short and obese is an endocrinal problem (Cushing's syndrome or hypothyroidism) while **tall and obese** is due to non-endocrinal disorders such as overnutrition, genetic syndromic or familial. Lethargy and facial puffiness is the hallmark of hypothyroidism. Early-onset hypothyroidism presents with developmental delay. Short proportionate stature with normal mentation is characteristic of Isolated growth hormone deficiency noticed often after the first two years of age.

Diabetes is the most common disorder but cannot be suspected by mere observation. However, it may be suspected in patients presenting with generalized weakness without any observation findings.

Observation in Skeletal Disorders

They may present as localized or generalized bony swelling or defects. One must observe whether the patient is sick or not, type and distribution of defects and other accompanied observational findings. Sick patient with localized bony swelling may indicate local osteomyelitis while in a comfortable patient, it may signify benign or slowly progressive malignant tumor. Generalized bony defects such as chest deformities (beading of costochondral junctions and Harrison sulcus), frontoparietal bossing of skull, epiphyseal widening at wrists, bowing of legs may denote rickets or chondrodystrophy such as achondroplasia. Rickets in a healthy infant or toddler suggests vitamin D deficiency while that in a malnourished and sick patient denotes resistant rickets commonly due to chronic renal tubular disorders or other genetic disorders. Generalized bony defect with abdominal distension, chest and spinal deformities and delayed development may suggest storage disorders such as MPS – mucopolysaccharidosis. Generalized bony swelling in a sick patient may suggest leukemia, histiocytosis or sickle cell disease. Care must be taken to differentiate bony swelling from joint involvement.

Though analysis of detailed history is able to pinpoint a system involved in the disease process, at times, it is not so easy. It is not uncommon that a presenting symptom nay represents any one of the systems discussed above. In such a case, the approach to observation may have to be based on basic knowledge genesis of symptoms. The following discussion covers the symptom-based observational approach.

Observation in Case of Tachypnea

Besides the respiratory system, cardiac, neurological and metabolic disorders may share this symptom. Moderate intercostal and/or subcostal chest retractions in not-so sick but anxious patient and often without fever would suggest cardiac tachypnea. Precordial pulsations and the site of apex impulse may help to define the cardiac disease. However, acute left ventricular failure (cardiac asthma) may simulate closely bronchial asthma on observation.

Tachypnea due to neurological disease (as in the case of respiratory muscle paralysis due to Guillain-Barre syndrome) is seen as shallow breaths without chest retractions and hypophonia or aphonia. So, it can easily be differentiated from pulmonary or cardiac diseases. Metabolic acidosis has deep and rapid breaths but the patient is not dyspneic which means there is no increase in work of breathing as evident by the absence of accessory muscles working. Thus, tachypnea without dyspnea is the observational diagnosis of metabolic acidosis.

Table

Sick look	Others	Resp rate	Chest retraction	Chest & others	Diagnosis
Yes	Normal	++	Intercostal	Fever	Pneumonia
Yes	Poor	++	Intercostal	Pulsations	CCF
Yes	Poor	+	None	Flattening	Chronic TB
Yes	Poor	+++	None	Deep breath	Met acidosis
No	Normal	+++	None	Shallow breath	Bronchiolitis
No	Normal	++	None	Fever	Pl effusion TB

Observation in Case of Jaundice

Besides hepatobiliary disorders, jaundice is also a manifestation of hemolytic anemia that is caused by unconjugated or indirect hyperbilirubinemia (has a lemon yellow tinge and usually mild jaundice) as against conjugated or direct hyperbilirubinemia (deep yellow or greenish tinge, often moderate to severe jaundice) in hepatobiliary disorders. Pallor is the main differential feature in hemolytic jaundice and is best observed with the prominent creases on the palms. Patient with hemolytic jaundice is mostly not sick and splenomegaly is more prominent than sickness in hepatobiliary disorders with hepatomegaly in prominence and often with ascites.

Table

Sick	Nutrition	Icterus	Pallor	Liver	Spleen	Diagnosis
Yes	Normal	++-	--	+	-	HAV hepatitis
Yes	Poor	++	+	+++	++	Cirrhosis
Yes	Normal	+++	--	--	--	Cholangitis
No	Normal	+	--	++	+/-	HBV hepatitis
No	Normal	+	+++	+	++	Hemolytic
No	Normal	+/-	+++	--	--	B12 deficiency

Observation in Case of Edema

Edema may be a feature of renal, hepatic, cardiac, nutritional or allergic disorders, localized edema may be due to local venous or lymphatic obstruction. Thus, one should note whether the edema is localized or generalized. The initial appearance of edema around the eyelids is characteristic of renal disorders and most of them are not acutely sick while cardiac diseases typically present with edema on dependent parts such as legs in a mobile patient and sacral edema in a bed-ridden patient. Such patients appear chronically sick. Edema in a chronic liver disease manifests as generalized abdominal distension due to ascites in addition to edema on the legs. Jaundice is not a feature of a compensated chronic liver disease and to a small extent may simulate chronic cardiac disease with hepatomegaly on observation. Lethargy and disinterest in routine play activities or eating and irritability when disturbed are characteristics of nutritional edema and may also present with skin and/or hair changes. Hepatomegaly is a common feature even in such a patient.

Angiedema is accompanied by signs of inflammation and itching and is often localized and hence never poses a challenge to diagnosis in case of edema.

Myxedema due to hypothyroidism also presents with puffiness of face but other features as lethargy helps to differentiate it from other causes.

Table

Sick look	Nutrition	Extent	Abdomen distension	Diagnosis
No	Normal	General ++	Flanks full	Nephrotic syndrome
No	Normal	Lips, eye ++	--	Allergy
Sick	Normal	Eyes +	--	Acute nephritis
Sick	Poor	Eyes, legs	Upper abd	CCF
Sick	Poor	Eyes, abd	Upper abd	Chronic liver disease
Sick	Poor	Eyes	Upper abd	Protein malnutrition
Sick	Normal	Localized limb	--	Venous/lymphatic obst

Observation in Case of Abdominal Distension

One should observe whether the patient is sick or not, localized or generalized abdominal distension, flank fullness or not, presence of significant pallor, edema, jaundice or increased peristalsis.

An acutely sick patient generally represents an acute surgical problem as in the case of intestinal obstruction or acute appendicitis. Rarely medical conditions simulate surgical problems as seen in a severely hypokalemic or toxic patient with paralytic ileus.

Chronically sick patients with abdominal distension may be due to chronic liver disease, storage disorders with multi-system involvement and malignant tumors. Generalized abdominal distension with the fullness of flanks denotes the presence of ascites and that in a non-sick patient suggests nephrotic syndrome. Partially treated nephrotic syndrome patient may present with the disappearance of generalized edema but ascites take time to resolve. Chronic constipation may present with abdominal distension and is usually due to a faulty diet. However, if present in a poorly nourished patient, it may be due to chronic intestinal obstruction as in case of congenital megacolon or at times due to IBD, celiac disease or intestinal tuberculosis.

Table

Sick look	Nutrition	Abd distension	Pallor	Icterus	Other	Diagnosis
Sick	Normal	General	--	--	Peristalsis	Int obstruction
Sick	Poor	General	--	--	--	Malnutrition
Sick	Poor	Flanks	+	++	--	Cirrhosis
Sick	Normal	Flanks	--	--	Edema	Dengue fever
Sick	Poor	Upper	++	--	Multisystem	Storage disorder
No	Normal	Flanks	+	--	Edema	Nephrotic syn.
No	Normal	General	--	--	Feces +	Constipation

Observation in Case of Pallor

As discussed in the section of hematological observation, the sick patient indicates mostly bone marrow disease, one with abdominal distension (hepatosplenomegaly) is infiltrative marrow disease while one without abdominal distension is due to marrow aplasia. If patient is not sick but with abdominal distension, it is likely to be hemolytic anemia with or without jaundice but one without abdominal distension is mostly due to deficiency anemia. Observation of other accompanying features can further narrow down the diagnostic probability.

Table

Sick look	Nutrition	Icterus	Abdominal distension	Other	Diagnosis
Sick	Normal	--	--	Purpura	Marrow aplasia
Sick	Normal	--	Upper	Purpura	Leukemia
Sick	Normal	+	Spleen +	--	Ac hemolytic
No	Normal	+	Spleen ++	Facies	Con hemolytic
No	Normal	--	Spleen ++	Stunted	Thalassemia
No	Normal	--	--	Koilonychia	Iron def
No	Normal	--/+	--	Pigmentation	B12 def

Observation in Case of Short Stature

As discussed in the section of endocrine diseases, short stature with poor weight and a sick patient represent chronic malnutrition either primary or secondary. Proportionate short stature otherwise normal is due to isolated GH deficiency, genetic or constitutional problem. Those with body defects are due to rickets of various types and chondrodystrophy.

Table

Sick look	Nutrition	Body proportion	Abdomen distension	Other	Diagnosis
Sick	Poor	Normal	General	Edema	Malnutrition
Sick	Poor	Normal	Upper	Multisystem	Storage disease
No	Obese	Abnormal	General	Facies	Hypothyroid
No	Normal	Normal	--	Web neck	Turner syndrome
No	Normal	Normal	General	Bony defects	Rickets
No	Normal	Abnormal	--	Bony defects	Achondroplasia
No	Normal	Normal	--	--	GH deficiency

Observation in Case of Obesity

Short and obese is endocrinal – hypothyroidism, adrenal disorder or syndromic as Prader-Willi syndrome. Tall and obese are generally due to exogenous causes – wrong lifestyles, genetic or familial.

Table

Sick look	Obese	Height	Other features	Diagnosis
Sick	++	Short	Hypertension	Adrenal tumor
No	+	Short	Facies, MR	Hypothyroid
No	+++	Normal	--	Exogenous, genetic

In summary, the power of observation guided by analysis of detailed history leads to narrowing down the clinical diagnostic probability. One must be committed to observing based on critical thinking of what history has suggested. However, when there is no clue, as does happen at times, one must observe every part of the body closely because there would be a clue hiding somewhere. Other parts of physical examination finetune the diagnostic process. This would pave the way to very specific and fewer laboratory tests to confirm the final diagnosis if need be. The beauty of bedside clinical medicine is the ability to practice medicine rationally which offers joy and a thrill to a doctor and blessings from a satisfied patient.

PREFACE TO PART 4

Advancing technology and easy availability of investigatory modalities including imaging, genetic and immunological tests have made many doctors depend on them for diagnosis of diseases, avoiding detailed history and physical examination. Test results must be correlated with clinical impression and hence are not meant to diagnose diseases but only to confirm, support or rule out the provisional clinical diagnosis. Test results are not always right and dependable. A positive test may be seen without an active disease and a negative test may not rule out the disease. Without a provisional diagnosis, test results could add to confusion besides wasting time and money. There is nothing like "routine tests". Doctors must know what they expect out of a test rather than treat what they see in the test results. **We should not treat test results but treat the disease**. Rationality demands minimum and appropriate tests based on provisional clinical diagnosis. Hence, there is a need for **"Testing a test"**.

Dr. Y. K. Amdekar

Part 4
Testing a Test

Section 1
General View

80 General View

Introduction

In evidence-based modern medicine, ideally, clinical bedside diagnosis should be confirmed by relevant laboratory tests. However, it may not be necessary for every patient and it may not be possible for various reasons. Rational practice demands provisional clinical diagnosis before ordering relevant laboratory tests. Tests are not meant to search the diagnosis but just to confirm, support or rule out clinical bedside provisional diagnosis. Test results must be correlated with clinical profile and not considered in isolation. Test results are at times confusing and there may be a disparity between test results and clinical judgment that must be cautiously addressed. Hence, **a test must be tested** for its worth in a given situation.

Clinical bedside diagnosis of any disease consists of four components – anatomy (site of disease), pathology (type of disease), etiology (cause of disease) and functional status of an affected organ (normal, compensated or decompensated function). The tests should be planned accordingly to confirm either or all the components of the diagnosis as per the need.

Tests for Anatomical Diagnosis

A particular system or organ involved in the disease is often evident clinically but further localization may not be clear. For example, symptoms of respiratory disease may arise from the airways, lung parenchyma, interstitium or pleura. Imaging modalities help in the evaluation of microanatomy. Images must be interpreted in correlation with a clinical profile which is often not shared with a radiologist.

Abdominal USG is commonly ordered in case of vague abdominal symptoms. The presence of lymph nodes and fluid in the peritoneal cavity in an abdominal USG are normal findings but the size and other characteristics of lymph nodes and the amount of peritoneal fluid decide whether they are abnormal. Besides, normal abdominal USG may not rule out an abdominal disease. The same is true about other imaging modalities such as X-ray, CT or MRI scans. Normal images don't exclude diseases as imaging modalities show only the structural changes and diseases do exist with functional deterioration without obvious structural abnormalities. Video imaging modalities are able to study the function of an affected organ as in the case of swallowing incoordination.

An abnormal image may be an artifact, a normal variant and hence needs cautious interpretation. A 2D echocardiogram is commonly used in the diagnosis of heart diseases and may also evaluate heart functions besides structural changes. Similarly, liver disease may be localized either to hepatocyte, biliary tract, venous system or reticuloendothelial system. Selective biochemical tests may be able to pinpoint the microanatomy of liver disease. The same is true about other organs. Thus, it may be necessary to confirm the microanatomical diagnosis by relevant tests.

Tests for Pathological Diagnosis

Imaging modalities may help to a certain extent to guess the pathology such as edema, caseation, necrosis, fibrosis, consolidation, emphysema or tumor etc. Histology of a biopsied or an aspirated sample detects pathology more clearly as in case of inflammation, caseation or atrophy and helps in the probable etiological diagnosis. Histopathology is most important in the diagnosis of tumors. All such test results have to be correlated with clinical profile to make a certain etiological diagnosis as many pathological abnormalities are shared by different etiology. For example, histopathology of tuberculosis and lymphoma may not be easy to differentiate and at times, both diseases may coexist.

Biopsied or aspirated samples can also be subjected to etiological diagnosis of infections. Neutrophilic leukocytosis suggests inflammation but fails to define the cause. Urinalysis can reveal glomerular inflammation as in case of nephritis and stool microscopy can show mucous or blood as evidence of inflammation. But they do not give etiological diagnosis. Acute phase reactants as ESR or CRP are also markers of inflammation and stool calprotectin of intestinal inflammation. Intra-cellular enzymes leak out into the blood when cells are damaged as happens with hepatocyte damage leading to an increase in ALT/AST. The level of increase corresponds with the degree and acuity of damage. The same is true about muscle damage that leads to an increase in CPK – creatine phosphokinase or LDH denoting cellular damage.

Tests for Etiological Diagnosis

Infection is the common cause of diseases in routine practice. Culture must be attempted in bacterial infections that may also reveal antibiotic sensitivity against a causative organism. This assumes far more importance in the case of infections that carry a high risk of antibiotic-resistant strains as in the case of tuberculosis, UTI or typhoid fever. However, culture may not be possible in every infection for genuine reasons. For example. Brucella, leptospirosis or rickettsia are difficult to culture. If etiology cannot be confirmed in such infections, at least, supportive tests should strengthen the possible diagnosis as done by antibody tests in these infections.

Antibody tests are not ideal because they continue to be positive well after the disease is cured. IgM antibody suggests recent infection and IgG antibody the past infection. Even IgM antibodies may persist in the blood for a few months and hence by themselves, do not suggest active infection.

However, confirmative or supportive tests may not be necessary for every infection as in classical acute tonsillitis, acute bacillary dysentery or common viral infections such as measles or varicella. It is because clinical diagnosis is near certain and progress of such a disease is possible to monitor clinically. On the other hand, laboratory tests are mandatory when the choice of drugs depends on accurate etiological diagnosis or progress and complete control of the disease cannot be monitored clinically as in the case of UTI (urinary tract infection), meningitis or tuberculosis. It is clear that antibiotics should not be prescribed without confirmation of an infection, for which provisional diagnosis is a must prior to testing, the exception being an emergency situation as in a very sick patient.

Rapid antigen tests are substitutes for culture but have limitations. The antigen may persist for a long time after the disease has been cured and it detects both live and dead organisms and hence may not suggest active infection. The advantage of an antigen test is the fact that the test results are available immediately and prior antibiotic therapy does not interfere with the test results. PCR – polymerase chain reaction – is a molecular test that can detect infection in an early stage when organisms are small in number and the test is available now. It is most accurate and hence more useful. PCR is also used in the diagnosis of genetic disorders. A blood smear may pick up malarial parasites and also LD bodies in kala azar, which are confirmative tests. Similarly, stool microscopy can confirm the diagnosis of amebiasis or giardiasis and other intestinal parasitic infections.

Bone marrow examination can pick up leukemia and further special tests can diagnose the type of disease. Diagnosis of autoimmune disorders can be supported by antibody tests and immune deficiency diseases can be diagnosed by specific tests of immune functions. Obviously, such diseases demand accurate diagnosis by laboratory tests to an extent possible prior to starting specific therapy, though the exact etiology of many diseases remains obscure. While the etiological diagnosis should always be attempted, it may not be always possible for genuine reasons and in such cases, supportive tests must be ordered.

Tests for Functional Diagnosis (To Assess Functional Integrity)

Functional impairment of an organ may exist without structural changes and are therefore not evident on routine imaging or histopathology but are detected with biochemical abnormalities. Commonly employed blood tests include blood sugar, LFT (liver function tests), RFT (renal function tests), thyroid profile, intestinal absorptive functions, electrolytes and acid-base, ABG (arterial blood gas). 2D echocardiogram and pulmonary function tests are also commonly used. EEG (electroencephalogram) for epileptic focus and EMG (electromyogram) and nerve conduction for neuromuscular disorders, BERA (brainstem evoked response auditory) for hearing assessment and VER (visual evoked response) for visual acuity are some other tests used in special situations. Degree of functional abnormality correlates with the severity of the disease to differentiate between organ dysfunction and organ failure.

Tests for Monitoring the Progress of Diseases

When clinical improvement alone cannot guarantee a complete cure, laboratory tests are necessary. ESR or CRP are often used in such situations. In the case of Rheumatic fever, the patient becomes asymptomatic within a few days but aspirin is continued for a few more weeks till ESR comes down to normal indicative of control of inflammation. In acute bacterial infections such as typhoid, fever may continue longer in which case, the appearance of eosinophils in CBC would suggest an improving condition and rule out antibiotic resistance. (Absence of eosinophils is characteristic of active infection). Similarly, a patient suffering from meningitis may improve clinically but antibiotics may have to be continued longer if repeat CSF has not come back to normal. Chronic infections such as tuberculosis, chronic organ dysfunctions and other chronic diseases such as malignancy need repeat tests to ensure desired control or cure of the disease.

Concept of Sensitivity and Specificity

It is important to measure the reliability of a given test in terms of accurate prediction of a suspected disease. "Gold standard" is one where the test is 100% reliable. Detection of a malarial parasite in a blood smear is "gold standard" for the diagnosis of malaria and the reliability of every other test would be compared with this gold standard test.

Sensitivity refers to the ability of a positive test to predict the presence of disease accurately while specificity is the ability of a negative test to predict the absence of disease accurately. Thus, a positive test with 80% sensitivity can diagnose 80% of patients accurately but misses the diagnosis in 20% of patients. Similarly, a negative test with 80% specificity rules out the disease accurately in 80% of the patients but the other 20% may have a disease. Ideally, the test should be 100% sensitive and 100% specific but no test is that accurate. Thus, the physician must keep in mind the probability of false +ve or false -ve test results and should always correlate the test result with the clinical profile. For example, a positive bacterial culture may be due to contamination of a sample or the presence of a commensal organism – one that is normally present but not the cause of the disease as happens in the case of alpha or non-hemolytic streptococci reported in throat culture. It is the beta-hemolytic streptococci that are pathogenic. AFB – acid-fast bacilli (tubercle bacilli) in sputum can be detected only if the number of bacilli in the sample is as high as 5000-10000, culture is positive if the number of bacilli are between 50-100 while GeneXpert can detect even 5 bacilli in the sample. Blood thick smear should be screened thoroughly for the presence of malarial parasites and then a thin smear can differentiate between vivax and falciparum. However, as parasites are present in the blood for a short time that may coincide with the onset of high fever and then disappear from the blood into the spleen. Thus, the timing of a blood smear may influence detection. That is why all the laboratory reports end with a statement "please correlate clinically" especially when a blood smear does not show malarial parasite.

In summary, modern medical science has evolved with advances in the field of diagnostics. Evidence-based medicine demands proof of the diagnosis for rational treatment. However, there are many limitations of investigatory modalities. Laboratory tests should be used to confirm, support or rule out the provisional diagnosis made on the bedside and should not be used to search the diagnosis. Unfortunately, tests are being misused in place of clinical bedside medicine which is vanishing fast. This trend must be reversed and judicious use of modern technology is the need of the hour.

MCQs

1. Generalised weakness (feeling tired) may be a result of this system (anatomical diagnosis)

A) Hematological
B) Cardiac
C) Respiratory
D) All of the above

2. Chest X-ray is not ideal to diagnose the disease involving this anatomical site

A) Lungs
B) Pleura
C) Bronchi
D) Mediastinum

3. Laboratory tests fail to diagnose this condition

A) Alzheimer disease
B) Irritable bowel syndrome
C) Migraine
D) All of the above

4. This test is not diagnostic of active disease

A) Mantoux test for tuberculosis
B) Reducing substance (sugar) in stool for lactose intolerance
C) Rapid antigen test for malaria
D) All of the above

5. Which of the following statement is WRONG? Positive blood culture may

A) Suggest active disease
B) May indicate recently cured disease
C) May be a commensal
D) May be a contaminant

Answers to MCQs

Correct answers as follows:

Q1 D	Q2 C	Q3 D	Q4 D	Q5 B

Section 2

Commonly Ordered Tests

81 ABC of CBC

Back to Basics

Complete blood count includes estimation of hemoglobin and hematocrit, number of red blood cells, white blood cells (neutrophils, lymphocytes, monocytes, basophils and eosinophils) and platelets. It is not enough to count the number of different blood cells but equally important is to study the characteristics of the cells in terms of size, shape, color, maturity including abnormal cells in **peripheral blood smear (PS).** It is an important part of CBC. In fact, cell count must be corroborated with peripheral smear. PS is used to screen various types of diseases such as infections and blood disorders and monitor their progress.

RBCs (Erythrocytes) and Hemoglobin

Normal RBC count is 4.5 to 5.5 million/ ml and Hb 12-15 Gm%. Normal value of RBC count and hemoglobin vary as per the age, especially in early life. Hemoglobin level at birth is as high as 16-18 Gm% which gradually comes down to 10 Gm% at about 3 months of age and then increases to around 12 Gm% at one year of age. Thus, degree of anemia in infants must be correlated with normal values at that particular age. Low level suggests anemia.

RBCs contain hemoglobin that carries oxygen to the tissues that turns into energy to keep the body healthy and also help in eliminating carbon-dioxide from the body via lungs. RBCs do not have nucleus that makes them change shape which helps smooth travel through blood stream. Anemia is mainly due to deficiency of iron or B12 / folate but may also be due to hemolysis of RBCs or deficient production by bone marrow. RBC indices would indicate type of anemia. Polycythemia refers to increased hemoglobin level and is seen in severe hypovolemia as in case of capillary leak syndrome triggered by dengue viral infection and also in cyanotic heart diseases due to chronic hypoxia.

Hematocrit

It refers to packed cell volume. Normal level is 35-45%, varies a little with age and gender. Low hematocrit means less number of RBCs.

WBCs (Leukocytes)

Normal WBC count is between 4500–11,000/ml. Differential WBC count consists of 50-60% neutrophils, 30-40% lymphocytes, 2-8% monocytes, 2-4% eosinophils and 0-1% basophils. WBCs are the part of immune system as they fight against infections and defend the body against foreign material. Neutrophils are the first to respond to bacterial or viral infection. Eosinophils fight against parasitic infections and also respond to foreign material such as pollen or dust mite. Thus, it has a role in allergic disorders. Basophils produce non-specific immune response and also play a role in asthma. Lymphocytes are of two types – B cell and T cell. B cells are responsible for humoral immunity by producing antibodies while T cells kill the organisms. Monocytes are like garbage trucks as they help clearing the dead cells.

Neutrophilic leukocytosis suggests acute inflammation that may result from acute bacterial infection, acute viral infection during initial 1-2 days and acute non-infective inflammation as in case of rheumatological disorders. However, typhoid fever, brucella and rickettsia are acute bacterial infections that present with leukopenia. Leukopenia is also a feature of acute viral infections beyond initial 1-2 days. Lymphocytosis is seen in acute viral infection beyond initial 1-2 days, typhoid fever (also monocytosis), chronic infections including pertussis, tuberculosis and lymphatic leukemia and also during recovering bacterial infections. Eosinopenia is seen in acute infections including typhoid fever and normalization of eosinophil count indicates recovery from such infections. Eosinophilia denotes allergic disorders including in case of worm infestations.

Platelets (Thrombocytes)

Normal platelet count is 1–4 lakhs/ml. Thrombocytopenia is a feature of typhoid fever, vital infections and malaria while thrombocytosis is seen in severe inflammation. Platelets play a major role in control of bleeding by clamping together to form a clot that plugs the site of bleeding. In case of severe inflammation with oozing of blood, platelet count increases (thrombocytosis) as happens in autoimmune disorders and also in severe destructive bacterial infections. In typhoid, viral infections and malaria, platelet count goes down to moderate level (thrombocytopenia). However, as quality of platelets is good, usually there is no bleeding in such cases. When platelets are reduced to very low level (usually < 50000), there exists a risk of bleeding while when they are increased, there is a risk of thrombosis obstructing blood flow.

Thrombocytopenia results either from defective production as in case of bone marrow diseases or excessive peripheral destruction as in hypersplenism or antibody mediated destruction as in immune thrombocytopenia (ITP).

Thrombocytosis is seen in iron deficiency anemia, malignancy or severe inflammation.

Methods of Cell Counting

Hemocytometer is a counting chamber (Neubauer counting chamber) that was used commonly in clinical practice that involved manual counting. Automated counters are now-a-days used in most laboratories. They provide quick and smooth counting. These counters recognize blood cells by their size – WBCs are larger than RBCs in size, which are larger than platelets. Thus, if RBCs are smaller than normal as in case of iron deficiency anemia, counter counts such small RBCs as platelets and hence platelet count is reported to be high. On the other hand, if there is a small blood clot in the sample, platelets are consumed and platelet count reported to be low. Such technical issues must be considered in the interpretation. Ideally, in case of doubt (when clinical profile does not match with the result), results of platelet count as reported by the counter should be checked with peripheral blood smear. Roughly, number of platelets counted manually in one high power field multiplied by 10,000 should be total platelet count. Automated counters also cannot differentiate monocytes, basophils and eosinophils and they are clubbed together as others. Technician studies peripheral smear and assigns approximate value to these three types of WBCs. Latest generation of automated counters are now available that can recognize all types of WBCs. Besides blood cell count, automated counters evaluate more than 50 parameters either directly or indirectly by calculating the values such as hematocrit and RBC indices.

MCQs

1. CBC / PS should be ordered on D1 of fever in this condition

A) Acute tonsillitis
B) Pneumonia
C) Malaria
D) All of the above

2. Ideal time to order CBC in case of undiagnosed fever is on

A) First day
B) After 2-3 days
C) Either of the two
D) Only after D 4

3. Which of the following statement is WRONG? Bacterial infection may present with

A) Leukocytosis
B) Leukopenia
C) Normal WBC count
D) None of the above

4. Eosinopenia is a feature of

A) Malaria

B) Tuberculosis

C) Rheumatological disorders

D) Typhoid

5. Automated counter may mislead in case of

A) RBC count

B) WBC count

C) Hemoglobin

D) Platelets

Answers to MCQs

Correct answers as follows:

Q1 C	Q2 B	Q3 D	Q4 D	Q5 D

82 CBC in Short Duration Fever

Basics Revisited

CBC is the most common test ordered in routine practice in case of fever. Ideally, it should be ordered 48 hours after onset of fever as it takes some time for the bone marrow to respond appropriately. Therefore, it is important to consider the timing of the test in relation to the duration of the fever. Results must be correlated with clinical profile and not interpreted in isolation. Clinical profile of the disease for interpretation of CBC report includes age, nutritional and immune status of the patient, drugs administered prior to the test and severity of the disease. Provisional differential diagnosis is a prerequisite to ordering any tests. Random testing without probable clinical diagnosis is likely to confuse more than help in the final diagnosis.

Besides total WBC count, differential cell count assumes importance. It is not only neutrophils and lymphocytes, but eosinophils and platelet count are relevant for interpretation. A peripheral blood smear may also offer clues to the diagnosis. It is important to realize that CBC results can be variable even in the same disease and may have a different interpretation. For example, an acute bacterial infection often presents with neutrophilic leukocytosis but typhoid fever or worsening severe bacterial infection may suppress bone marrow with resultant leukopenia. Similarly, eosinopenia is a feature of acute infection but in a child with an allergy who has increased eosinophils, it may not reveal eosinopenia and confuse the doctor about interpretation. Thus, every part of CBC needs careful assessment and clinical correlation is vital.

Following case scenarios will help in the rational interpretation of CBC report. Note abnormalities, correlate with clinical profile to arrive at a probable diagnosis and find answers at the end.

Case 1

2 year old child presented with a high fever, no other complaints for 3 days. Physical examination showed a sick look, high fever, no other localizing signs
Hb 10 Gm%, WBC 18000 P 75 L 23 M 2 E 0 Pl 2.8 L

Case 2

2 year old child presented with high fever and cold for a day. Physical examination showed no localizing signs.
Hb 9 Gm%, WBC 16000 P 70 L 27 M 3 E 0 Pl 1.1 L

Case 3

6 year old child presented with high fever for 3 days, no other complaints. Physical examination showed no localsing signs.
Hb 10 Gm%, WBC 18000 P 78 L 16 M 3 E 3 Pl 2.9 L

Case 4

8 year old child presented with fever for 4 days, no other complaints. Physical examination showed sick look with high fever, no other signs
Hb 11 Gn%, WBC 3200 P 42 L 48 M 10 E 0 Pl 0.8 L

Case 5

4 year old child presented with high fever for 3 days, no other complaints. Physical examination showed not a sick child, no abnormality.
Hb 7 Gm% WBC 7400 P 52 L 43 M 2 E 3 Pl 0.8 L

Answers with Explanation

Case 1

High fever without localization on D3 in a younger child, neutrophilic leukocytosis (acute inflammation – either infective or non-infective) eosinopenia (acute infection), normal platelets (unlikely acute viral infection), sick child without localization (hidden acute bacterial infection)

Diagnosis – look for **acute UTI** (confirm with urine culture)

Case 2

High fever and cold (nasal symptom) on D1 in a younger child, neutrophilic leukocytosis, (acute inflammation – infective or non-infective) eosinopenia (acute infection), thrombocytopenia (likely viral infection), nasal symptoms favor viral infection.

Diagnosis – **acute viral infection**. Note that neutrophilic leukocytosis on D1may also be an acute viral infection that may change to lymphocytic response and leukopenia over next 2-3 days.

Case 3

High fever without localization on D3 in an older child, mild anemia, neutrophilic leukocytosis (acute inflammation – infective or non-infective), normal eosinophils (unlikely an acute infection), normal platelets (unlikely viral infection)

Diagnosis – **systemic inflammatory disease**. Note the difference in terms of normal eosinophils that makes acute infection unlikely. Systemic inflammatory disease may show increasing neutrophilic leukocytosis with thrombocytosis and often decreasing hemoglobin.

Case 4

High fever without localization on D4 in an older child, leukopenia, lymphocytosis monocytosis, eosinopenia and thrombocytopenia. All these findings may suggest acute viral infection, However, most vital infections improve over 3-4 days and those who don't improve present with other symptoms and signs. Besides, this child looks sick on D4 that is more likely to be acute bacterial infection. Thus, it may be type of acute bacterial infection that responds with leukopenia.

Diagnosis – **Typhoid fever**

Case 5

High fever in non-sick child without localizing signs on D3, low hemoglobin (anemia), normal WBC and differential count (rules out acute inflammatory diseases – both infective and non-infective) thrombocytopenia.

Diagnosis – **Malaria,** It should be confirmed with peripheral blood smear

Following table summarizes interpretation of CBC in the diagnosis of common diseases

Hb	TC	P	L	E	Pl	Disease
d	N	+++	+++	0	N	Acute bacterial infection
N	++	++		0	N	Acute viral infection
N	+++	+++		N	High	Systemic inflammation
N	Low		++	0	Low	Typhoid fever
N	+/-	+/-	+/-	N	N	Chronic infection or N
Low	+/-	+/-	+/-	N	Low	Malaria
Low	+++		+++	N	Low	Acute leukemia
High	++		++	0	Low	Dengue capillary leak

83 Laboratory Diagnosis of Anemia

Basics Revisited

Hemoglobin concentration in health differs in relevance to age, gender and hydration state. Hb less than the lower limit of normal for a particular age denotes anemia. In neonates, Hb is 16-17 Gm% which slowly reduces to around 10 Gm% by the age of 3 months. It rises slowly over the next few years to attain a normal level of 13-15 Gm% in children > 5 years of age and adults, Hb between 11.9-10 Gm% is considered as mild anemia, between 9.9-7 Gm% as moderate and < 7 Gm% as severe anemia. Anemia may be caused by deficiency of major nutrients (iron, B12, folate), hemolysis of RBCs (congenital or acquired) or bone marrow disorders (aplasia or infiltration). One or more of these three factors are responsible for anemia of chronic infections, inflammatory diseases and chronic organ disorders (renal, liver, thyroid). Chronic persistent hemorrhage presents as deficiency anemia while acute severe hemorrhage manifests as shock. RBC indices and peripheral blood smear examination help to narrow down the probable type of anemia. Further tests are necessary to pinpoint final diagnosis.

RBC indices measure MCV (mean corpuscular volume – ratio of hemoglobin % and RBC count – normal value 80-100 femtoliter), MCH (mean corpuscular hemoglobin – ratio of hemoglobin in Gm and RBC count – normal value27-31 picogram/cell), MCHC (mean corpuscular hemoglobin concentration – hemoglobin in Gm and hematocrit – normal value 32-36 grams/decilitre) and RDW (red cell diameter width – ratio of MCV and standard deviation of the mean cell size – range of red blood cell volume – normal value 12-16%)

MCV and RDW together can help diagnosis of type of anemia.

Low MCV N RDW – thal trait, anemia of chronic disease

Low MCV, H RDW – iron def, thal major, other hemolytic anemias, vit C, E deficiency, copper deficiency

H MCV, N RDW – aplastic anemia, bone marrow disease, liver disease, hypothyroidism

H MCV, H RDW – megaloblastic anemia

Increased RDW indicates active bone marrow and so also increased platelet distribution width.

Low MCV, MCH and MCHC in iron deficiency anemia, High MCV,MCH and normal MCHC in megaloblastic anemia, High MCHC in spherocytosis, sickle cell and autoimmune hemolytic anemia.

Peripheral Blood Smear

It is an important test in hematological disorders that reveals abnormalities, if any in various blood cells. Test results can be altered by technical issues such as delay in making a smear, extremes of temperature exposure, clotted blood or inexperienced technician. Even prior blood transfusion does alter test results.

RBCs

It gives information about size (anisocytosis – normal, microcytes or macrocytes), shape (poikilocytosis – normal, spherocytes, sickle-shaped) and color (pink or pale) of RBCs, It can reveal premature cells such as normoblasts, if more than 1% indicating hyperactive bone marrow as in hemolytic anemia, burr cells in renal disease, fragmented RBCs - schistocytes in microangiopathic hemolytic anemia, tear-drop cells in myelofibrosis and myeloproliferative disorders, acanthocytes or spur cells with thorny projections in liver disease, helmet cells in intravascular hemolysis, rouleaux formation meaning stack of RBCs stuck together as in connective tissue disorder, multiple myeloma, diabetes and allergic diseases, Howell-jolly bodies in splenectomy and B12 / folate deficiency, Heinz bodies denoting denatured Hb clumped in RBCs. A confirmative test for malaria is demonstrating the parasite in RBCs, a thick smear helps to pinpoint the diagnosis and a thin smear can recognize the type of parasite – vivax or falciparum. It can also indicate severity by calculating the parasitic index.

WBCs

Observed band cells are a premature form of polymorphonuclear cells and if increased > 10% in peripheral smear indicates acute bacterial infection, also referred to as "shift to left". Band cells have curved nuclei as against oval in neutrophils. Toxic granules in neutrophils indicate acute bacterial infection. Hypersegmented neutrophils (increase in a number of lobes) denote B12 deficiency anemia, myelofibrosis, chronic renal or liver disease or leukemia. Premature WBCs – atypical lymphocytes > 5% are seen in EB viral infection, blast cells are seen in leukemia. Basophilic stippling is seen in lead poisoning.

Platelets

It is ideal to count the number of platelets in one high power field in a blood smear and correlate it with the platelet count reported by the automated counter. Roughly, the number of platelets in one high power field multiplied by 10,000 should be the expected total platelet count. Such a correlation takes care of technical issues in counter-reporting. Large size platelets – mega platelets suggest hyperactive bone marrow. Immature platelet fraction is the ratio of immature platelets to the total number of platelets and increases in IPF suggests recovering thrombocytopenic condition.

Clinical Application in the Diagnosis of Anemia

Here are a few laboratory reports for you to interpret. Answers with explanations are given at the end.

Case 1

Hb 8 Gm%, RBC 3.7 PS – microcytic hypochromic, MCV 60, MCH 22, MCHC 27, RDW 18%, WBC 7800, platelet 4.5

Case 2

Hb 8 Gm%, RBC 3.5 PS – macrocytic hypochromic, MCV 110, MCH 22, MCHC 34, RDW 18% WBC 3200, hypersegmented neutrophils, platelet 0.7 lakh

Case 3

Hb 6 Gm%, RBC 2.7, PS – microcytic hypochromic, normoblasts, target cells, MCV 62, MCH 23, MCHC 25, RDW 24%, WBC 18,000, platelet 2.3 lakh

Case 4

Hb 7 Gm%, RBC 2.9, PS – microcytic, hyperchromic, spherocytes, MCV 72, MCH 28, MCHC 40, RDW 12% , WBC N, platelet N

Case 5

Hb 8 Gm%, RBC 3.4, PS – macrocytic hypochromic, MCV 110, MCH 33, MCHC 34, RDW 14%, WBC 2500, platelet 0.7 lakh

Answers with Explanation

Case 1

Microcytic hypochromic anemia, RBC indices are low except RDW is high. Platelets are high because microcytes (small size RBCs are counted as platelets by automated counter)

Diagnosis – **iron deficiency anemia**

Case 2

Macrocytic hypochromic, high MCV and RDW, hyper segmented neutrophils are characteristic of megaloblastic anemia, low WBC and platelet count – pancytopenia is due to suppressed bone marrow that is due to lack of DNA maturation as B12 is necessary for DNA maturation,

Diagnosis – **B12 deficiency anemia.** It simulates aplastic anemia except RDW is high in B12 deficiency while normal in aplastic anemia.

Case 3

Microcytic hypochromic, all RBC indices are low and RDW is very high, normoblasts suggest hyperactive bone marrow denoting hemolytic anemia, WBC count is high because normoblasts are bigger than RBCs and hence counted as WBCs by automated counter (it is necessary to calculate corrected WBC count by subtracting normoblast percentage from total RBCs)

Diagnosis – **Thalassemia Major**

Case 4

Microcytic hyperchromic, high MCHC, spherocytes, normal WBC and platelets

Diagnosis – **hereditary spherocytosis**

Case 5

Macrocytic hypochromic, high MCV but normal RDW, low WBC and platelet count – pancytopenia

Diagnosis – **aplastic anemia**

84 Acute Phase Reactants (ESR, CRP, PCT)

Back to Basics

Acute phase reactants are markers of inflammation that are evident by the change in their serum concentration during inflammation. ESR is an exception as it is not measured in serum, it depends on the sedimentation rate of erythrocytes. Cytokines such as IL6 (interleukin 6), IL1, tumor necrosis factor-alpha (TNF-alpha) and gamma interferon (IFN-gamma) induce the production of acute-phase reactants. Thus, the more the cytokines produced, the higher will be acute phase reactants.

Acute phase reactants are classified as positive (increased concentration) or negative (decreased concentration). Positive acute phase reactants include commonly used CRP, PCT (procalcitonin) and also ferritin, fibrinogen, ceruloplasmin. Negative acute phase reactants include albumin, transferrin, antithrombin.

ESR

It is measured by mounting blood in a vertical standing tube and allowing RBCs to settle down. During inflammation, RBCs clump together and so descend fast to the bottom. The higher the distance they travel within an hour, the higher the ESR at the end of one hour. Normal value 0-20 mm/at the end of one hour. It is not a good screening test except a three-digit value that suggests serious disease - severe bacterial infection, inflammation or malignancy. ESR depends on fibrinogen level and RBC rouleaux formation. It is increased in case of increased fibrinogen level and macrocytic anemia. ESR is low in case of low levels of fibrinogen (as in HLH), microcytosis, polycythemia, hypergammaglobulinemia, hyperviscosity and high WBC counts. Females tend to have higher ESR up to 20 mm, in men up to 15 mm. There are technical problems such as tilted tube causes elevation of ESR while less anticoagulant with clotting of blood leads to low ESR. ESR rises slowly and has too many variables dependent on it. ESR may have some value as a sickness index - prognosis in a suspected disease. High ESR in an otherwise normal person needs repeat tests after some time before embarking on other tests.

CRP

Normal value is < 10 mg/L. It is produced by the liver in response to IL6, it starts rising between 4-12 hours of stimulation and peaks by 24-48 hours. It has a long half-life and so it takes several days to come to a baseline after the stimulus has disappeared. It has a wide range of reference values, thus sequential records are more useful than a single value. Several factors decide CRP polymorphism - such as genetic and phenotypic variables besides environmental and lifestyle issues. Including dietetic factors. Such as high transfat consumption increases CRP level, amount and type of carbohydrates, fiber, protein especially from meat and micronutrients also affect CRP. Different cytokines exert variable triggers to CRP, IL 8 releases CRP from hepatocytes the most. It is elevated in many conditions including traumatic conditions, infarctions, serotonin syndromes (caused by interaction with some drugs that increase serotonin levels). If a high CRP level does not come down within 3 days of treatment, the situation needs a review. The higher the elevated CRP, the more is the likelihood of a bacterial infection. CRP in viral infection is mildly increased. Low platelet with high CRP is seen in malaria, low platelet with normal CRP in dengue viral disease.

In SLE (systemic lupus erythematosus), ESR is high but CRP is low. This is because of the development of antibodies against CRP. While in diseases with low fibrinogen such as HLH (hemolymphocytic phagocytosis), CRP is high but ESR is low. Thus, in specific conditions, both ESR and CRP are important.

Procalcitonin

Normal level 0.05 ng/ml. It is attenuated by interferon-gamma in response to viral infections and hence it is low in viral infection and is a specific marker of bacterial infection. The level of PCT correlates with the severity of the bacterial infection and also decreases as infection comes under control. It is detectable within 3-4 hours of infection and peaks at 6-12 hours and has a half-life of 12 hours. In health, it is < 0.05 microgram/L, infection and is unlikely if PCT is between 0.1 to 0.5, local infection is often seen with PCT between 0.5 to 2. However, besides likely infection, trauma, surgery and shock of other types are likely to produce such a response. Systemic infection typically results in PCT between 2-10 microgram/L and if > 10 it suggests sepsis and septic shock. In localized infections including empyema or subacute bacterial endocarditis, PCT may be normal. PCT is used for initiation, withdrawal or escalation of antibiotic therapy. In primary care, PCT > 0.25 microgram/L justifies antibiotic therapy.

MCQs

1. This is the earliest detectable acute phase reactant

A) ESR
B) CRP
C) Procalcitonin
D) All of the above

2. CRP level peaks at this time

A) Between 12-24 hours
B) Between 24-48 hours
C) Between 48-96 hours
D) Beyond 96 hours

3. ESR is a parameter to stop drug treatment in this disease

A) Acute bacterial pneumonia
B) Tuberculosis
C) Rheumatic fever
D) Nephrotic syndrome

4. This test is commonly used at birth

A) ESR
B) CRP
C) Procalcitonin
D) Any of the above

5. ESR is high but CRP is low in this disease

A) Tuberculosis
B) Rheumatic fever
C) Nephrotic syndrome
D) SLE (systemic lupus erythematosus)

Answers to MCQs

Correct answers as follows:

Q1 C	Q2 B	Q3 C	Q4 B	Q5 D

85 Urinalysis

Macroscopic (volume, color, odor, transparency), chemical (urine strips for pH, specific gravity, glucose, proteins (picks up only albumin), bilirubin, nitrites, ketones, RBCs, leukocyte esterase enzyme denoting WBC in urine – 10 or more WBCs/c.mm is pyuria, the intensity of color change proportionate to the concentration of each compound) and microscopic (cells – RBCs in infections, WBC casts in interstitial nephritis and severe infections, tumor, stone, pyuria in infections, RBC casts in nephritis, granular casts in acute tubular necrosis, waxy casts in chronic renal disease, fatty casts in nephrotic syndrome (lipid particles seen in the protein matrix), crystals in stones, organisms – done on the centrifuged sample under light microscopy but can be done under phase-contrast microscopy that offers more details and also fluorescence flow cytometry) analysis. Also included are urinary electrolytes, drugs and poison testing, pregnancy test and microbiological cultures.

Volume of Urine

In routine practice, one depends on history by asking a patient or parent of a child whether usual amount of urine is passed or not. However, one may have to measure the exact volume in extreme conditions such as oliguria or polyuria. < 0.5 ml per kg of body weight per day is considered as oliguria and > 4 ml per kg of body weight per day as polyuria. Urine volume is not easy to measure and may need collection by catheterization in young children or sick adults. Unless it is likely to offer information that would change the management, it should be avoided due to fear of infection. Older children and adults can collect urine during 24 hours. Oliguria results from dehydration and glomerular diseases while polyuria is commonly due to diabetes mellitus or diabetes insipidus as well as due to renal tubular disorders.

Proteinuria

Normally proteins are not filtered by the kidney and if small molecular proteins leak out through glomeruli, they are reabsorbed by tubules. Thus, a very small amount of protein (< 150 mg/day) is present in urine. Transient proteinuria may be present in dehydration, fever or intense exercise. Strongly acidic urine and concentrate urine gives false +ve results while alkaline urine and dilute urine gives false -ve results. 24 hour urinary protein estimation is most reliable and can be assessed in a spot sample by urinary protein creatinine ratio – normal < 0.2, abnormal > 0.5 and nephrotic range > 2. Orthostatic or postural proteinuria refers to elevated protein excretion in standing position but not in lying down position and is due to compression of renal vein between aorta and left superior mesenteric artery. Ideally first morning fresh sample must be examined.

Hematuria

Red urine may be due to hemoglobinuria or myoglobinuria, drugs like rifampicin or methyldopa and beetroot consumption. Frank red color suggests bleeding from collecting system as in case of renal stone (fresh RBCs) while cola-colored urine indicates glomerular disease such as nephritis (crenated RBCs). Few RBCs may be seen in urine due to fever or use of ibuprofen. However one must follow this finding to rule out any significant renal pathology. Endothelial glomerular disease (acute post-streptococcal nephritis) presents with mild edema, oliguria and hypertension in a mildly sick child besides Hematuria while interstitial glomerular disease presents with isolated Hematuria. Epithelial glomerular disease per se does not produce Hematuria unless pathology has extended to endothelium.

Urine Culture

Urinary tract infection should be confirmed by urine culture because increased WBCs in urine may also result from non-infective inflammatory conditions such as renal stone, tumor or nephritis. Ideally, mid-stream specimen must be collected after cleaning external part and if possible, the sample should be collected in the laboratory itself so as to avoid contamination and delay in processing. Colony count > 10^5 is considered significant of UTI.

Here are a few laboratory reports for you to interpret. Answers with explanations are given at the end.

Case 1

Small volume, urine macroscopy – cola colored, chemical examination - proteins +, urine protein / creatinine ratio 0.3 microscopy – RBCs +, crenated, RBC casts +, WBCs 4-5/HPF

Case 2

Normal volume, urine microscopy - bright red-colored, chemical examination – proteins +, urine protein / creatinine ratio 0.4, microscopy – RBCs ++, fresh cells, no casts, WBCs 6-8/HPF

Case 3

Urine macroscopy – N, chemical – proteins +++, urine protein/creatinine ration 4.5, microscopy – fatty casts

Case 4

Turbid urine, chemical examination of urine – proteins +, urine protein / creatinine ratio 0.6, nitrites and leukocyte esterase enzyme + on a urinary strip, microscopy – WBCs 50-60/HPF, RBCs +, culture -ve

Case 5

Urine macroscopy – N, chemical – proteins +, urine protein / creatinine ratio 0.7, microscopy – WBCs 4-5/HPF, culture E.coli colony count > 10^6

Answers with Explanation

Case 1

Cola colored urine suggests the glomerular endothelial or interstitial origin of blood, PC ratio (protein/creatinine) is normal (no significant proteinuria), crenated RBCs and RBC casts suggest glomerular endothelial pathology

Diagnosis – **glomerulonephritis**

Case 2

Bright red color suggests fresh blood coming from collecting system and not kidneys, no significant proteinuria, a high number of fresh RBCs without casts, WBCs in small number that is not significant of pyuria

Diagnosis – **ureteric (stone) or bladder (tumor) pathology**

Case 3

Macroscopy N, protein-creatinine ratio 4.5 suggests severe proteinuria of nephrotic range, fatty casts denote increased lipids in urine

Diagnosis – **Nephrotic syndrome** (proteinuria and hypercholesteroemia)

Case 4

Turbid urine suggests probable infection, no significant proteinuria, nitrites and leukocyte esterase enzyme +ve on urine strip denotes probable infection, a high number of WBCs with few (insignificant) RBCs indicate severe pyuria indicating probable infection. However, culture is -ve.

Most probable diagnosis – **UTI**

UTI can be confirmed only with +ve urine culture. When culture is -ve, one must look at clinical presentation (high fever, sick child, backache suggestive of upper UTI, frequency and burning of micturition indicative of lower UTI) and if highly suggestive of UTI, one may consider repeating the culture and start an antibiotic. Negative culture may be a technical error or may also be due to prior antibiotic therapy.

Case 5

Macroscopy, chemical examination and microscopy are all normal but culture is +ve (significant colony count)

Diagnosis – **asymptomatic bacteriuria.** In such a situation, one must look at the clinical profile and if normal, the best way is to repeat urine culture as the previous result could be due to technical error. However, asymptomatic bacteriuria should not be treated with antibiotics but the patient should be closely observed for any new symptoms or signs.

86 Stool Examination

It is mainly indicated in gastrointestinal disorders such as infections, non-infective inflammatory disorders such as inflammatory bowel disease, bleeding disorders due to local causes and maldigestion or malabsorption. A stool sample is collected in a clean container and sent to the laboratory without delay. Tests include macroscopic examination (color, consistency, odor, volume, presence of mucous or blood), microscopic examination (RBCs, WBCs, macrophages, ova or cyst of parasites, fungal spores, fat globules), chemical analysis (guaiac test for occult blood, reducing substance for sugar malabsorption, calprotectin for inflammation, stool pH - acidic in sugar malabsorption) and culture for bacteria or fungi. Rectal swab for stool culture is reserved for specific conditions such as immune deficiency or chronic persistent diarrhea.

Clinical Application

Stool Examination in Acute Diarrhea

In routine practice, it is rarely justified. Viral diarrhea is usually a small intestinal infection, seen in young children and presents as a large volume of watery stools often resulting in dehydration. Bacterial infection is usually a large intestinal infection and presents as frequent but small volume stools with mucous and / or blood with abdominal pain and high fever. So the distinction between viral and bacterial acute diarrhea is clinical and there is no need for stool examination. Rarely, acute watery diarrhea may be due to cholera – that is rare now. It presents as a large volume of frequent watery stools and the patient mostly presents in shock due to severe dehydration. Hanging drop preparation is necessary to confirm cholera.

Stool Examination in Chronic Diarrhea

It is strongly indicated. Chronic diarrhea may be caused by chronic infections (bacterial, parasitic or fungal), especially in immune-compromised patients in whom malabsorption of multiple nutrients (carbohydrates, proteins and fats besides vitamins and minerals), allergy (especially to animal proteins), bile acid irritation and drug toxicity are additional factors. Thus, chronic diarrhea in such a situation is multifactorial. Besides stool microscopy, one may need chemical tests, tests for malabsorption and culture for various organisms.

Stool Examination for Malabsorption

Fat malabsorption

Stool is greasy or oily in case of fat malabsorption and is typically a feature of cystic fibrosis. Stool microscopy shows fat globules in other pancreatic disorders and also in case of excess of fat consumption. In giardiasis. The stool appears to be greyish white, is large in quantity and has a very foul smell. Ideally, excretion of stool fat over 24 hours in 1-3 days period after ingestion of measured amount of fat can be studied to judge the degree of fat malabsorption. It may assume importance to differentiate various conditions resulting in fat malabsorption. For example, bile acid deficiency and bacterial overgrowth in the intestines may result in a small excess of fat in stools, a moderate amount of fat is lost in stools in celiac disease and severe steatorrhea is seen in pancreatic diseases. Though routinely such tests are not required and mere microscopic presence of stool fat globules in conjunction with clinical profile serves the purpose.

Carbohydrate malabsorption

It presents as watery stools with perianal excoriation due to acidic stools and stool shows the presence of reducing substance evident of sugar malabsorption. It is important to realize that reducing substances in the stool should not be tested in case of acute diarrhea. This is because lactase is an enzyme in the most superficial layer of the intestinal mucosa and is the first to be destroyed in case of any intestinal insult. When lactase enzyme is not available, lactose is not absorbed and it is seen as a reducing substance in the stool sample. In acute diarrhea, such a change is very transient and self-limiting. It does not call for a change in diet. The same is true in a breast-fed infant in whom, as breast milk contains a large amount of lactose, reducing substance in stool has no relevance and so should not be tested. However, in chronic diarrhea, it is not only lactose but also other carbohydrates that are not absorbed and hence test for reducing substance in stool is relevant.

Other tests

Other tests may be necessary to substantiate intestinal malabsorption. D-xylose absorption test measures xylose in urine and blood after oral consumption and a low level would suggest intestinal malabsorption of sugar. Specific lactose malabsorption may be found by hydrogen breath test.

Unabsorbed lactose enters the colon where it is absorbed and resultant hydrogen is excreted in the breath. Similarly, the Schilling test is used for vitamin B12 malabsorption. Protein malabsorption is evident by low serum protein levels. However low serum protein may be caused by many other diseases and hence not specific to protein malabsorption. Barium study of intestines or other imaging modalities may offer a non-specific clue to intestinal malabsorption. Endoscopy and intestinal biopsy may help in confirming specific diagnosis such as celiac disease or inflammatory bowel disease.

Intestinal tuberculosis rarely presents with diarrhea because the disease affects submucosa and not intestinal mucosa. Once the healing starts either naturally or induced by treatment, it results in subacute intestinal obstruction due to scarring and presents as constipation as the main symptom.

Stool examination in stools with mucous and / or blood

Such a condition may be of short duration as in case of acute bacillary dysentery or of long duration as in case of parasitic infections (commonly amebiasis and giardiasis) or inflammatory bowel disease. Blood in the stool may not be visible by the naked eye. Microscopic examination may pick up blood (also by guaiac test) besides ova or cysts of parasites. Calprotectin in stool is a marker of inflammation. Rectal bleeding may occur without loose stools and it may result from hard stools as in severe constipation. It may also be a result of hemorrhoids, intestinal polyps, diverticulosis, vascular malformations or abnormal gastric mucosa in the small intestine as in Meckel's diverticulum. For small bleeders in the intestine, radioactive technetium study may be necessary. Refractory anemia is often a presentation of such occult intestinal bleed.

MCQs

1. This microscopic finding differentiates bacillary dysentery from other non-infective causes

A) RBCs
B) WBCs
C) Macrophages
D) All of the above

2. Microscopic stool examination is normal in this acute bacterial infection

A) Tuberculosis
B) Dysentery
C) Typhoid fever
D) Cholera

3. Stool must be checked for reducing substance in this condition

A) Viral diarrhea
B) Every case of diarrhea
C) Chronic diarrhea
D) All of the above

4. Stool must be checked for fat globules in this condition

A) Liver disease

B) Pancreatic disease

C) Intestinal disease

D) All of the above

5. Stool culture is indicated in this condition

A) Bacillary dysentery

B) Chronic persistent diarrhea

C) Typhoid fever

D) Tuberculosis

Answers to MCQs

Correct answers as follows:

Q1 C	Q2 D	Q3 C	Q4 D	Q5 B

87 Antibody, Antigen and PCR

Back to Basics – Antibody Tests

The body responds to infection by producing antibodies to fight infection. IgM antibody is the initial response that may appear in the first 5-7 days and disappears over the next few weeks (IgM antibodies against dengue and brucella may remain for 2 months, CMV for 4 months, toxoplasma and rickettsia for many months) followed by long-lasting IgG antibodies for a variable time (months or years). Though detection of IgM antibody suggests recent infection, the test may be negative early in the course of the disease and the test may remain positive well after the disease is cured.

Besides, there is a possibility of cross-reacting antibodies to other infections. Fourfold rise of antibodies over 7-10 days from the initial level offers high sensitivity but for which one has to wait for that length of time and so it is impractical. IgG antibodies occur a few weeks after infection and persist for a long time hence they indicate past infection. The presence of antibodies also depends on the patient's ability to mount an appropriate response. Thus, the antibody test is less dependable for diagnosis and test results need cautious interpretation. There are different methods of antibody testing such as agglutination or Elisa, the latter being more reliable. It is ideal to prove infection with culture, antigen detection or molecular test and only when it is not possible that antibody test is an alternative. However, culture must be ordered prior to starting antibiotic therapy. Organism captured on culture may be a contaminant or a commensal and not responsible for the disease. Antigen tests are also available, the results of which are not interfered with by prior antibiotic therapy but they can't differentiate between active and dead organisms. Molecular diagnosis has high sensitivity and specificity but is costly and may not be available. Finally, clinical correlation is important for rational interpretation.

Indications for Antibody Tests

Those viral infections that have a non-specific clinical profile and have a short viraemic period are best diagnosed with IgM antibodies. While PCR can detect viral infections but results may take time and it is not cost-effective. Thus, the IgM antibody test is commonly used to detect viral infections such as EBV, herpes, dengue, chikungunya, CMV as well as measles, rubella and mumps. Few bacterial infections such as leptospirosis, rickettsia and brucella are also detected by specific IgM antibody tests as these organisms are difficult to culture.

Commonly Employed Antibody Tests and their Limitations

Widal test

It is widely used in clinical practice though single test result is not dependable and detection of the four-fold rise of antibody though diagnostic is impractical.

Theoretically, O antibody suggests recent infection while H antibody denotes past infection. Prior typhoid vaccine may alter results unless the vaccine uses Vi antigen. The tube test is better than the slide test, thus, the Typhidot test is not recommended, it should not be used for the diagnosis of typhoid fever. Besides, many other intestinal gram-negative organisms also show cross-reaction to widal test and even malarial parasites also cross-react. Thus, blood culture is the only way to confirm the diagnosis of typhoid.

Antibody tests for hepatitis

IgM HAV strongly supports the diagnosis of active hepatitis A infection but IgG antibody denotes past infection or immunization with HAV vaccine. Hepatitis B virus has three antigens, two of them (S and E) in blood and C antigen in the liver. IgM HbC (antibody to core antigen) denotes active infection while antibody against S and E antigen indicates recovering or past infection. Antibody to S alone in absence of HbS antigen is due to prior vaccination. The presence of S antigen suggests of infection that may be active or silent while e antigen represents high infectivity. Other viruses such as CMV, EBV or HIV can also be detected by antibody tests.

ASLO (Anti-streptolysin O) antibody test –

It has similar limitations in that positive test suggests recent or prior exposure to such an infection. Streptococcal infections are so common in the community and it is necessary to know antibody titer in the community. Unless the test shows a very high titer compared to one that is prevalent in the community, the diagnostic value of this test remains limited. In fact, a negative test may rule out recent as well as past streptococcal infections

Leptospira, Rickettsia and Brucella antibody tests

These tests also have similar limitations but as these organisms are difficult to culture, antibody tests are widely used in conjunction with clinical correlation.

Dengue antibody test

IgM antibody becomes positive only after the first few days and so not useful for early diagnosis. However, the presence of both IgG and IgM antibodies in febrile child suggest a second episode of dengue with a risk of immune-mediated complications.

TB antibody test

It should never be used. Even Mantoux test and Interferon-gamma assay such as Gold test are not recommended for diagnosis as they only suggest exposure to infection anytime in the past but not necessarily a recent disease.

Antibody tests for rheumatological and immune disorders

Such tests are specialized tests, rarely ordered in routine practice and should not be used randomly, best left to specialists. They are often not very specific with the exception of Anti-dsDNA (part of ANA) that is diagnostic of SLE (systemic lupus erythematosus). ANA may be normal in 5% of the population and per se is not diagnostic of any disease. Similarly, RA factor is present in polyarthritis in older female child and should not be ordered in every joint disease. Absence or low level of IgG or IgA deficiency denotes immune deficiency disorder.

Antigen Tests

These tests are more specific and useful than antibody tests. They have the advantage of quick results available in minutes that are not interfered by prior antibiotic therapy but cannot differentiate live from dead bacilli and antibiotic sensitivity cannot be assessed. Dengue NS1 antigen test is routinely used but may not be positive during the first 24 hours of the illness. A throat swab showing strep antigen may be reliable to diagnose bacterial pharyngitis but is not representative of pneumonia. Urinary antigen tests have been tried in the diagnosis of respiratory infections including pneumonia but have not been found to be reliable. Antigen tests on CSF samples are also used in the diagnosis of bacterial meningitis

Rapid antigen test for malaria

Though blood smear microscopy is the gold standard for the diagnosis of malaria, it needs skill and patience to perform the test. In absence of such feasibility, a rapid antigen test is useful. Glutamate dehydrogenase test and lactase dehydrogenase test is positive in case of active infection by either vivax and falciparum and histidine rich protein test is positive only in falciparum but cannot differentiate live from dead parasites. Antigen test may remain positive for a month or more even after control of infection.

NS1 antigen test for dengue virus

This test is useful for early diagnosis as it is positive in first 24-48 hours. Though, in 5% of patients, it may be negative in the initial days. It is more specific for the diagnosis of dengue fever as compared to antibody tests.

Rapid antigen test for streptococcal throat infection

It is a fairly reliable test, the result of which is available in few minutes as against the culture that takes 2-3 days. However, this test is specific only to streptococcal infection and antibiotic sensitivity is not available. As viral infections are common, this test can decide the need for antibiotic therapy.

Rapid antigen test for pneumonia

Sensitivity and specificity of such a test is not high and result also depends on the collected sample (blood or urine).

Rapid antigen test for meningitis

Latex particle agglutination test (LPA) in CSF is considered to be a useful test in the diagnosis of meningitis as compared to gram staining and culture. Test can screen common organisms causing meningitis such as streptococcus pneumoniae and hemophilus influenza.

Antigen test for Covid 19 infection

They are less sensitive as compared to PCR but test result is available immediately. However, in a symptomatic patient, positive antigen test may be used for diagnosis.

PCR – Polymerase Chain Reaction (also known as real time PCR or reversed transcription PCR – rtPCR, quantitative PCR)

The test detects DNA (genetic material that contains information for all living things) or RNA (information copied from DNA and involved in making proteins) of an infectious agent or abnormal cells in the sample. PCR besides being accurate, becomes positive in very early stage of the disease, even before symptoms appear, when there are not enough existing pathogens or antibodies for detection. Test employs multiplication of small amount of genetic material several times known as amplification that makes it easy to detect.

PCR is useful in detection of infectious diseases, genetic disorders and malignancy. Test can be done on any tissue including blood or saliva. The sample will show DNA besides patient's own DNA. Polymerase enzyme is added to the sample to produce copies of existing genetic material and the process is repeated several time to produce large number of copies that helps detection of abnormal DNA.

Certain viruses are made up of RNA instead of DNA. In such cases, RNA has to be changed into DNA before copying (rtPCR). Amount of genetic material can be counted in the same sample (qPCR). Multiplex PCR can screen several pathogens at a time in a given sample and is used in the etiological diagnosis of pneumonia or meningitis.

False -ve results in PCR may be due to insufficient sample, very small pathogen load and their dynamics and variability in techniques. However, chance of false -ve test results is extremely small. False +ve results are negligible, though may be caused by contamination.

GeneXpert test for TB

Test is ideally done on a sputum sample but lymph node or other biopsied tissues can also be subjected to this test. Positive yield from CSF sample in TB meningitis is low and further lower in pleural fluid in TB pleural effusion. CB-NAT – cartridge based nucleic acid amplification test is used in India. The test also detects rifampicin resistance, if any. The test is positive even if a sample has 10-15 bacilli per ml as against culture that needs 50-100 bacilli per ml while smear needs 5000-10000 bacilli per ml in the sample. Besides, test also picks up dead bacilli and so test may be positive in recently treated patient. GeneXpert Ultra is a further modification that can detect even small number of bacilli in the sample. However, as sensitivity increases, specificity goes down a bit and so there can be false +ve results.

MCQs

1. IgM antibody denoting recent infection may persist for
A) 4-5 days
B) 1-2 weeks
C) 2-3 months
D) Any of the above

2. This disease is diagnosed in routine practice only by antibody tests
A) Typhoid fever
B) Corona virus
C) Leptospirosis
D) Malaria

3. Typhoid fever may be confirmed by
A) Typhidot test
B) Widal slide test
C) Widal tube test
D) None of the above

4. Streptococcal antigen test for pharyngitis is not used in India because
A) It is not reliable
B) Clinical diagnosis is certain
C) It is not cost-effective
D) None of the above

5. **Which of the following statement is WRONG?. GeneXpert test for tuberculosis can be done on this sample**

A) Sputum

B) Gastric aspirate

C) Blood

D) Lymph node

Answers to MCQs

Correct answers as follows:

Q1 D	Q2 C	Q3 D	Q4 C	Q5 C

88 Liver Function Tests

Back to Basics

Liver is one of the largest organs in the body and is unique in terms of ability to react to damage and repair as well as regenerate. It performs multiple functions such as synthesis of plasma proteins such as albumin and clotting factors, production of bile, excretion of bile, cholesterol, hormones and drugs, metabolism of proteins, fats and carbohydrates, enzyme activation, storage of glycogen, vitamins and minerals, detoxification and purification of blood. In routine clinical practice, few blood tests are commonly used in the evaluation of liver diseases.

Initial Screening Tests

Urinalysis

High colored urine with presence of bile salts and pigments suggests direct bilirubinemia.

Blood tests

These tests include bilirubin (decides the **extent** of the disease), – conjugated and unconjugated fractions, proteins – albumin and globulin (evaluates **chronicity** of the disease), enzymes (assesses **acuity** of the disease) – SGOT (AST), SGPT (ALT), alkaline phosphatase and gamma-glutamyl transferase (**GTT – specific to bile duct disease)** and prothrombin time (estimates **seriousness** of the disease).

Serum bilirubin

Normal level 0.2-1.2 mg%, of which direct (conjugated) fraction is < 0.3 mg%. Generally, icterus is not visible in the eyes unless total bilirubin is > 2 mg%. In case of increased bilirubin level, if direct fraction is > 20% of the total bilirubin, it is considered as conjugated bilirubinemia. In such a case, urine is high colored (dark yellow) and chemical examination of urine shows bile salts and bile pigments. If direct fraction is < 20% of the total bilirubin, it is considered as indirect (unconjugated) bilirubinemia. In such a case, urine is not high colored (pale yellow) due to urobilinogen. Increased direct bilirubin is due to liver cell (hepatocyte) disease or biliary tract disease. Itching in a non-sick child with higher degree of jaundice is characteristic of biliary tract disease as compared to sick child with proportionately lesser degree of jaundice suggests hepatocyte disease. Increased unconjugated bilirubinemia is due to hemolysis of RBCs that generates bilirubin in amount that liver cannot conjugate and hence retained in the blood. It is not water soluble and so cannot be excreted in urine. Besides, hepatocyte or biliary tract disease and hemolysis of RBCs, congenital enzyme defects may also result in jaundice – either conjugated (Dubin-Johnson or Rotor syndrome) or unconjugated (Criggler-Najjer or Gilbert syndrome). Such enzyme defects are benign except Criggler-Najjer type 1 that may result in brain damage. They manifest with jaundice without abnormal liver functions or anemia.

SGOT / SGPT (AST / ALT)

Normal level 5-40 units. SGPT is more specific to liver pathology while SGOT is raised in muscle diseases including heart muscle and also intestinal mucosa and high WBC count. When both are increased but SGOT is higher than SGPT, it suggests systemic disease (typhoid, malaria) involving multiple organs in which liver is also diseased while SGPT is higher than SGOT denotes primarily liver disease (viral A hepatitis). Marked increase in thousands denotes acuity of hepatocyte damage as seen typically in viral A hepatitis while moderate increase is seen in many other hepatocyte diseases. Enzymes may be very low if most of the hepatocytes are already destroyed as happens in late stages of liver failure, however, by then all other liver functions are severely abnormal.

Alkaline phosphatase and gamma-glutamyl transferase

Normal Alkaline phosphatase is up to 150 IU (varies with laboratories) and GTT up to 40 IU. Alkaline phosphatase is increased in hepatic/biliary tract and bone diseases but gamma GT is more specific to biliary tract disease.

Serum albumin and globulin

Normal total protein 6-7 Gm% of which albumin is 3.5-4 Gm% and remaining is globulin. A low level of albumin with normal or increased globulin (reversal of albumin-globulin ratio) suggests chronic hepatocyte disease.

Prothrombin time

Normal 11-13 seconds. Most of the time, result is given as INR (international normalised ratio – calculation based on PT), normal value is between 1 and 1.5. Increased INR suggests liver cell failure.

Other Tests

Blood tests

Glucose and ammonia are considered in suspected liver cell failure. Infection can be proved by serological tests such as IgM HAV for acute hepatitis A disease and so also other infections (hepatitis B and C, CMV, EBV). Extra-hepatic infections may also result in hepatitis (typhoid, leptospirosis, malaria) for which specific tests may be necessary. Diseases caused by inborn errors of metabolism require relevant tests (serum ceruloplasmin for Wilson disease or hypoglycemia in glycogen storage disease and specific metabolic tests as in case of tyrosinosis).

Imaging study

USG helps to evaluate hepatomegaly and liver cell architecture, gall bladder and biliary tract, portal venous system, splenomegaly and ascites. MRI can assess degree of iron overload and fibrosis as well as fat in the liver.

Liver biopsy

Helps to diagnose cirrhosis and offer clues in support of inflammatory disorders (autoimmune hepatitis and other types of hepatitis) and storage disorders.

In summary, urinalysis for bile salts and pigments along with serum bilirubin, proteins, enzymes and INR can evaluate micro-anatomy and pathology of the disease as well as functioning level of liver cells. Specific tests would be necessary for further etiological workup.

MCQs

1. **Total bilirubin is 2 mg%, Direct fraction is 0.8 mg%, indirect fraction is 1.2 mg%. It is suggestive of**

A) Indirect bilirubinemia
B) Direct bilirubinemia
C) Both together
D) Any of the above

2. **Total bilirubin 4 mg%, Direct 3 mg%, SGPT 1200, SGOT 400 Serum proteins 6.5 Gm% Alb 3.8 Gm%. It mostly suggests**

A) HAV
B) HBV
C) HBC
D) Any of the above

3. **Total bilirubin 4 mg%, Direct 3 mg%, SGPT 300, SGOT 450 Serum proteins 6 Gm% Alb 3.5 Gm%, Alkaline phosphatase 30 units. Hb 7 Gm% It mostly suggests**

A) Hepatitis B
B) Cholangitis
C) Malaria
D) None of the above

4. Total bilirubin 32 mg%, Direct 22 mg%, SGPT 30, SGOT 40, Alkaline phosphatase 40, Serum proteins 5 Gm%, Alb 2.2 Gm%, INR 2.8. It is most suggestive of

A) Acute hepatitis
B) Acute hepatitis with failure
C) Chronic hepatitis
D) Chronic liver disease with failure

5. Total bilirubin 12 mg%, Direct 10 mg%, SGPT 50, SGOT 30, Alkaline phosphatase 600, Serum proteins 6.5 Gm%, Alb 4 Gm%, INR 1.8. It is mostly suggestive of

A) Acute hepatitis with failure
B) Chronic hepatitis with failure
C) Biliary obstruction
D) Any of the above

Answers to MCQs with Explanation

Q 1 B – Direct bilirubin level more than 20% of the total or more than 2 mg% is considered direct bilirubinemia.

Q 2 A – Markedly increased SGPT suggests acute liver disease such as hepatitis A. Such a high SGPT does not indicate serious disease. In fact, mild increase in bilirubin in this child suggests mild disease.

Q 3 C – SGOT > SGPT suggests extra-hepatic disease that has caused hepatitis. Low Hb level may denote malaria as possible cause. Such findings are also seen in typhoid but not low Hb.

Q 4 D – Markedly high bilirubin level suggests severe disease, low proteins and albumin indicates chronic disease, high INR denotes liver cell failure in which as liver cells are destroyed, there is no more enzymes available to leak out in blood. It is important to note that higher bilirubin with increased INR with normal enzymes suggest bad prognosis.

Q 5 C – Moderate increase in bilirubin with marked increase in alkaline phosphatase and normal protein level suggests primary biliary tract obstructive disease.

89 Renal Function Tests

Back to Basics

Kidney has four major functions. They include **filtration** (cells, proteins and large molecules are retained), **reabsorption** (water and small molecules), **excretion** (waste products) and **secretion** (H+, K+, NH_3, urea, creatinine, histamine, drugs like penicillin, hormones such as renin, erythropoietin, calcitriol). These functions maintain homeostasis in the body. Filtration is the glomerular function and reabsorption the tubular function.

Initial Screening Tests

Urinalysis is a simple and useful screening test. Macroscopic, microscopic and chemical examination offer a clue to a probable diagnosis. (Details of urinalysis can be found in another chapter). GFR – glomerular filtration rate – tests filtration function and serum urea and creatinine reflect the same. Serum proteins – albumin and globulin, calcium and phosphorus may represent abnormal urinary loss and so also serum electrolytes and blood gas. In most of the renal diseases, glomerular dysfunction goes hand in hand with tubular functions. Isolated tubular dysfunction needs special tests but it is not common in routine practice.

eGFR

Estimated GFR is a rough measure of glomerular filtration function but is adequate for monitoring progress in slowly progressive renal diseases. It is calculated by the following formula.

eGFR = 0.55 X height in cm divided by serum creatinine in mg% (0.55 as a constant is used > one year of age, in neonate it is 0.35 and in infants 0.45). Normal eGFR varies between 80 and 120 ml/min. eGFR < 60 ml/min suggests renal disease.

Serum creatinine

It is a measure of glomerular filtration. Normal value varies a lot with age. Most laboratories have a printed normal value that represents adult value in which 1.2 mg% is considered a higher limit of normal. For practical purposes, three-fourths of height in cm is a number that should be considered as a higher limit of normal serum creatinine with change in decimals. For example, if a child's height is 100 cm, then three-fourths is 75 and so the normal level of serum creatinine in such a child should be < 0.75 mg%. It is important to realize that serum creatinine increases beyond the normal limit only when eGFR decreases to less than 30 ml/min. Thus, abnormal serum creatinine is a late sign of renal disease and eGFR should be used for monitoring chronic progressive glomerular disease.

Blood urea nitrogen (BUN)

It is a product of dietary protein metabolism as against creatinine is a product of muscle protein metabolism. Blood urea includes nitrogen and other molecules and is approximately double the amount of BUN. The normal level of BUN is 7-10 mg%. Both BUN and serum creatinine (Cr) are increased in renal dysfunction. The normal ratio of BUN / Cr varies between 12-20. If > 20, it suggests prerenal disease (dehydration or hypoperfusion). This is because BUN is reabsorbed by tubules in prerenal conditions. If the ratio is < 12, it may be due to renal disease or liver disease (ammonia is not converted into urea) or malnutrition due to protein deficiency.

Serum proteins – albumin and globulin

Albumin is lost in the urine in case of glomerular epithelial disease, such as nephrotic syndrome. It results in hypoalbuminemia and compensatory increase in alpha-2 macroglobulin to maintain osmotic pressure in the blood. Thus, albumin–globulin ratio is reversed. (It is also reversed in chronic liver disease).

Other blood tests

Excessive loss of electrolytes in urine results in lower level while abnormal retention leads to higher level. Results are corroborated with urinary electrolytes. Such tests include serum sodium, potassium, chlorides, bicarbonate, ammonia, calcium, phosphorus, uric acid etc. Anion gap is the difference between (Na + K) and (Cl + HCO_3). Arterial blood gas detects disturbance in acid-base metabolism. Low anion gap metabolic acidosis is seen in renal diseases and also in diarrhea while high anion gap metabolic acidosis is seen in diabetes and sepsis.

Imaging tests

Structural abnormalities are picked-up by abdominal USG as in obstructive uropathy. Micturating cystourethrogram (MCU) detects vesico-ureteric reflux. CT, MRI, angiography and radionuclide scans are other imaging modalities used for specific purposes.

Renal biopsy

It may be necessary in chronic medical renal diseases that helps planning therapy and monitoring progress.

In summary, urinalysis including microscopy, chemical examination and bacterial culture along with blood urea nitrogen and serum creatinine are basic investigations for diagnosis of common renal diseases. Abdominal USG is useful for diagnosis of surgical renal disorders and occasional medical renal diseases.

MCQs

1. eGFR is an ideal test in this condition

A) Acute nephritis
B) Nephrotic syndrome
C) Obstructive uropathy
D) None of the above

2. Higher limit of serum creatinine in a normal 4 year old child is

A) 0.4 mg%
B) 0.5 mg%
C) 0.6 mg%
D) 0.7 mg%

3. Ratio of blood urea and serum creatinine > 20 suggests

A) Prerenal disease
B) Acute renal disease
C) Chronic renal
D) Post-renal disease

4. Arterial blood gas is an important test in

A) Glomerular disease
B) Tubular disease
C) Either of them
D) Both of the them

5. These imaging tests are necessary in an infant suffering from urinary tract infection

A) Abdominal USG
B) Radionuclide scan
C) Micturating cystourethrogram
D) All of the above

Answers to MCQs

Correct answers as follows:

Q1 C	Q2 D	Q3 A	Q4 B	Q5 D

90 Hormonal Tests

Back to Basics

The thyroid function test is routinely used in office practice. Other hormonal tests are selectively used such as growth hormone, sex hormones, adrenal and parathyroid hormones. Hypothalamus-pituitary axis controls the production of thyroid, parathyroid and adrenal hormones while the pituitary itself generates growth hormone and anti-diuretic hormone besides LH and FSH.

Initial Screening Tests

Thyroid function tests

It includes T3, T4 , FT4 and TSH. Normal–TSH 0.5-5 mu/L, T3 80-200 nanogram/dL, T4 5-12 microgram/dL, FT4 07-1.5 microgram/dL Most of T3 and T4 are both bound to different proteins and so interpretation of their value should consider available protein binding sites. As T4 is converted into T3, free T4 is considered as the early indicator of hypothyroid state. TSH is increased in the hypothyroid state and decreased in the hyperthyroid state. The incidence of iodine deficiency has decreased with the use of iodised salt though it still exists in some parts of our country. It presents as an endemic goiter with low T4 but high T3 as a result of an adaptive response of conversion of T4 and TSH s often normal. Congenital hypothyroidism is seen in 1 out of 3500-4000 neonates and leads to developmental delay if diagnosed late. Hence neonatal screening is strongly recommended. TSH is estimated in cord blood as a screening test for congenital hypothyroidism.

Growth hormone

It is a pulsatile hormone-dependent on many variables and hence a single estimation is of no use. IGF 1 – insulin-like growth factor 1 level in blood correlates well with growth hormone and hence used in clinical practice. Growth hormone can be estimated by a challenge test in which its production is stimulated by other factors such as insulin. In case of the absence of an expected increase, GH deficiency is diagnosed.

Adrenal functions

Cortex produces steroids (glucocorticoids, mineralocorticoids, progestins, androgens and estrogens) while medulla produces adrenaline and noradrenaline. Urine steroid profile, serum electrolytes, ACTH stimulation test and imaging studies help to diagnose adrenal disorders.

Parathyroid function

It helps to maintain calcium homeostasis by increasing absorption from intestines, retention of calcium by kidneys and maintaining blood level of calcium by moving calcium from bones. Initial screening test includes serum calcium, phosphorus and alkaline phosphatase and serum parathormone (PTH). X-ray of bone helps to define rarefaction if any.

91 Blood Glucose

Back to Basics

When demand for glucose and energy is met, the remaining glucose is converted into glycogen by insulin and stored in the liver. Glycogenolysis can provide glucose only for a few hours and if fasting continues, the brain uses ketone bodies formed from the breakdown of fatty acids to provide energy.

Initial screening test

Normal fasting blood sugar < 100 mg%, post-prandial < 140 mg% A1C < 5,7 and fasting insulin < 25mIU/L which comes back to the same level at the end of 3 hrs during glucose tolerance test. C-peptide is another hormone produced by the pancreas and its normal level is between 0.5-2 nanogram/mL and it correlates well with insulin level. Thus, C-peptide level is used to differentiate between type 1 (insulin deficiency and so low C-peptide level) and type 2 (insulin resistance so high C-peptide)

Hyperglycemia (fasting blood sugar > 125 mg%) can result from insulin deficiency or resistance. Hypoglycemia (less than 55 mg%) may be caused by hyperinsulinism, failure of glycogenolysis or neoglucogenesis and defective fatty acid metabolism.

92 Chest X-ray

Back to Basics

A chest X-ray is not much useful in primary airway disorders as well as interstitial diseases and hence the general dictum "more the cough, lesser is the need for chest X-ray". A chest X-ray can help in the diagnosis of diseases of lung and pleura as well as cardiac disorders. Besides respiratory and cardiac disorders, a chest X-ray can detect lesions arising from other mediastinal structures and thoracic bony cage. Ideally, a radiologist must be informed about the provisional diagnosis so that he can choose the right type of view and exposure to get the best interpretation. Usually, a chest X-ray should be taken in the upright position with full inspiration (PA and lateral view) but in infants and young children, one may be forced to take it in a lying down position (AP view). In AP view, the normal heart appears to be falsely large, the scapula is seen within lung fields, ribs are more parallel and vertebrae are visible through the heart shadow. In PA view, which is a gold standard, the scapula is drawn away from lung fields, ribs are more oblique, vertebrae appear less dense and heart size is appropriately normal. In a chest X-ray, air appears black, fat dark grey, soft tissue grey and bone white.

How to Read a Chest X-ray

A chest X-ray must be technically proper in terms of position, exposure and phase of respiration for correct interpretation. Rotational film in expiration as well as underexposed or overexposed films give an erroneous impression. One must look at all the areas systematically as described below.

A – Airways
B – Bones
C – Cardiac
D – Diaphragm
E – Exposure and edges (borders)
F – Fissures
G – Gastric bubble
H – Hilum
I – Intercostal spaces

One must be able to ascribe a shadow to the anatomical part. Lateral or decubitus films help in defining the exact site. Decubitus film in particular is useful to pick up pleural fluid. Silhouette sign refers to the loss of normal borders between thoracic structures. It is usually caused by an intrathoracic mass that touches the border of the heart or aorta.

It is important to correlate radiological findings with clinical profile as suggested by history and physical examination. A chest X-ray does not offer an etiological diagnosis though typical radiological findings may be ascribed to a specific etiology.

Section 3
Other Tests

93 Tests for Musculoskeletal Disorders

Back to Basics

Muscle disorders may be inflammatory (myositis), degenerative (myopathy and muscular dystrophy), neurological (paresis).
The most common skeletal disorders are vitamin D deficiency (rickets in children and osteomalacia in adults) and osteoporosis. Other disorders include inflammatory (osteomyelitis, arthritis), tumors and skeletal dysplasia.

Initial Screening Tests

CPK - creatine phosphokinase

Normal value 20-120 U/L High value is seen when muscles are damaged as the enzyme leaks out into the blood and it could be as high as thousands. However, as the muscle damage increases, CPK level goes down as there are not many muscles left for the enzyme to leak out. CPK may increase even with a prick while collecting a blood sample.
Other tests include electromyography, muscle biopsy and genetic tests.

Vitamin D

It is important for bone health and also contributes to immune function and helps other organs. The best source of vitamin D is sunlight (Ideally half an hour between 11 am and 1 pm with open body surface as much as possible) though some of the food items such as fish, egg, cheese etc do provide a small amount. Hence in western countries, many food items including milk are fortified with vitamin D. Deficiency is supported by high alkaline phosphatase and low phosphorus in blood and X-ray of bones but may be confirmed by low blood level of 1:25 OH cholecalciferol. However, normal value of 1.25 OH D > 18 picogram/mL

Other tests include DEXA scan for estimating bone density and imaging modalities. Rheumatological disorders need specific antibody tests and HLA B12 for spondyloarthritis.

94 Tests for Bleeding Disorders

Back to Basics

In case of injury, the blood clot is formed at the site to stop bleeding through the interplay between many clotting factors and platelets. Deficiency of any of these factors or platelets results in excessive bleeding. Besides, vasculitis may also lead to the oozing of blood out of the blood vessels.

Initial Screening Tests

Bleeding time, platelet count, PT- prothrombin time and aPTT – partial thromboplastin time help to differentiate between platelet and coagulation factor deficiencies. Bleeding time is prolonged in platelet disorders (thrombocytopenia, DIC, Won Willebrand disease and late stage of liver cell failure). PT is prolonged in vitamin K deficiency, early stage of liver cell failure and DIC) and aPTT is prolonged in hemophilia, late stage of liver cell failure and DIC.

95 Pulmonary Function Test

Back to Basics

Airways are responsible for ventilation (moving air in and out) and lung parenchyma helps in oxygenation and removal of carbon dioxide. Oxygen diffuses from the alveolar membrane into the blood and carbon dioxide diffuses back into the alveoli. In health, all segments of the lungs are ventilated and perfused by blood to facilitate the transfer of gases.

Initial Screening Tests

Tests for ventilation

Spirometer is used to assess ventilatory function. It assesses lung volume, lung capacity, rate of flow. It can differentiate (FEV1 / FVC) between obstructive and restrictive airway disease. Bronchodilator challenge can show reversibility of airway obstruction. The peak flow meter can measure peak expiratory flow rate (PEFR) and is used to monitor the improvement of obstructive airway disease on treatment.

Tests for gas exchange

Arterial blood gas measures PaO_2 and $PaCO_2$ and evaluates acid-base disturbances. Alveolar-arterial oxygen gradient (A-a O_2 gradient) can be calculated that evaluates the presence of a shunt, if any (difference between ventilation and perfusion). The pulse oximeter is a part of clinical bedside measurement that estimates oxygen saturation in capillary blood. Such a measurement has limitations but is an easy non-invasive method.

96 Immune Function Test

Back to Basics

We are born with innate immunity that consists of mechanical barriers such as skin, mucous membranes, stomach acidity as well as neutrophils, monocytes, macrophages and natural killer cells (NK cells). Adaptive immunity is provided by B lymphocytes through the production of antibodies and T lymphocytes through cellular immunity. IgM antibody is an initial response but short-lived while IgG antibody develops later but lasts long. IgA antibodies work at the mucosal level.

Initial Screening Tests

T cell function is assessed by CBC (absolute lymphocyte count), flow cytometry (CD 4 and CD 8 cells), Mantoux test and ADA – adenosine deaminase and molecular tests B cell function is evaluated by serum immunoglobulins (IgG, IgM, IgA, IgE), flow cytometry (CD 19 and CD 20) Phagocyte function is assessed by CBC (neutropenia), NBT (nitro blue tetrazolium) and DHR (dihydrorhodamine) Leukocyte adhesion defect presents with leukocytosis with non-healing ulcer without pus formation.

Complement function is evaluated by CH 50 (classic pathway) or AH 50 (alternate pathway)

www.ingramcontent.com/pod-product-compliance
Ingram Content Group UK Ltd.
Pitfield, Milton Keynes, MK11 3LW, UK
UKHW062005290726
14090UKWH00022B/1409